Recent Advances in Cardiothoracic Surgery

Recent Advances in Cardiothoracic Surgery

Edited by Daniel Willson

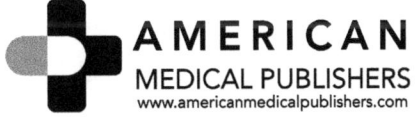

AMERICAN
MEDICAL PUBLISHERS
www.americanmedicalpublishers.com

American Medical Publishers,
41 Flatbush Avenue,
1st Floor, New York,
NY 11217, USA

Visit us on the World Wide Web at:
www.americanmedicalpublishers.com

ISBN: 978-1-63927-495-6

Cataloging-in-Publication Data

Recent advances in cardiothoracic surgery / edited by Daniel Willson.
      p. cm.
Includes bibliographical references and index.
ISBN 978-1-63927-495-6
1. Heart--Surgery. 2. Chest--Surgery. 3. Cardiovascular system--Surgery.
4. Surgery, Operative. I. Willson, Daniel.
RD598 .R43 2022

617.412--dc23

Table of Contents

Permissions

List of Contributors

Index

Preface

It is often said that books are a boon to mankind. They document every progress and pass on the knowledge from one generation to the other. They play a crucial role in our lives. Thus I was both excited and nervous while editing this book. I was pleased by the thought of being able to make a mark but I was also nervous to do it right because the future of students depends upon it. Hence, I took a few months to research further into the discipline, revise my knowledge and also explore some more aspects. Post this process, I begun with the editing of this book.

Cardiothoracic surgery is the surgery that deals with the treatment of diseases affecting organs within the thorax, which includes organs like heart, great vessels, lungs, esophagus, thymus, etc. Cardiothoracic surgery is usually used to treat complications of heart diseases such as valvular heart disease, endocarditis, ischemic heart disease, rheumatic heart disease and many more. Neurological damage is one of the major concerns and risks in cardiothoracic surgery and there are other risks of having infections such as myo- or pericarditis, bloodstream infections, cardiac device infection, endocarditis, pneumonia and empyema. Some of the modern cardiothoracic surgery includes modern beating heart surgery, minimally invasive surgery and lung volume reduction surgery. This book covers in detail some existent theories and innovative concepts revolving around cardiothoracic surgery. It also traces the progress of this field and highlights some of its key concepts and applications. It is a vital tool for all researching or studying cardiothoracic surgery as it gives incredible insights into emerging trends and concepts.

I thank my publisher with all my heart for considering me worthy of this unparalleled opportunity and for showing unwavering faith in my skills. I would also like to thank the editorial team who worked closely with me at every step and contributed immensely towards the successful completion of this book. Last but not the least, I wish to thank my friends and colleagues for their support.

Editor

Right anterolateral thoracotomy: an attractive alternative to repeat sternotomy for high-risk patients undergoing reoperative mitral and tricuspid valve surgery

Hailong Cao, Qing Zhou, Fudong Fan, Yunxing Xue, Jun Pan and Dongjin Wang[*]

Abstract

Background: Reoperative cardiac valve surgery via sternotomy is associated with a substantial morbidity and mortality. This study evaluated the right anterolateral thoracotomy for high-risk patients undergoing mitral and tricuspid valve redo procedures.

Methods: Out of a series of 173 patients undergoing redo cardiac valve surgery, 24 patients were reoperative via the right anterolateral thoracotomy as the high-risk group on the basis of the proximity of the heart and great vessels to the sternum and the presence and location of patent bypass grafts.

Results: In all cases, sternotomy was avoided. The mitral valve and tricuspid valve were replaced in 4 and 19 patients and repaired in 1 and 2 patients, respectively. Moreover, left atrial folding was performed in 5 patients. Mortality was 8.3%. All other patients had uneventful outcomes and normal valve function at follow-up.

Conclusions: Reoperative cardiac valve surgery can be performed safely using the right anterolateral thoracotomy in high-risk patients. It offers enough exposure. It minimizes the need for cardiac dissection, and thus, the risk for injury. Avoiding a high-risk resternotomy increases patients comfort and safety of redo mitral and tricuspid valve surgery.

Keywords: Right anterolateral thoracotomy, Reoperation, Mitral and tricuspid valve surgery, High-risk

Background

Reoperative cardiac valve surgery through a median sternotomy continues to be a common surgical approach but is technically challenging. It has several associated risks including injury to the right ventricle, injury to patent coronary artery bypass grafts and bleeding, thereby increasing operative morbidity and mortality [1]. In the setting of reoperative cardiac surgery, the redo-sternotomy had been proven to be one of the most dangerous phases of the operation, particularly for patients with huge heart or firm and gapless adhesion [1, 2].

Several protective strategies have been described for reoperative cardiac valve surgical procedures, including femoral vessel exposure before sternotomy [3], prophylactic initiation of cardiopulmonary bypass [1], and a right thoracotomy approach [4–6]. Routine computed tomography scanning is performed to visualize the relationship of the mediastinal contents to the sternum and to identify the patients at risk for injury during reentry [7]. However, it still cannot rule out accidental injury during sternotomy [3]. Moreover, potential postoperative complications, such as mediastinitis, sternal dehiscence, and phrenic nerve injury, have been reported [8]. Therefore, we herein present our experience that reoperative mitral and tricuspid valve surgery can be performed safely using the right anterolateral thoracotomy in high-risk patients.

* Correspondence: gldjw@163.com; shuqu_1982@sina.com
Department of Thoracic and Cardiovascular Surgery, the Affiliated Drum Tower Hospital of Nanjing, University Medical School, 321 Zhongshan RD, Nanjing 210008, China

Methods

Patient enrollment

From December 2012 to July 2016, 173 patients underwent redo cardiac valve surgery at department of thoracic and cardiovascular surgery in the Affiliated Drum Tower Hospital of Nanjing University Medical School. All of these patients had at least one prior operation that had been performed via a median sternotomy. All included patients had given written informed consent for their detail clinical data. Twenty four high-risk patients were chosen the right anterolateral thoracotomy, others were reoperative via the primary median sternotomy. The study was conducted according to the Helsinki Declaration and approved by the ethics committee of Nanjing University.

Definition of high-risk patients

(1) proximity (<5 mm) of right atrium or ventricle to the sternum (Fig. 1a, b); (2) previously placed bypass graft crossing midline with <1 cm distance from the posterior surface of the sternum, or fixed to the sternum (lack of movement on angiography); (3) proximity of ascending aorta to the sternum (<5 mm); (4) history of mediastinitis, >2 sternotomies, chest radiation; (5) severe pulmonary hypertension, severe dilated right ventricle; (6) reoperation within 6 months from the last operation [2].

Operation technique

Under general anesthesia with a single or dual lumen endotracheal tube, the patients were positioned in a 30° anterior oblique positionafter the fourth rib has been marked anteriorly. External defibrillation pads were placed. After the right anterolateral thoracotomy was performed through the right fourth intercostalspace via an approximate 12 cm incision (Fig. 1c), cardiopulmonary bypass was initiated using cannulation through right femoral artery, right femoral vein and superior vena cava under transesophageal echocardiography guidance. In case of pleural adhesions due to prior surgery, the right lung had to be dissected from the pericardium. The operative field was filled with carbon dioxide gas at the rate of 5 L/min throughout the surgery. After beginning cardiopulmonary bypass, dissection of the ascending aorta for conventional aortic cross-clamping was initially attempted in all patients. Twenty two patients underwent cardiopulmonary bypass with a mild hypothermia (32 °C to 34 °C), antegrade cold blood high potassium cardioplegic arrest. Two patients were cooled to 24 °C and induced ventricular fibrillation to perform the surgery under continued retrograde perfusion via coronary sinus for failure to dissect the ascending aorta.

Statistical analysis

Statistical analysis was performed using SPSS, version 15.0 (SPSS, Chicago, IL). Continuous variables are expressed as mean ± SD. Categoric variables are presented as number and proportions.

Results

Patient characteristics

The demographic data of the patients are shown in Table 1. We studied 24 patients from this series (11

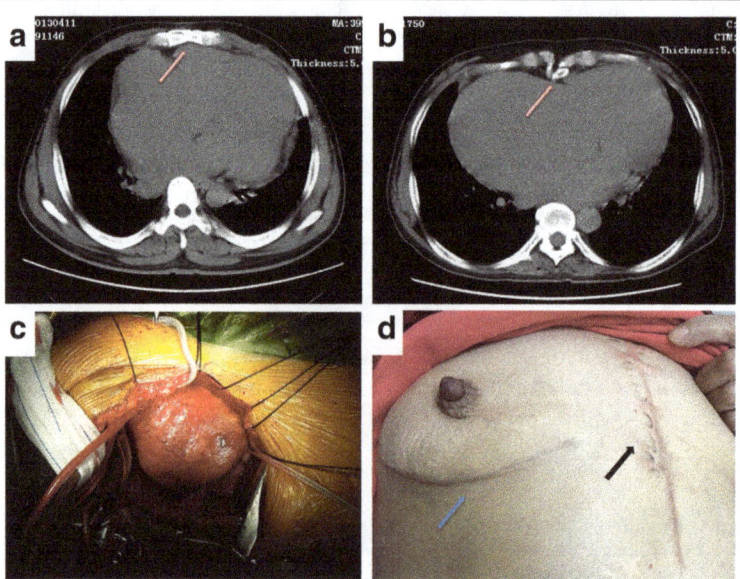

Fig. 1 a CT scan shows the firm adhesion between the right ventricle and the sternum in high-risk patients; **b** CT scan shows the firm adhesion between the right atrium and the sternum in high-risk patients; **c** The exposure by the right anterolateral thoracotomy after beginning of cardiopulmonary bypass; **d** The primary incision (black arrow) and the redo incision (blue arrow)

Table 1 Patients' demographic and preoperative clinical data

Variable	Mean ± SD or Number (%)
Age(years)	51.3 ± 8.6
Gender (n)	
Male	13 (54.2%)
Female	11 (45.8%)
Perivous operation time (n)	
1	22 (91.7%)
2	2 (8.3%)
Primary operation (n)	
Mitral valve repair	2
Mitral valve replacement	18
Aortic valve replacement	7
Atrial septal defect repair	3
Tricuspid valvuloplasty	9
Coronary artery bypass grafting	3
New York Heart Association class (n)	
Class III	15 (62.5%)
Class IV	9 (37.5%)
Mitral valve insufficiency (n)	5
Tricuspid valve insufficiency (n)	21
Atrial fibrillation (n)	22
Left ventricular ejection fraction (%)	47.5 ± 13.2
Left atrial diameter (mm)	79 ± 3.1
Right atrial diameter (mm)	72 ± 25
Cardiothoracic ratio (%)	69 ± 18

Table 2 Summary of Operative Variables

Variable	Mean ± SD or Number (%)
Category of operation (n)	
Mitral valve repair	1
Mitral valve replacement	4
Tricuspid valvuloplasty	2
Tricuspid valve replacement	19
Left atrial folding	5
Total surgery (min)	268 ± 89
Cardiopulmonary bypass (min)	133 ± 49
Cross-clamp (min)	67 ± 34
Blood loss during operation (ml)	238 ± 116
Blood transfusion during operation (ml)	325 ± 246
Incision length (cm)	12.6 ± 2.3

Outcomes and follow-up

Postoperative data was shown in Table 3. The chest drainage volume of the first 24 h was 225 ± 87 mL, and there was no postoperative blood transfusion in 17 patients. There were 8 patients whose duration of mechanical ventilation exceeded 24 h and 12 patients whose intensive care unit stay time exceeded 3 days. Six patients received continuous renal replacement therapy for acute renal failure or oliguresis. Extracorporeal membrane oxygenation was performed in 4 patients for low output syndrome (3 patients) and severe hypoxemia. Two patients died for low output syndrome causing multisystem organ failure and lung hemorrhage causing uncontrollablepulmonary infection. The left 22 patients' postoperative hospital stay was 16.4 ± 7.9 days.

Postdischarge follow-up information was obtained by follow-up clinc and telephone interview. The duration of follow-up ranged 6 to 42 months and follow-up rate was 100%. All the patients were surviving at the time of follow-up and willing to personally provide information regarding their functional status. There were no late deaths or cardiovascular accident during the follow-up.

females, 13 males, mean age 51.3 ± 8.6 years) who underwent redo mitral and tricuspid valve surgery via right anterolateral thoracotomy. Two patients had already undergone two previous cardiac operations. Table 1 lists all primary operations. Five and Twenty one patients had mitral and tricuspid valve insufficiency, respectively. Twenty two patients had atrial fibrillation. Fifteen patients were in New York Heart Association Class III, and left 9 were in Class IV. Mean left ventricular ejection fraction was 47.5% and mean cardiothoracic ratio was 69%. Left and right atrial diameter were 79 ± 3.1 and 72 ± 25, respectively.

Operative characteristics

Table 2 lists all category of operations. Most patients received tricuspid valve replacement. The patients were in the operating room for a mean of 268 min, and had an average duration of cardiopulmonary bypass and cross-clamp of 133 and 67 min, respectively. Moreover, the blood loss during operation was 238 ± 116 ml, and the blood transfusion was 325 ± 246 ml. The incision length was 12.6 ± 2.3 cm (Fig. 1d). The intraoperative course was uneventful and no patient was converted to a full sternotomy.

Table 3 Postoperative data of all patients

Variable	Mean ± SD or Number (%)
Drainage at the first day (mL)	225 ± 87
Ventilator >24 h (n)	8 (33.3%)
Intensive care unit stay >3 day (n)	12 (50%)
Continuous renal replacement therapy (n)	6 (25%)
Extracorporeal membrane oxygenation (n)	4 (16.7%)
Low output syndrome (n)	3 (12.5%)
Lung hemorrhage (n)	2 (8.3%)
Postoperative hospital stay (days)	16.4 ± 7.9
Mortality (%)	2 (8.3%)

Discussion

More and more minimally invasive techniques for cardiac valve surgery have been proven comparable results to conventional techniques [9]. Therefore, there is a greater interest in less invasive approaches to the heart, especially when these alternative access routes decrease the surgical risk and also do not compromise the quality of surgery via the standard approach. Due to these findings, we performed redo mitral and tricuspid valve surgery through a less invasive right anterolateral thoracotomy in high-risk patients. This series documented 24 patients undergoing the less invasive technique for redo cardiac valve procedures.

As a result, the right anterolateral approach offered excellent visualization of the mitral and tricuspid valve structures due to a direct-line view [10]. Median sternotomy for access in reoperations of cardiac valve requires more extensive and time-consuming dissection of adhesions. Reentry via a sternotomy bears the potential risk of direct injury to the right atrium and ventricle and is associated with bleeding complications and blood transfusion requirements [1]. In case of previous coronary artery bypass conduits, venous and especially internal mammary artery grafts (in our series, three patients) are prone to injury during reintervention. Hemorrhage from the heart or great vessels during sternotomy for cardiac reoperations has been reported to occur in 3.6% to 4.3% of cases [2]. Approximately one third of these patients die [2]. Our current data have not reported any major hemorrhage or mortality associated with dissection of adhesions via right thoracotomy. In our group, indeed, which patients with a severe dilated atrium or ventricle or the location of patent bypass grafts, it was believed that this risk was even higher via a sternotomy [11].

However, the dissection of the ascending aorta to achieve aortic cross-clamping is a major concern in patients via the right anterolateral thoracotomy. In the present two cases, dissecting the ascending aorta for aortic cross-clamping was not possible due to severe adhesion or location of patent bypass graft. We therefore decided to apply a strategy involving hypothermic fibrillatory arrest without an aortic cross-clamp, which is known as the no-touch technique [12]. Adequate myocardial protection against both ischemic and distention injuries and reducing the risk of stroke are generally major concerns in left heart surgery performed under fibrillatory arrest [13]. In order to achieve successful myocardial protection, we opened the left atrium immediately upon fibrillation in order to keep the left ventricle decompensated. Moreover, carbon dioxide gas was infused into the operative field to ensure that air did not enter the systemic circulation, and the mean arterial perfusion pressure was maintained at over 30 mmHg in order to keep the aortic valve closed. Transesophageal echocardiography confirmed that no intracardiac air was present before cardioversion.

Moreover, poor exposure of the ventricles requires specific strategies regarding de-airing, pacing-wire insertion, and defibrillation. It is mandatory to allow the left heart to fill with blood before the atrial septum is closed completely. Only the aortic root is de-aired before the aortic cross-clamp is opened. The ventricular pacing wire is inserted on the empty heart during cardiopulmonary bypass. Defibrillation can be performed with preoperatively fixed external paddles.

Isolated reoperative tricuspid valve surgery is considered to be associated with high operative risk [4]. Although the operation may not be technically complicated, the increased risk is usually due to the fact that patients are referred for surgery late in their disease process. Such patients often have evidence of right heart failure and associated complications. It is unknown whether poor postoperative outcome is related to the severity of tricuspid regurgitation itself or to the poor overall status of such patients. In previous studies, hospital mortality ranged from 0% to 37% [14, 15]. However, mortality of our study was lower than that of previous studies, and prognosis of present study was better than that of previous studies. It was convincing that prevention of dissection of the right ventricle, is additionally protective against dilatation of the right ventricle after surgery that would result in poor right heart function. Our policy is to use bioprosthetic valves (Medtronic Hancock II or Carpentier-Edwards Perimount) for tricuspid valve replacement in all patients to avoid excessive anticoagulation, regardless of patient age or presence of a previously implanted mechanical prosthesis in the aortic and/or mitral position.

In this series, we found that a dual lumen endotracheal tube was necessary. There were two cases of pulmonary hemorrhage in our group at the early stage by using a single lumen intubation. It was caused by excessively compressing lung during dissecting adhesions of right atrium and ascending aorta. After that, we used a double lumen endotracheal tube to avoid excessive lung injury. As a result, there was no pulmonary hemorrhag by the double lumen endotracheal tube. Severe pulmonary dysfunction, as determined by the PO2/FiO2 ratio [16], is also a relative contraindication to the right thoracotomy approach. In the present series, two patients had preoperative severe pulmonary dysfunction. One died of lung hemorrhage causing uncontrollable pulmonary infection, another weaned from the ventilator required tracheostomy but recovered fully.

The blood loss and transfusion are denitely less using this approach, probably because of the avoidance of sternotomy. The added advantage of totally eradicating the risk of deep sternal infection is invaluable. Phrenic nerve damage, which is especially attributed to right anterolateral thoracotomy, was not seen in our series. Since the nerve is always easily visible, there should not be incidental damage. Moreover, the intact thorax offers earlier mobilization and return to daily life activities [6].

Limitations

The current study has some limitations. First, our patient population is small because of the rarity of patients requiring a redo cardiac valve surgery with a high-risk resternotomy. Second, the heterogeneity of this group of patients with regard to demographics, prior surgery, preoperative cardiac function, and comorbid conditions makes risk adjustment impossible, so we did not do a case–control study between the right anterolateral thoracotomy and the resternotomy. Moreover, we accept that different valve reoperations provide different surgical challenges, the preoperative status of the patient can have a profound influence on the surgical outcome [17].

Conclusion

The right anterolateral thoracotomy has become a standard approach for redo mitral and tricuspid valve surgery in high-risk patients at our institution. It avoids a high-risk resternotomy, and can be performed safely and reduces the possibility of injury to the heart.

Acknowledgements
We thank Dr. Yonghong Liu for collecting clinical data for this study.

Funding
This work was supported in part by Jiangsu Provincial Medical Youth Talent [QNRC2016034], Jiangsu Province Health Department Program Grant [Z201411], Key Project supported by Medical Science and technology development Foundation, Nanjing Department of Health [JQX14006].

Authors' contributions
HC participated in the design of the operation and drafted the manuscript. QZ did most operations and helped to draft the manuscript. FF participated most operations and performed the statistical analysis. YX participated most operations and interpreted the data. JP did some operations and revised the paper. DW conceived of the study and participated in the design of the operation. All authors read and approved the final manuscript.

Competing interests
The authors declare that they have no competing interests.

References

1. Park CB, Suri RM, Burkhart HM, Greason KL, Dearani JA, Schaff HV, et al. Identifying patients at particular risk of injury during repeat sternotomy: analysis of 2555 cardiac reoperations. J Thorac Cardiovasc Surg. 2010; 140:1028–35.
2. Ghoreishi M, Dawood M, Hobbs G, Pasrija C, Riley P, Petrose L, et al. Repeat sternotomy: no longer a risk factor in mitral valve surgical procedures. Ann Thorac Surg. 2013;96:1358–65.
3. Roselli EE, Pettersson GB, Blackstone EH, Brizzio ME, Houghtaling PL, Hauck R, et al. Adverse events during reoperative cardiac surgery: frequency, characterization, and rescue. J Thorac Cardiovasc Surg. 2008;135:316–23.
4. Pfannmüller B, Moz M, Misfeld M, Borger MA, Funkat AK, Garbade J, et al. Isolated tricuspid valve surgery in patients with previous cardiac surgery. J Thorac Cardiovasc Surg. 2013;146:841–7.
5. Arcidi JM Jr, Rodriguez E, Elbeery JR, Nifong LW, Efird JT, Chitwood WR Jr. Fifteen-year experience with minimally invasive approach for reoperations involving the mitral valve. J Thorac Cardiovasc Surg. 2012;143:1062–8.
6. Romano MA, Haft JW, Pagani FD, Bolling SF. Beating heart surgery via right thoracotomy for reoperative mitral valve surgery: a safe and effective operative alternative. J Thorac Cardiovasc Surg. 2012;144:334–9.
7. Chaikriangkrai K, Maragiannis D, Belousova T, Little S, Nabi F, Mahmarian J, et al. Clinical Utility of Multidetector Computed Tomography in Redo Valve Procedures. J Card Surg. 2016;31:139–46.
8. Gammie JS, Sheng S, Griffith BP, Peterson ED, Rankin JS, O'Brien SM, et al. Trends in mitral valve surgery in the United States: results from the Society of Thoracic Surgeons Adult Cardiac Surgery Database. Ann Thorac Surg. 2009;87:1431–7.
9. Lamelas J, Nguyen TC. Minimally Invasive Valve Surgery: When Less Is More. Semin Thorac Cardiovasc Surg. 2015;27:49–56.
10. Guedes MA, Pomerantzeff PM, Brandão CM, Vieira ML, Grinberg M, Stolf NA. Mitral valve surgery using right anterolateral thoracotomy: is the aortic cannulation a safety procedure? Rev Bras Cir Cardiovasc. 2010;25:322–5.
11. Imran Hamid U, Digney R, Soo L, Leung S, Graham AN. Incidence and outcome of re-entry injury in redo cardiac surgery: benefits of preoperative planning. Eur J Cardiothorac Surg. 2015;47:819–23.
12. Kitamura T, Stuklis RG, Edwards J. Redo mitral valve operation via right minithoracotomy—"no touch" technique. Int Heart J. 2011;52:107–9.
13. Petracek MR, Leacche M, Solenkova N, Umakanthan R, Ahmad RM, Ball SK, et al. Minimally invasive mitral valve surgery expands the surgical options for high-risks patients. Ann Surg. 2011;254:606–11.
14. Bernal JM, Morales D, Revuelta C, Llorca J, Gutiérrez-Morlote J, Revuelta JM. Reoperations after tricuspid valve repair. J Thorac Cardiovasc Surg. 2005;130:498–503.
15. McCarthy PM, Bhudia SK, Rajeswaran J, Hoercher KJ, Lytle BW, Cosgrove DM, et al. Tricuspid valve repair: durability and risk factors for failure. J Thorac Cardiovasc Surg. 2004;127:674–85.
16. Braxton JH, Higgins RS, Schwann TA, Sanchez JA, Dewar ML, Kopf GS, et al. Reoperative mitral valve surgery via right thoracotomy: decreased blood loss and improved hemodynamics. J Heart Valve Dis. 1996;5:169–73.
17. Murzi M, Miceli A, Di Stefano G, Cerillo AG, Farneti P, Solinas M, et al. Minimally invasive right thoracotomy approach for mitral valve surgery in patients with previous sternotomy: a single institution experience with 173 patients. J Thorac Cardiovasc Surg. 2014;148:2763–8.

2

Modified double patch repair with infarct exclusion technique for ventricular septal perforation

Takuma Yamasaki* (ID), Shuhei Fujita, Yuji Kaku, Junko Katagiri and Takeshi Hiramatsu

Abstract

Background: Ventricular septal perforation (VSP) after acute myocardial infarction (AMI) is accompanied by the worsening of rapid hemodynamics, resulting in a poor prognosis. In our department, infarct lesions are preoperatively detected with electrocardiogram (ECG)-synchronized contrast computed tomography, and the scope of approach and exclusion is determined. Furthermore, to effectively prevent a residual shunt, modified double patch repair and infarct exclusion techniques were used in combination to preserve left ventricular (LV) function. This method is reported because it considers both techniques as a surgical procedure that can be accomplished relatively easily and simultaneously.

Case presentation: We targeted two consecutive VSP patients who underwent this procedure. It took an average of 1 day from the onset of VSP to surgery. We performed double patch and infarct exclusion for VSP using bovine pericardium via an LV incision. Two patches were marked with a skin pen to anastomose eight mattresses equally. In addition, a one piece-coupled patch was made for infarct exclusion. The two patients were extubated on the day after surgery and intra-aortic balloon pump assistance was also withdrawn. Without perioperative complications, they could leave the intensive care unit after 6.5 days on average. Early postoperative ECG and magnetic resonance angiography showed good LV wall contraction, except at the infarcted area, with no evidence of a residual shunt.

Conclusion: The modified double patch repair with infarct exclusion technique is more effective for preventing a residual shunt and maintaining postoperative cardiac function than either of the techniques alone.

Keywords: Acute myocardial infarction, Ventricular septal perforation, Double patch repair, Infarct exclusion

Background

Ventricular septal perforation (VSP) after acute myocardial infarction (AMI) is accompanied by the worsening of rapid hemodynamics, resulting in a poor prognosis. Arnaoutakis et al. reported on the largest and most recent database of The Society of Thoracic Surgeons in 2012 [1]; operative mortality was found to be 54.1% if repair was attempted within 7 days of AMI. On the other hand, Lundblad et al. reported that the 30-day mortality rate of VSP closure using the infarct exclusion technique was 16.7%, which was significantly better than that of patch closure [2]. Caimmi et al. reported that the 30-day mortality rate of VSP closure using the double patch technique was 18.8%, and it showed good results when

no postoperative residual shunt was observed [3]. However, there are no established views on the approaches and surgical techniques because VSP is a rare disease [4]. In our department, infarct lesions are preoperatively detected with electrocardiogram (ECG)-synchronized contrast computed tomography (CT) and the scope of the approach and exclusion is determined. Furthermore, in order to prevent a residual shunt, the modified double patch repair and the infarct exclusion techniques were used in combination to preserve left ventricular (LV) function. We report on our experiences of this technique and review the existing literature.

Case presentation

We targeted two consecutive VSP patients who underwent this procedure from September to December 2015. Case 1 was a 71-year-old man with AMI onset 7 days prior. The diameter of VSP was 12 mm, the responsible

* Correspondence: takuma360j@gmail.com
Department of Cardiovascular Surgery, Japanese Red Cross Kyoto Daini Hospital, Kamanza-Dori, Marutamachi-Agaru, Kamigyo-Ku, Kyoto 602-8026, Japan

lesion occurred in the left anterior descending artery (LAD) #7–99% delay, the pulmonary blood flow/systemic blood flow (Qp/Qs) was 3.6, and the pulmonary capillary wedge pressure (PCWP) was 22 mmHg. Emergency surgery was performed under artificial respiration management.

Case 2 was a 78-year-old woman with AMI onset 3 days prior. The diameter of VSP was 18 mm, the responsible lesion occurred in the LAD #7-total, the Qp/Q s was 2.6, and PCWP was 20 mmHg. Emergency surgery was performed under intra-aortic balloon pumping (IABP).

ECG-synchronized contrast CT was performed before surgery to identify the infarct area and to set up a surgical strategy (Fig. 1). A median sternotomy incision approach was employed, establishing extracorporeal circulation by ascending aorta and right atrial cannulation. A longitudinal transinfarction incision was performed in the LV myocardium parallel to and 1.5 cm away from the interventricular septum while the heart was beating, and the location of the septal defect was identified. After grasping the boundary between the normal myocardium and the infarcted myocardium manually, antegrade cold blood cardioplegia was infused to arrest the heart. The fragile myocardium surrounding the VSP was excised. A bovine pericardium patch (10 × 15 cm) was trimmed to make a perfect circle with a diameter of 4.5 to 5.5 cm to be used as the 1st patch. Two pieces of patch marked with a skin pen were made to sandwich the septum evenly with an 8-needle mattress. The 2nd patch on the LV side was combined with a patch for infarct exclusion (Fig. 2a). 3–0 polypropylene sutures were concentrically conducted on the 1st patch on the right ventricular (RV) side with an 8-needle mattress; the needle thread was penetrated from the RV side to the LV side into the relatively healthy septal muscle around the VSP. Three needles on the upper edge of the circular patch were inserted into the RV free wall. The 1st patch led to the

RV via the VSP (Fig. 2b). A set of needle threads penetrating the ventricular septum were passed through the 2nd patch and gelatin-resorcin-formalin (GRF) glue (Cardial, Technopole, Sainte-tienne, France) or BioGlue (Cryolife Inc., Kennesaw, Georgia, USA) was injected between patches. After completion of the double patch (Fig. 2c), the patch for infarct exclusion was threaded with mattress sutures clockwise from the lower edge of the circular patch. The patch was appropriately trimmed so as not to apply tension to the patch and to exclude infarcted muscle and the double patch from the LV cavity (Fig. 2d). The LV incision line was double suture-closed with the felt sandwich method by using 3–0 polypropylene sutures. Finally, a coronary bypass anastomosis was added to the LAD and the operation was completed (Fig. 2e). In both cases, the anterior LV wall approach was used on the infarcted myocardium side, and coronary artery bypass grafting (CABG) was performed. The average operation time was 290 min, the average aortic cross clamp time was 115 min, and the average extracorporeal circulation time was 192 min. Both patients were extubated on the day after surgery and IABP assistance was also withdrawn. Without perioperative complications, these patients could leave the intensive care unit after 6.5 days and be discharged from hospital after 33.5 days on average. Early postoperative ECG and magnetic resonance angiography showed good LV wall contraction, except at the infarcted area, with no evidence of a residual shunt (Fig. 3), and coronary bypass graft was also patent on coronary artery CT. No symptoms of heart failure occurred, and the patients were discharged without complications.

Discussion

Acute phase VSP is often difficult to treat surgically because of the unstable circulatory dynamics and fragile myocardium around the VSP. In this report, an intra-

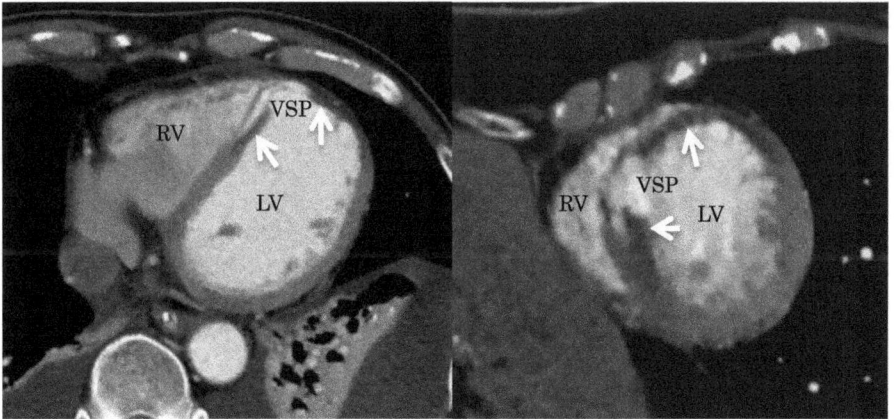

Fig. 1 Preoperative computed tomography shows the myocardium having poor contrasting that became light thickness (white arrows)

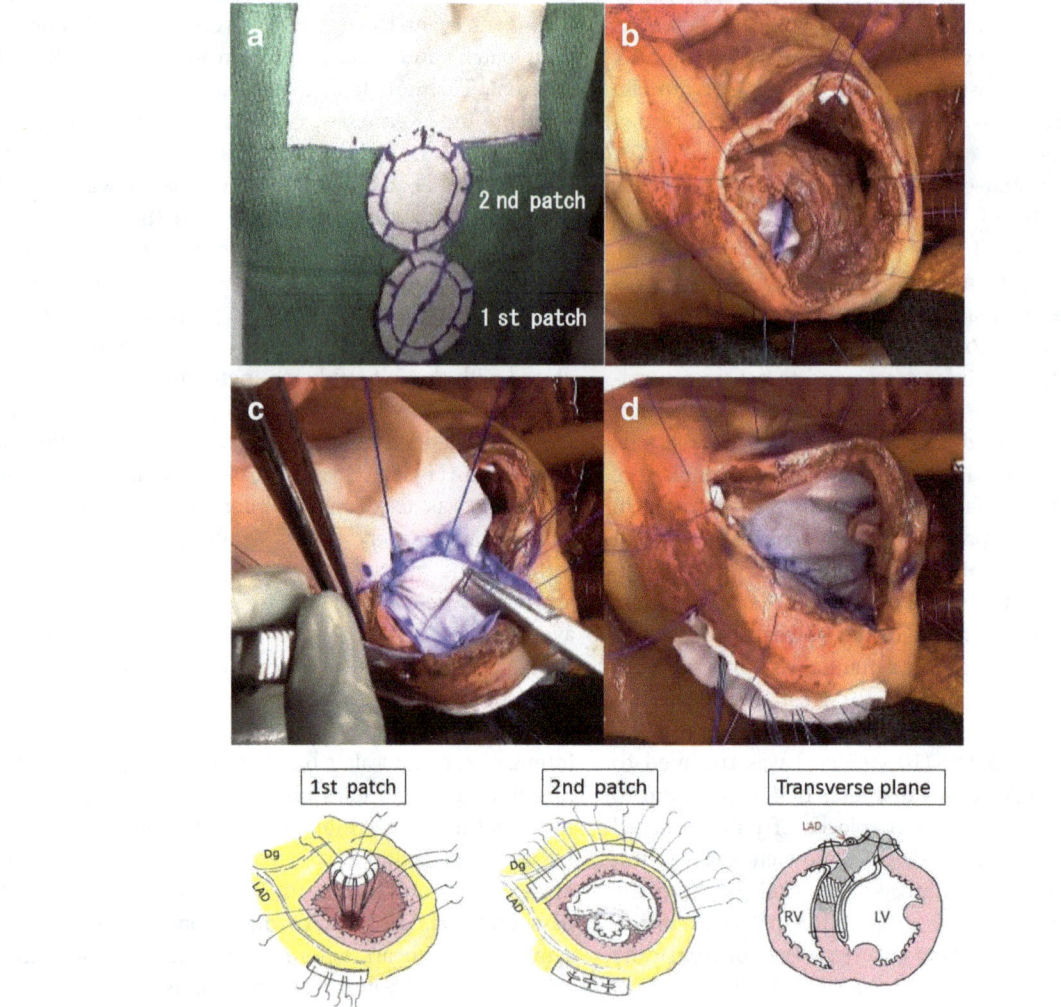

Fig. 2 a Two patches were made in order to sandwich the septum evenly with an 8-needle mattress. **b** The 1st patch led to the right ventricle via VSP. **c** A set of needle threads penetrating the ventricular septum was passed through the 2nd patch. **d** The patch was appropriately trimmed to exclude the infarcted muscle from the left ventricular cavity. **e** Schema of the modified double patch repair with infarct exclusion technique

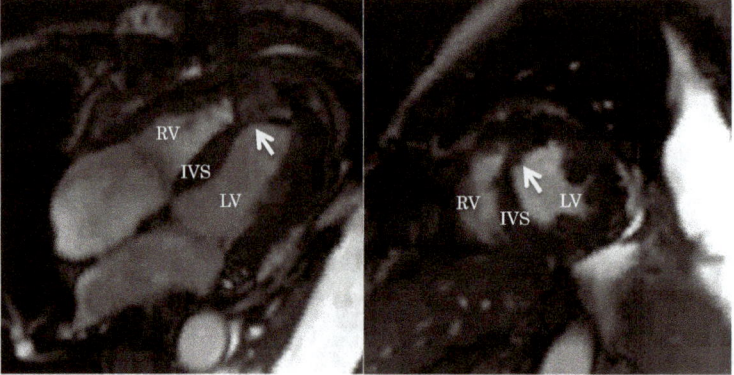

Fig. 3 Postoperative magnetic resonance angiography shows the double patch with infarct exclusion (arrow) without residual shunt

aortic balloon pumping was inserted before surgery in one case, and artificial respiration management was needed in the other case as the respiratory and circulatory dynamics had deteriorated; surgery in the acute phase was then judged to be necessary. In this study, we approached from the anterior wall of the LV, the side of the infarcted myocardium, in order to minimize the damage to the non-infarcted myocardium. In addition, to reliably prevent the remaining shunt and maintain cardiac function after surgery, the VSP was closed in both cases by using the modified double patch repair with infarct exclusion technique. This technique can simultaneously achieve the advantages of both the double patch technique and the infarct exclusion technique; therefore, it is considered a useful and effective technique.

Surgical treatment for VSP was greatly improved by the infarct exclusion method reported by Komeda and David et al. They claimed that their technique, which does not resect any part of the RV, could be beneficial in reducing the risk of further RV dysfunction, and that it improved surgical results [5]. However, the hand movement to the LV outflow tract and the LV rear wall at the time of sewing the patch requires considerable ingenuity and skill because the operative field is deep and the posterior papillary muscle is present. As a result, a postoperative shunt remains, requiring reoperation, and results in death from heart failure in many cases [6].

On the other hand, many good results of the double patch method, in which VSP is sandwiched between two patches, have been reported. The advantages of the double patch method for VSP are that it is easy to approach the ventricular lumen from one side and that the procedure can be easily performed. In this method, two patches are uniformly sandwiched between eight needles of mattress nodules so as to sandwich the infarcted septal muscle from the LV and RV; the LV pressure is diffused, thus suturing disintegration can be reduced [7]. In addition, it is possible to increasingly prevent a residual shunt by compensating with glue paste, such as GRF and BioGlue, between patches [8]. Also, in the long term, the double patch method has been reported to alleviate wall motion abnormalities in the ventricular septum [3]. Hosoba et al. reported mid-term results of the extended sandwich patch technique through right ventriculotomy and achieved good results when neither severe septal dyskinesia nor aneurysmal change in the LV was observed [9]. However, in the double patch method based on the RV approach to VSP caused by myocardial infarction in the LAD region, right heart failure due to RV incision may be a problem after surgery [10]. Therefore, we believe this to be a novel procedure as it prevented the residual shunt more effectively by decreasing the LV pressure to the double patch,

controlled bleeding from the LV incision line, and prevented postoperative LV aneurysm and rupture. Furthermore, identification of the infarct range with preoperative CT and infarct exclusion with a correctly sized patch can prevent LV remodeling at the remote stage and maintain LV function. By using a 2nd patch as a series of patches, it is relatively easy to perform both the double patch method and infarct exclusion method. However, if the preoperative condition is more imminent, it is difficult to image the CT and identify the infarct range, and similarly, it is considered to be difficult in the case of a more extensive infarction or posterior VSP.

Conclusion

This modified double patch repair with infarct exclusion technique is more effective than either technique alone for preventing a residual shunt and bleeding of the incision sutures, and can be effective for maintaining postoperative cardiac function.

Abbreviations
AMI: Acute myocardial infarction; CABG: Coronary artery bypass grafting; CT: Computed tomography; ECG: Electrocardiogram; GRF: Gelatin-resorcin-formalin; IABP: Intra-aortic balloon pumping; ICU: Intensive care unit; LAD: Left anterior descending artery; LV: Left ventricle; PCWP: Pulmonary capillary wedge pressure; Qp/Qs: Pulmonary blood flow/systemic blood flow; RV: Right ventricle; VSP: Ventricular septal perforation

Acknowledgements
We would like to thank Editage (www.editage.jp) for English language editing.

Funding
None.

Authors' contributions
TY performed surgery, analyzed the data, wrote the manuscript, and obtained informed consent from the patients; SF provided the figures; YK contributed to analysis; JK collected the data; and TH assisted in the preparation of the manuscript. All authors have read and approved the final manuscript.

Competing interests
The authors declare that they have no competing interests.

References
1. Arnaoutakis GJ, Zhao Y, George TJ, Sciortino CM, McCarthy PM, Conte JV. Surgical repair of ventricular septal defect after myocardial infarction: outcomes from the society of thoracic surgeons national database. Ann Thorac Surg. 2012;94:436 44.

2. Lundblad R, Abdelnoor M. Surgery of postinfarction ventricular septal rupture: the effect of David infarct exclusion versus Daggett direct septal closure on early and late outcome. J Thorac Cardiovasc Surg. 2014;148:2736–42.

3. Caimmi PP, Grossini E, Kapetanakis EI, Boido R, Coppo C, Scappellato F, et al. Double patch repair through a single ventriculotomy for ischemic ventricular septal defect. Ann Thorac Surg. 2010;89:1679–81.

4. Asai T. Postinfarction ventricular septal rupture: can we improve clinical outcome of surgical repair? Gen Thorac Cardiovasc Surg. 2016;64:121–30.

5. David TE, Dale L, Sun Z. Postinfarction ventricular septal rupture: repair by endocardial patch with infarct exclusion. J Thorac Cardiovasc Surg. 1995;110:1315–22.

6. Kawada N, Kurosawa H, Suzuki K, Okuyama H, Ishii S, Nomura K, et al. Modified Komeda-David operation for postinfarction ventricular septal perforation. Kyobu Geka. 2005;58:289–93.

7. Balkanay M, Eren E, Keles C, Toker ME, Guler M. Double-patch repair of postinfarction ventricular septal defect. Tex Heart Inst J. 2005;32:43–6.

8. Musumeci F, Shukla V, Mignosa C, Casali G, Ikram S. Early repair of postinfarction ventricular septal defect with gelatin-resorcin-formol biological glue. Ann Thorac Surg. 1996;62:486–8.

9. Hosoba S, Asai T, Suzuki T, Nota H, Kuroyanagi S, Kinoshita T, et al. Mid-term results for the use of the extended sandwich patch technique through right ventriculotomy for postinfarction ventricular septal defects. Eur J Cardiothorac Surg. 2013;43:e116–20.

10. Kitamura S, Mendez A, Kay JH. Ventricular septal defect following myocardial infarction: experience with surgical repair through a left ventriculotomy and review of literature. J Thorac Cardiovasc Surg. 1971;61:186.

3

Development and in vivo validation of tissue-engineered, small-diameter vascular grafts from decellularized aortae of fetal pigs and canine vascular endothelial cells

Xu Ma[1†], Zhijuan He[2†], Ling Li[3], Guofeng Liu[1*], Qingchun Li[1], Daping Yang[1], Yingbo Zhang[1] and Ning Li[1]

Abstract

Background: Tissue engineering has emerged as a promising alternative for small-diameter vascular grafts. The aim of this study was to determine the feasibility of using decellularized aortae of fetal pigs (DAFPs) to construct tissue-engineered, small-diameter vascular grafts and to test the performance and application of DAFPs as vascular tissue-engineered scaffolds in the canine arterial system.

Methods: DAFPs were prepared by continuous enzymatic digestion. Canine vascular endothelial cells (ECs) were seeded onto DAFPs in vitro and then the vascular grafts were cultured in a custom-designed vascular bioreactor system for 7 days of dynamic culture following 3 days of static culture. The grafts were then transplanted into the common carotid artery of the same seven dogs from which ECs had been derived (two grafts were prepared for each dog with one as a backup; therefore, a total of 14 tissue-engineered blood vessels were prepared). At 1, 3, and 6 months post-transplantation, ultrasonography and contrast-enhanced computed tomography (CT) were used to check the patency of the grafts. Additionally, vascular grafts were sampled for histological and electron microscopic examination.

Results: Tissue-engineered, small-diameter vascular grafts can be successfully constructed using DAFPs and canine vascular ECs. Ultrasonographic and CT test results confirmed that implanted vascular grafts displayed good patency with no obvious thrombi. Six months after implantation, the grafts had been remodeled and exhibited a similar structure to normal arteries. Immunohistochemical staining showed that cells had evenly infiltrated the tunica media and were identified as muscular fibroblasts. Scanning electron microscopy showed that the graft possessed a complete cell layer, and the internal cells of the graft were confirmed to be ECs by transmission electron microscopy.

Conclusions: Tissue-engineered, small-diameter vascular grafts constructed using DAFPs and canine vascular ECs can be successfully transplanted to replace the canine common carotid artery. This investigation potentially paves the way for solving a problem of considerable clinical need, i.e., the requirement for small-diameter vascular grafts.

Keywords: Vascular endothelial cells, Decellularized aortae of fetal pigs, Scaffold, Tissue-engineered small-diameter vascular grafts

* Correspondence: FennyL789@163.com
†Equal contributors
[1]Department of Plastic Surgery, The Second Affiliated Hospital of Harbin Medical University, 246 Xuefu Road, Nangang District, Harbin, Heilongjiang 150086, China
Full list of author information is available at the end of the article

Background

Coronary artery and peripheral arterial diseases have high rates of mortality and morbidity and so represent a massive economic and clinical burden to healthcare worldwide [1]. The most promising approach to solving this vascular problem and thus reducing the morbidity associated with these diseases is the use of small-diameter (<6 mm) vascular grafts [2]. Although autologous vessels (e.g., saphenous veins) represent the gold standard grafts for small-diameter vessels, many patients do not have veins suitable for grafting [3]. Thus, there is a considerable clinical need for small-diameter vascular grafts.

Tissue engineering has emerged as a promising alternative for producing small-diameter vascular grafts [4]. Tissue engineering strategies consist of three main components: scaffolds that house the cells and support cellular growth and activity; seed cells, which preserve the specific function of the tissue; and a nurturing environment [5]. Scaffolds provide temporary or permanent support to damaged tissues, and scaffold materials can be generally divided into two categories: native biological materials and synthetic polymeric materials [6]. Compared with synthetic polymer-based scaffolds, natural polymers present a biologically active environment to cells and promote excellent cell adhesion and growth [7]. However, numerous studies have also reported on the poor mechanical properties of natural polymers [7–9]. Recently, decellularized tissue-engineered vascular grafts have been widely used as natural scaffolds to produce arterial conduits that provide ideal biomechanical properties and cell compatibility [10, 11]. For instance, Böer et al. showed that intensified decellularization of equine carotid arteries generated highly suitable matrix scaffolds for vascular tissue engineering [12]. However, the in vivo application of tissue-engineered vascular grafts has not been widely investigated.

Recently, Liu et al. studied the mechanical properties of decellularized aortae of fetal pigs (DAFPs) and conducted an assessment of cell adhesion and compatibility by seeding with porcine aortic endothelial cells (ECs) and performing subdermal implantation in adult male Sprague Dawley rats [13]. Their results showed that DAFPs exhibited minimal calcification and exhibited almost no immunological reaction during the entire follow-up period [13]. In this study, small-diameter vascular grafts were constructed with DAFPs and by seeding with canine vascular ECs. These vascular grafts were then implanted into the same dogs from which ECs had been derived. The aim of this study was to determine the feasibility of using DAFPs to construct tissue-engineered small-diameter vascular grafts and to test the performance and application of DAFPs as tissue-engineered vascular scaffolds in the canine arterial system.

Methods

Experimental animals

Fetal pigs of 100-day gestational age were delivered by cesarean section. Adult mongrel dogs were used as both vascular EC donors and graft recipients. All animals received humane care in compliance with the Guide for Care and Use of Laboratory Animals published by the National Institutes of Health (NIH publication No. 85-23, revised 1996).

Preparation of fetal pig aorta

Pregnant sows were intravenously anesthetized with 1% pentobarbital sodium (10 mg/kg) and delivered by cesarean section. After removal of fetuses, sows were euthanized by excessive anesthesia. Fetal pigs with crown-rump lengths of 25–30 cm were selected and 5-cm sections of aorta were excised under sterile conditions. These specimens werecryopreserved immediately transported to the laboratory with a warm ischemia time of <30 min [14].

Preparation of DAFPs

Fetal pig aortae with an outer diameter of 4 mm and a length of 6 cm were selected. After removal of surrounding tissues under sterile condition, the blood vessels were washed with sterile saline several times to remove residual blood. DAFPs were prepared by continuous enzymatic digestion using trypsin, DNase, and RNase as previously described [15] with few modifications. Aortae were first digested with a solution containing 0.1% trypsin/0.02% EDTA in phosphate-buffered saline (PBS) (without Ca^{2+} and Mg^{2+}) for 36 h (all reagents from Sigma, St. Louis, Mo., USA), and the solution was changed every 12 h. The aortae were then decellularized with 20 µg/mL RNase and 200 µg/mL DNase (Boehringer, Mannheim, Germany) for 4 h at 37 °C under a humidified atmosphere of 5% CO_2 and 95% air with constant gentle shaking. DAFPs were then washed with sterile PBS several times to remove the digestion residue. Following DAFP preparation, approximately 3 mm of the tissue at the end of each decellularized specimen was taken and cut into two semi-rings. Half of the tissue was examined following conventional hematoxylin–eosin (HE) staining, and the other half was used for DNA quantification [16]. Finally, DAFPs were subjected to vacuum freeze-drying and ethylene oxide sterilization.

Culture and identification of canine vascular ECs

Seven domestic dogs aged 6 months and weighing 25 kg were used. Intravenous administration of 1% pentobarbital sodium (10 mg/kg) was used for anesthesia. Approximately 10 cm of the left external jugular vein was excised under aseptic condition as previously described [17]. Primary vascular ECs were obtained by enzymatic digestion as previously described [18]. In brief, the outer membrane layer of the vessel was removed and the vessel was cut longitudinally to form a sheet. The intima layer was flattened on the culture dish. A solution of 0.2% collagenase A (Boehringer Mannheim, Germany) in PBS with Ca^{2+} and Mg^{2+} was injected beneath the inner membrane surface and subsequent digestion performed in an incubator for 15 min. The digested EC suspension was collected and centrifuged at 1000 rpm for 5 min. The EC pellet was resuspended and cultured in medium 199 (GIBCO) supplemented with 10% fetal bovine serum, 100 units/mL penicillin (Sigma), 100 mg/mL streptomycin (Sigma), 0.25 mg/mL amphotericin B (Sigma), 5 ng/mL endothelial growth factor (Boehringer Mannheim) and 1% L-glutamine (Sigma). Cells were passaged using trypsin digestion and the fourth generation was used as seed cells (the number of vascular seed cells in the fourth generation was sufficient for seeding purposes, and ECs still possessed abundant proliferative capacity at this passage). Cells were confirmed to be vascular ECs by morphology as well as by immunohistochemistry and immunofluorescence to detect the endothelial marker von Willebrand factor (vWF) as previously described [19].

Construction of tissue-engineered, small-diameter vascular grafts

Vacuum freeze-dried DAFP material was soaked in sterile PBS for 24 h. Vascular ECs were seeded onto DAFPs by rotational precipitation. Briefly, ECs were trypsinized to form a cell suspension and the EC concentration was adjusted to 3×10^6 cells/mL. Both ends of DAFP tubular stents were clamped and the cell suspension was injected into the arterial lumen using a syringe. The arteries were then rotated 120° after standing for 10 min and seeding was completed after a total rotation of 360°. The grafts were transferred to a vascular bioreactor system for 7 days of dynamic culture following 3 days of static culture. A vascular bioreactor system was designed and produced by our research group as depicted in Fig. 1. This bioreactor system was driven by a peristaltic pump [20] and specimens were placed in the processing chamber (Fig. 1b). The liquid flow in the system was gradually increased by adjusting the speed of the peristaltic pump so that the perfusion rate increased from 20 to 60 mL/min (the perfusion rate was 20 mL/min on the first day of dynamic culture and increased by 10 mL/min daily to 60 mL/min on the fifth day of dynamic culture, at which point the perfusion rate was maintained at 60 mL/min through to the seventh day). The static pressure due to height differences of the culture solutions was 10 mmHg, and the dynamic pressure generated by the peristaltic pump was 60 mmHg. After culture completion, the fixed ends (lacking ECs) were removed and then the grafts were used for surgical implantation into the same dogs from which ECs had been derived.

Surgical implantation of vascular grafts

The same seven dogs from which left external jugular veins were harvested to obtain ECs received general anesthesia. Routine preoperative preparation was followed and the right common carotid artery was

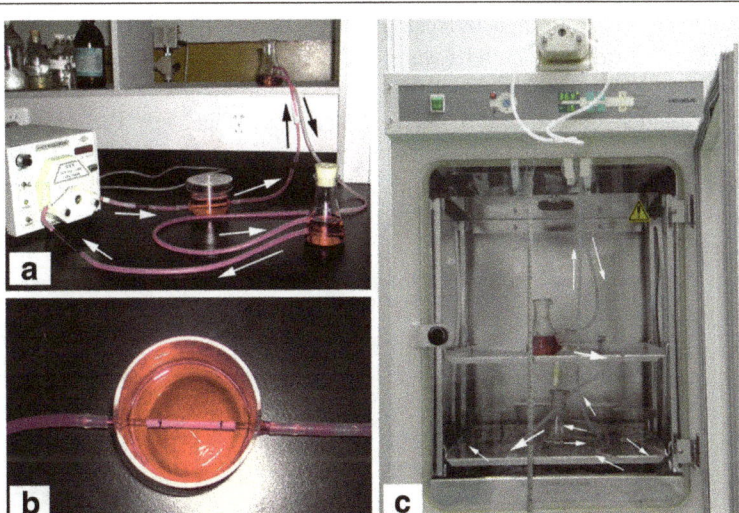

Fig. 1 A custom-designed and -produced vascular bioreactor system. **a**, the design of the vascular bioreactor system. **b**, the processing chamber used for specimen fixation. **c**, operation of the dynamic vascular bioreactor system. The dynamic vascular bioreactor system was placed into a tissue culture incubator. The height difference between culture solutions was regulated to control the static pressure within the vascular grafts. A controlled peristaltic pump regulated the dynamic pressure within the vascular grafts and the flow rate variation of the culture solutions. The arrows show the operation of the dynamic vascular bioreactor system

exposed. A location of the carotid artery with an external diameter of approximately 4 mm at diastole was selected as the site for implantation of the tissue-engineered vascular grafts. Vascular clamps were placed on both sides of the selected position, and the artery (4 mm in diameter) was transected. The tissue-engineered vascular grafts were used to bridge the common carotid artery using microsurgical techniques. The incisions were closed, and routine intramuscular injection of heparin as well as intravenous injection of antibiotics were applied postoperatively. Doppler ultrasonography was conducted at 1, 3, and 6 months and contrast-enhanced CT at 6 months, following implantation. Vascular grafts were sampled for histological and electron microscopic examination after the dogs were sacrificed at 6 months post-implantation.

Doppler ultrasonography and enhanced CT examination

All experimental animals received general anesthesia prior to each procedure and neck skin preparation prior to ultrasonic examination. Bilateral common carotid artery ultrasound was performed using a Doppler ultrasound device. Animals were injected with contrast medium prior to three-dimensional CT angiography.

HE staining

DAFPs and sampled vascular grafts were fixed in 10% neutral-buffered formalin solution, embedded in paraffin, transversely sectioned (5 μm) and stained using HE for histological assessment of general morphology.

Electron microscopy

Specimen surface ultrastructure was examined by scanning electron microscopy (SEM). Briefly, specimens were sequentially fixed in 1% (v/v) buffered glutaraldehyde and 0.1% (v/v) buffered formaldehyde for 1 and 24 h, respectively, dehydrated with a graded ethanol series, and dried. Dried samples were mounted on aluminum chucks and sputter-coated with gold (Cressington 108; Cressington Scientific Instruments, PA, USA). An S-3400 N scanning electron microscope (Hitachi, Tokyo, Japan) was used for sample examination.

For transmission electron microscopy (TEM), specimens were fixed in 2.5% glutaraldehyde solution, rinsed with 0.1 M phosphate buffer, and then fixed in 1% osmic acid for 2 h. Subsequent rinsing in double-distilled water was followed by dehydration in a graded series of water–acetone solution. Specimens were then impregnated with Epon 812 resin, embedded, and polymerized. Semi-thin sections were counterstained with azure II and basic fuchsin and examined with light microscopy to determine orientation. Ultra-thin sections were stained with uranyl acetate and lead citrate and then examined with a Zeiss EM10 electron microscope (Zeiss, Oberkochen, Germany).

Results
Identification of canine vascular ECs and morphology of DAFPs

Immunohistochemistry and immunofluorescence showed positive vWF staining in most cells (Fig. 2).

Histological staining of fetal porcine aortae revealed a typical three-layer structure of the arteries (Fig. 3A-a), and SEM demonstrated a complete layer of ECs with a cobblestone phenotype (Fig. 3B-a, b). The DNA content of DAFPs was <0.1%. Histological staining of DAFPs showed that the extracellular matrix remained intact; however, no nuclei or intact cells were present (Fig. 3A-b). In addition, SEM examination showed that after decellularization, endogenous ECs were completely removed and the structure of the inner elastic membrane was clearly visible (Fig. 3B-c, d).

Characterization of tissue-engineered, small-diameter vascular grafts

After 1 week of dynamic culture in the custom-made dynamic vascular bioreactor system, vascular grafts were successfully constructed using DAFPs and canine vascular ECs (Fig. 4). The vascular grafts possessed a complete, intact EC layer. Histological findings showed that a continuous cell layer was present on the inner surface of the grafts (Fig. 3A-c), and SEM revealed that ECs were tightly connected, forming a continuous cell layer that completely covered the inner elastic membrane (Fig. 3B-e, f).

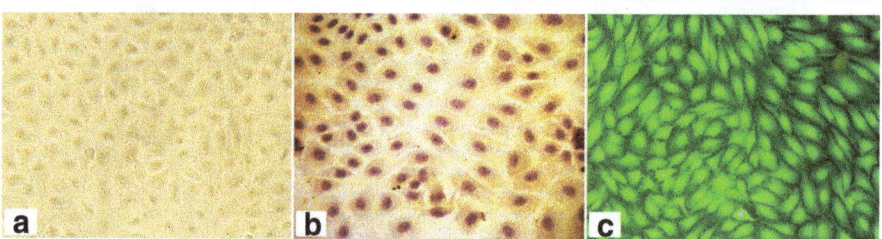

Fig. 2 Culture and identification of canine vascular endothelial cells (ECs). **a** optical microscopy image of ECs; **b** immunohistochemical staining for von Willebrand factor (vWF); **c** immunofluorescence of vWF. Most cells were vWF-positive

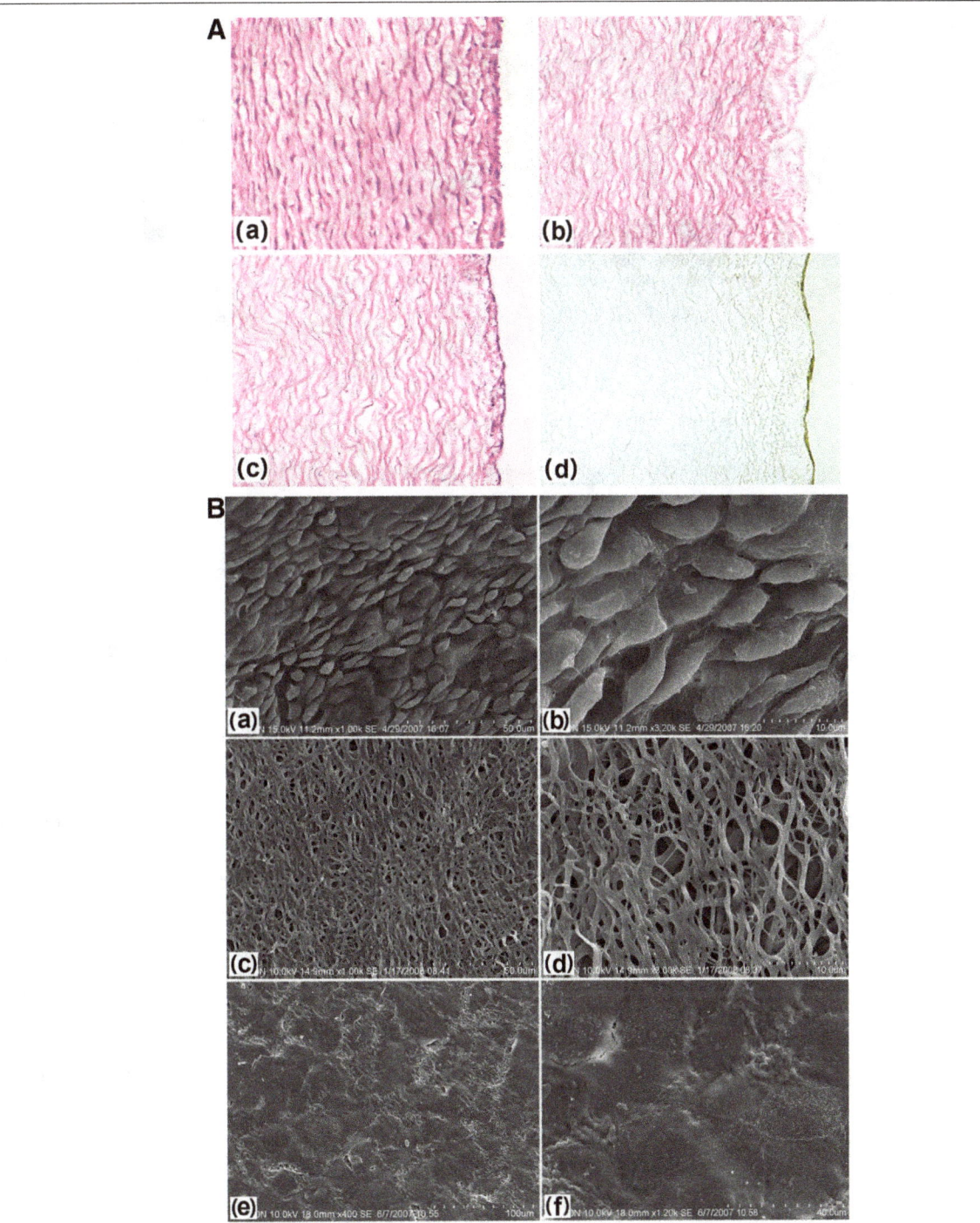

Fig. 3 Histological and immunohistochemical staining and scanning electron microscopy of specimens. **A**: **a**, histological staining of fetal pig aorta; **b**: histological staining of decellularized aortae of fetal pigs (DAFPs); **c**: histological staining of tissue-engineered vascular grafts with an EC layer; **d**: immunohistochemical staining of ECs of vascular grafts. **B**: **a**: fetal pig aortic EC layer at low magnification; **b**: fetal pig aortic EC layer at high magnification; **c**: the inner elastic membrane of DAFPs at low magnification; **d**: the inner elastic membrane of DAFPs at high magnification; **e**: the EC layer of tissue-engineered vascular grafts at low magnification; **f**: the EC layer of tissue-engineered vascular grafts at high magnification

Implantation and evaluation

Seven dogs were numbered and all were subjected to extensive postoperative evaluation (Table 1). Vascular diameter of the grafts matched that of the common carotid artery into which they had been implanted (Fig. 4). Following implantation, vascular grafts exhibited good patency and no obvious thrombi were found attached to the vascular wall, as assessed by Doppler

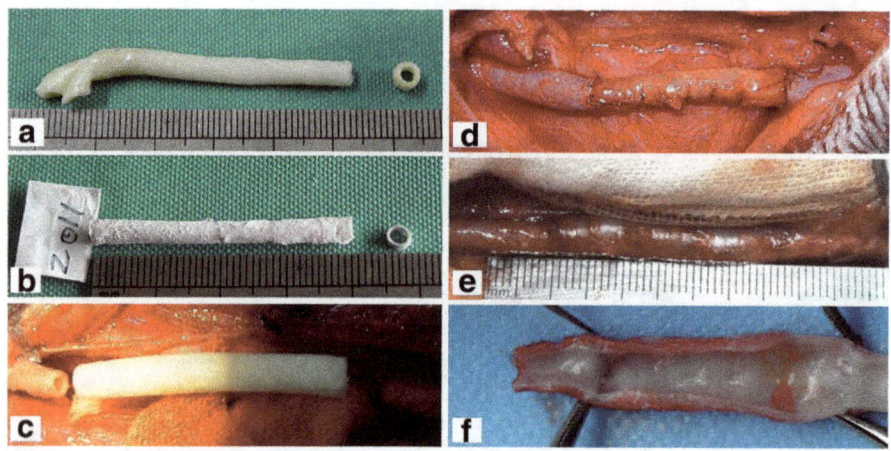

Fig. 4 General morphology of specimens. **a** general morphology of fetal pig aorta; **b** general morphology of vacuum freeze-dried DAFPs; **c** tissue-engineered vascular grafts after dynamic seeding of ECs; **d** the implantation of tissue-engineered vascular grafts in dogs; **e** general morphology of sampled vascular grafts at 6 months post-implantation; **f** the inner morphology of sampled vascular grafts at 6 months post-implantation

ultrasound and enhanced CT examination (Fig. 5). Six months after implantation, the grafts showed no obvious stenosis and expansion. Additionally, dynamic Doppler sonography revealed good graft compliance, and vascular grafts underwent spontaneous rhythmic vasodilation and contraction in synchrony with heartbeat.

Sampling results at 6 months post-transplantation showed that the tissue-engineered vascular grafts had smooth surface and no thrombi. As depicted in Fig. 6, histological staining showed that the grafts had been remodeled within the animals, and a continuous inner cell layer was identified. The tunica media was structurally dense and similar to natural arterial structure, and cells had evenly infiltrated and were identified as muscular fibroblasts by immunohistochemistry (smooth muscle actin expression was used as a classical marker for myofibroblasts). In addition, TEM examination of the inner cells showed that their surfaces were rich in finger, spherical, and villous protrusions and that they contained abundant cytoplasmic organelles, indicating that they were indeed ECs (Fig. 7). Moreover, Weibel–Palade bodies, which are membrane-enclosed rod-shaped organelles specifically found in ECs, were also identified.

Discussion

Extracellular matrix (ECM) scaffolds for vascular tissue engineering have mainly been derived from decellularized vascular matrix and decellularized small intestinal submucosa [21, 22]. Suitably decellularized blood vessels have the ideal shape and they possess biomechanical properties particularly suited for use as vascular grafts [23]. Li et al. have demonstrated that due to its low immunogenicity and optimal properties, decellularized fetal porcine vascular tissue could be used for tissue-engineered, small-diameter vascular grafts and as a potential alternative to xenogeneic transplantation [24]. Taking into account these studies, we hypothesized that

Table 1 Extensive evaluation of seven dogs at 6 months post-implantation of tissue-engineered vascular grafts

Number	Gross observations	Histological staining	Color Doppler ultrasonography and three-dimensional CT	Scanning electron microscopy	Transmission electron microscopy
1	No obvious expansion; smooth surface without thrombi when sampled	Similar to natural arterial structure; a continuous cell inner layer; dense tunica media	Good patency; no obvious thrombi; no obvious stenosis and expansion	Continuous endothelial cell layer; tight cell junctions	Confirmation of the continuous endothelial cell layer; identification of Weibel–Palade bodies
2	√	√	√	√	√
3	√	√	√	√	√
4	√	√	√	√	√
5	√	√	√	√	√
6	√	√	√	√	√
7	√	√	√	√	√

All dogs were tested in the same manner and "√" indicates the same positive findings

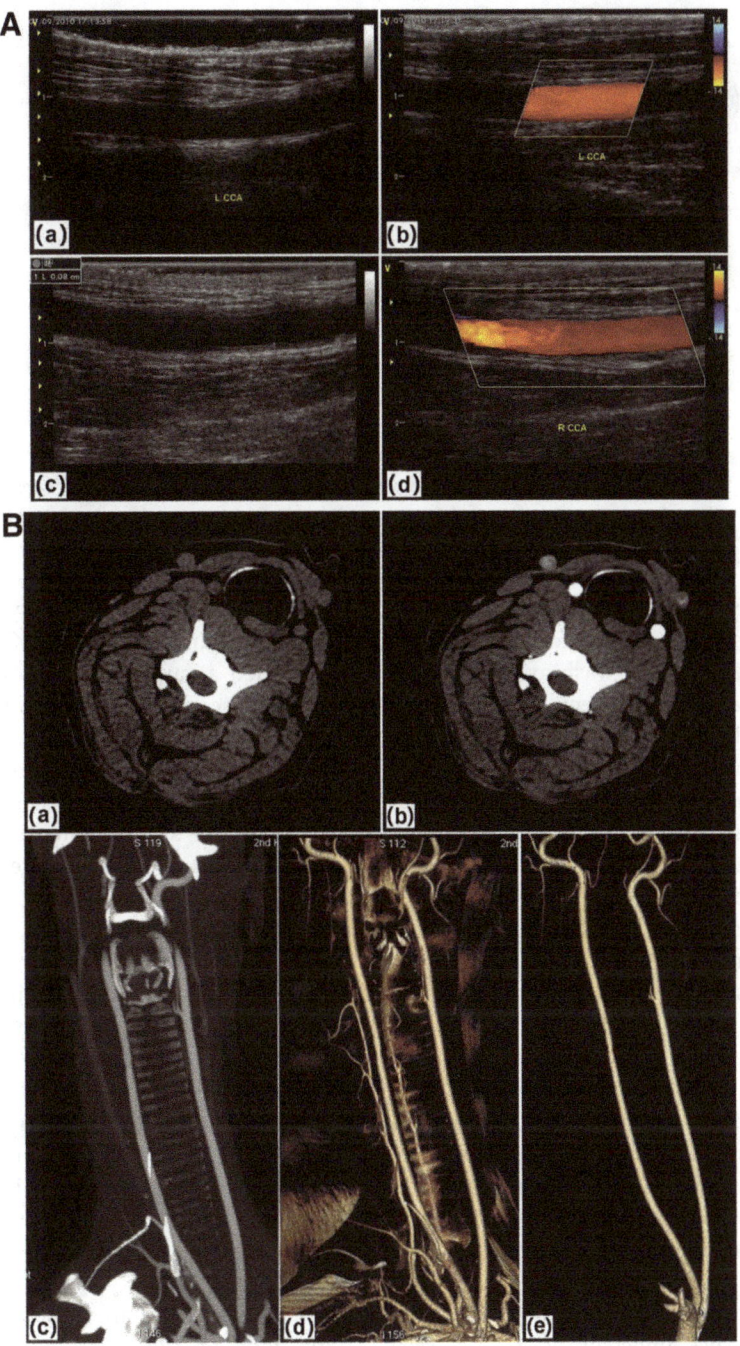

Fig. 5 Color Doppler ultrasonography and three-dimensional CT detection after the implantation of tissue-engineered vascular grafts into canine common carotid arteries. **A**: **a** and **b**, Color Doppler ultrasonography at 3 months post-implantation; **c** and **d**, 6 months post-implantation. **B**, three-dimensional CT detection at 6 months post-implantation. **a** and **b** are horizontal images; **c** is a coronal plane image; **d** and **e** are three-dimensional images

DAFPs could be used as a vascular tissue-engineered scaffold in the canine arterial system.

ECs seeded at the blood interface can prevent vascular grafts from being directly exposed to the bloodstream, consequently preventing thrombosis on the grafts, thus increasing their patency [25]. Cell-seeding methods include static seeding with biological glues and direct seeding [26]. Dynamic seeding can increase both cell-seeding efficiency and penetration of the scaffold [26]. In this study, a custom-designed and -produced vascular bioreactor system was used for dynamic seeding. This vascular bioreactor system

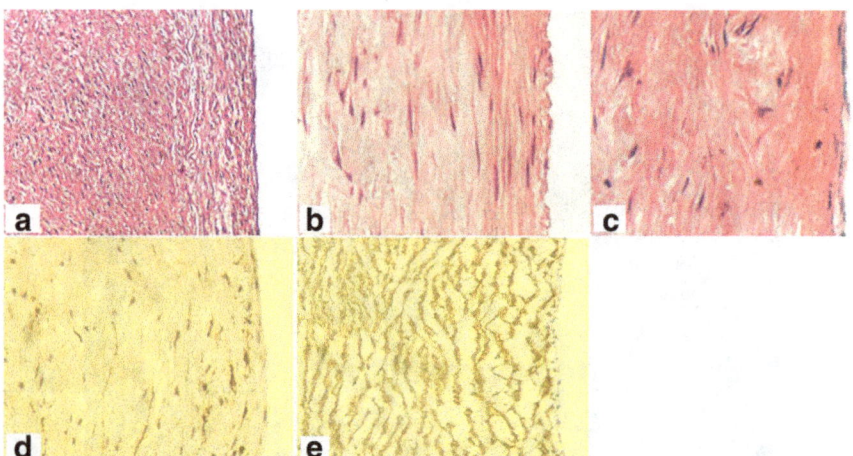

Fig. 6 Histological staining of tissue-engineered vascular grafts after implantation. **a**, **b**, and **c**, Hematoxylin–eosin staining of tissue-engineered vascular grafts at 6 months post-implantation; **d** smooth muscle actin (SMA) immunohistochemical staining of vascular grafts; **e** SMA immunohistochemical staining of fetal pig aorta as a positive control

can simulate the internal vascular mechanical environment, promote adhesion and proliferation of ECs, and prevent seeded ECs from washing away after transplantation into the arterial system. The results of the present study showed that dynamic seeding caused ECs to tightly attach to DAFPs.

ECs and smooth muscle cells are the main cellular components of the vasculature [27]. Vascular smooth muscle cells in the tunica media have important functional roles, for instance, regulation of vascular diameter, increase of vascular compliance, and secretion of ECM to affect the function of ECs [28]. Generating a functional smooth muscle layer is therefore important for successful vascular tissue engineering. A matching level of compliance between tissue-engineered, small-diameter vascular grafts and recipient vessels determines the long-term patency of blood vessels [29]. If a compliance mismatch occurs, fluid mechanical effects, such as the hydrodynamic shear stress of blood flow, result in graft wall thickening or expansion and formation of graft occlusions or aneurysms, ultimately leading to the failure of the implant [30].

However, the native architecture and low porosity of decellularized vessels have impeded efforts to seed smooth muscle layer into tissue-engineered blood vessels [31]. We also failed to seed smooth muscle cells into DAFPs due to the relatively compact structure of decellularized vessel matrix. Our laboratory is exploring effective methods for seeding smooth muscle cells into the acellular vascular matrix in vitro and trying to improve seeding efficiency using multi-needle, micro-needle injection. Thus, in this study, tissue-engineered DAFP scaffolds were only seeded with ECs. We found that the vascular grafts we constructed in this study possessed a complete EC layer, indicating that our

dynamic vascular bioreactor system meets the requirements of dynamic seeding of ECs.

We tried a variety of methods to label ECs in vitro to track seeded cells; however, our results were unsatisfactory and so cell-tracking experiments were not performed. We also implanted vascular grafts that had not been seeded with ECs in vitro, and this experiment is still ongoing. This ongoing investigation indicates that the patency of vascular grafts without seeded ECs is much lower (roughly no more than 60%) than those containing seeded ECs as described here (data not shown). The presence of an EC layer was confirmed in the vicinity of the anastomotic stoma of unobstructed vascular grafts, but the EC layer was notably absent in the middle of the grafts, indicating that ECs were migrating along the grafts from both sides of the normal blood vessel. Thus, it seems likely that in vitro seeded ECs in this study were involved in the reconstruction of the EC layer of vascular grafts. Taken together, it can be deduced that there were three sources of ECs in the inner layers of the vascular grafts: in vitro seeded ECs; normal vascular ECs migrating from both ends of the graft; and endothelial progenitor cells deposited by the blood.

The diameter of the tissue-engineered blood vessels constructed using DAFPs matched that of the canine common carotid artery. The implanted tissue vascular grafts exhibited good patency, and no obvious thrombi were found attached to the vascular walls by Doppler ultrasound and enhanced CT examination.. Taken together, our results indicated that these tissue-engineered blood vessels containing intact EC layers but no smooth muscle cell layers functioned well and were remodeled in vivo.

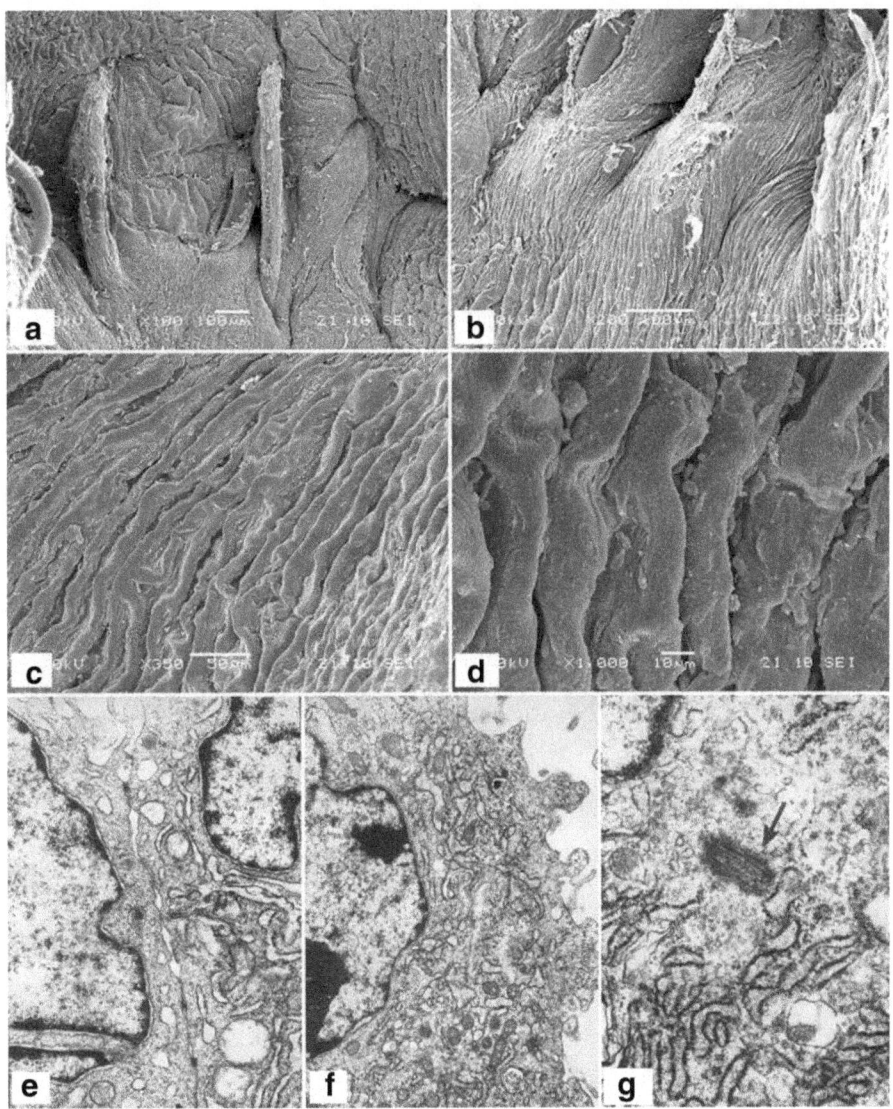

Fig. 7 Electron microscopy of tissue-engineered vascular grafts at 6 months post-implantation. **a–d**, the inner surface of vascular grafts by scanning electron microscopy; **e**, close connections between ECs were identified by transmission electron microscopy (TEM). **f**, the cell cytoplasm was rich in active organelles identified by TEM. **g** specific structures of ECs as seen at high magnification by TEM

In this study, we examined the feasibility of using DAFPs as a heterologous biomaterial. The ultimate goal of this work is to apply this technique to clinical practice. Following further improvements and refinement of the preparation method, vascular ECs from human patients could be seeded onto this heterologous scaffold material and cultured in vitro prior to implantation back into the cell donor. However, it is clear that much research must be conducted before this technology can be applied to humans. For example, the source of vascular ECs must be the recipient of vascular grafts to avoid transplant rejection [32]. However, obtaining adult ECs from recipients is not necessarily an ideal method because of the limited number of ECs that can be acquired and the adverse effects on the recipient of additional surgical trauma. Thus, the ideal source of seed cells for tissue-engineered vascular grafts is in vitro culture and induced differentiation of bone marrow stromal stem cells or circulating stem cells from the recipient.

There are many advantages of using pigs as heterologous organ donors in xenotransplantation research [33, 34]. Fetal pig was selected as the source of a tissue-engineered vascular scaffold in this study was selected. A more standardized DAFP material and convenient method of acquisition of autologous vascular seed cells in the future may make it easier to prepare tissue-engineered vascular grafts that have similar histological structures and physiological functions to human blood vessels. This investigation potentially paves the way to addressing the considerable clinical need for small-diameter vascular grafts. However, several limitations of our study should also be considered. First, the observation time was relatively short and a longer postoperative follow-up period would be desirable. Second, a control arm lacking EC seeding has not been reported here but is currently underway. Finally, the vascular bioreactor system in this study needs to be improved to better simulate the in vivo vascular mechanics of the arterial system and to improve culture efficiency of the grafts.

Conclusions

Tissue-engineered, small-diameter vascular grafts with an intact EC layer can be successfully constructed using DAFPs. These tissue-engineered blood vessels can be transplanted to replace the canine common carotid artery. Additionally, the grafts are structurally and functionally similar to normal artery after remodeling in vivo in animals. Therefore, DAFPs hold the potential for use in constructing tissue-engineered, small-diameter vascular grafts.

Abbreviations
DAFP: Decellularized aorta of fetal pigs; ECM: Extracellular matrix; ECs: Endothelial cells; HE: Hematoxylin and eosin; SEM: Scanning electron microscopy; SMA: Smooth muscle actin; TEM: Transmission electron microscopy; vWF: von Willebrand factor; W-P: Weibel-Palade

Acknowledgements
Not applicable.

Funding
None.

Authors' contributions
XM and ZH carried out the Conception and design of the research, participated in the Acquisition of data and drafted the manuscript. LL and GL carried out the Analysis and interpretation of data. QL and DY participated in the Statistical analysis. YZ and Ni participated in the design of the study and performed the statistical analysis. XM and ZH conceived of the study, and participated in its design and coordination and helped to draft the manuscript. All authors read and approved the final manuscript.

Competing interests
The authors declare that they have no competing interests.

Author details
[1]Department of Plastic Surgery, The Second Affiliated Hospital of Harbin Medical University, 246 Xuefu Road, Nangang District, Harbin, Heilongjiang 150086, China. [2]Department of Obstetrics and Gynecology, The First Affiliated Hospital of Harbin Medical University, 23 Youzheng Street, Nangang District, Harbin, Heilongjiang 150086, China. [3]Department of Cardiology, The Second Affiliated Hospital of Harbin Medical University, 246 Xuefu Road, Nangang District, Harbin, Heilongjiang 150086, China.

References
1. Kullo IJ, Rooke TW. Peripheral artery disease. N Engl J Med. 2016;374:861–71.
2. Adipurnama I, Yang MC, Ciach T, Butruk-Raszeja B. Surface modification and endothelialization of polyurethane for vascular tissue engineering applications: a review. Biomater Sci. 2016;5:22–37.
3. Gui L, Niklason LE. Vascular tissue engineering: building Perfusable vasculature for implantation. Curr Opin Chem Eng. 2014;3:68–74.
4. Wang W, Hu J, He C, Nie W, Feng W, Qiu K, et al. Heparinized PLLA/PLCL nanofibrous scaffold for potential engineering of small-diameter blood vessel: tunable elasticity and anticoagulation property. J Biomed Mater Res A. 2015;103:1784–97.
5. Grace NGJ, Soojung L, Robert BJ, Hwa JY, Eun YJ, Mi NB, et al. Trends in tissue engineering for blood vessels. J Biomed Biotechnol. 2012;2012: 956345.
6. Tibbitt MW, Rodell CB, Burdick JA, Anseth KS. Progress in material design for biomedical applications. Proc Natl Acad Sci U S A. 2015;112:14444–51.
7. O'Brien FJ. Biomaterials & scaffolds for tissue engineering. Mater Today. 2011;14:88–95.
8. Meng ZX, Wang YS, Ma C, Zheng W, Li L, Zheng YF. Electrospinning of PLGA/gelatin randomly-oriented and aligned nanofibers as potential scaffold in tissue engineering. Mater Sci Eng C. 2010;30:1204–10.
9. Zhao W, Jin X, Cong Y, Liu Y, Fu J. Degradable natural polymer hydrogels for articular cartilage tissue engineering. J Chem Technol Biotechnol. 2013; 88:327–39.
10. Mcfetridge PS, Daniel JW, Bodamyali T, Horrocks M, Chaudhuri JB. Preparation of porcine carotid arteries for vascular tissue engineering applications. J Biomed Mater Res A. 2004;70A:224–34.
11. Lopez-Ruiz E, Venkateswaran S, Peran M, Jimenez G, Pernagallo S, Diaz-Mochon JJ, et al. Poly(ethylmethacrylate-co-diethylaminoethyl acrylate) coating improves endothelial re-population, bio-mechanical and anti-thrombogenic properties of decellularized carotid arteries for blood vessel replacement. Sci Rep. 2017;7:017–00294.
12. Böer U, Hurtadoaguilar LG, Klingenberg M, Lau S, Jockenhoevel S, Haverich A, et al. Effect of intensified Decellularization of equine carotid arteries on scaffold biomechanics and Cytotoxicity. Ann Biomed Eng. 2015;49:2630–41.
13. Liu GF, He ZJ, Yang DP, Han XF, Guo TF, Hao CG, et al. Decellularized aorta of fetal pigs as a potential scaffold for small diameter tissue engineered vascular graft. Chin Med J. 2008;121:1398–406.
14. Abt PL, Praestgaard J, West S, Hasz R. Donor hemodynamic profile presages graft survival in donation after cardiac death liver transplantation. Liver Transpl. 2014;20:165–72.
15. Liao J, Joyce EM, Sacks MS. Effects of decellularization on the mechanical and structural properties of the porcine aortic valve leaflet. Biomaterials. 2008;29:1065–74.
16. Choi YC, Choi JS, Kim BS, Kim JD, Yoon HI, Cho YW. Decellularized extracellular matrix derived from porcine adipose tissue as a xenogeneic biomaterial for tissue engineering. Tissue Eng Part C Methods. 2012;18:866–76.
17. Falk J, Townsend LE, Vogel LM, Boyer M, Olt S, Wease GL, et al. Improved adherence of genetically modified endothelial cells to small-diameter expanded polytetrafluoroethylene grafts in a canine model. J Vasc Surg. 1998;27:902–9.
18. Aper T, Teebken O, Steinhoff G, Haverich A. Use of a fibrin preparation in the engineering of a vascular graft model. Eur J Vasc Endovasc Surg. 2004; 28:296–302.
19. Pratumvinit B, Reesukumal K, Janebodin K, Ieronimakis N, Reyes M. Isolation, characterization, and transplantation of cardiac endothelial cells. Biomed Res Int. 2013;2013:359412.

20. Xu J, Ge H, Zhou X, Yang D, Guo T, He J, et al. Tissue-engineered vessel strengthens quickly under physiological deformation: application of a new perfusion bioreactor with machine vision. J Vasc Res. 2005;42:503–8.

21. Badylak SF, Freytes DO, Gilbert TW. Extracellular matrix as a biological scaffold material: structure and function. Acta Biomater. 2009;5:1–13.

22. Cleary MA, Geiger E, Grady C, Best C, Naito Y, Breuer C. Vascular tissue engineering: the next generation. Trends Mol Med. 2012;18:394–404.

23. Peng H-F, Liu JY, Andreadis ST, Swartz DD. Hair follicle-derived smooth muscle cells and small intestinal submucosa for engineering mechanically robust and vasoreactive vascular media. Tissue Eng A. 2011;17:981–90.

24. Li Q, Huang C, Xu Z, Liu G, Liu Y, Xiao Z, et al. The fetal porcine aorta and mesenteric acellular matrix as small-caliber tissue engineering vessels and microvasculature scaffold. Aesthet Plast Surg. 2013;37:822–32.

25. Dudash LA, Kligman F, Sarett SM, Kottke-Marchant K, Marchant RE. Endothelial cell attachment and shear response on biomimetic polymer-coated vascular grafts. J Biomed Mater Res A. 2012;100:2204–10.

26. Villalona GA, Udelsman B, Duncan DR, McGillicuddy E, Sawh-Martinez RF, Hibino N, et al. Cell-seeding techniques in vascular tissue engineering. Tissue Eng B Rev. 2010;16:341–50.

27. Zhou R, Zhu L, Fu S, Qian Y, Wang D, Wang C. Small diameter blood vessels bioengineered from human adipose-derived stem cells. Sci Rep. 2016;6: 35422.

28. Qiu J, Zheng Y, Hu J, Liao D, Gregersen H, Deng X, et al. Biomechanical regulation of vascular smooth muscle cell functions: from in vitro to in vivo understanding. J R Soc Interface. 2014;11:20130852.

29. Fernandez CE, Achneck HE, Reichert WM, Truskey GA. Biological and engineering design considerations for vascular tissue engineered blood vessels (TEBVs). Curr Opin Chem Eng. 2014;3:83–90.

30. Stewart SF, Lyman DJ. Effects of a vascular graft/natural artery compliance mismatch on pulsatile flow. J Biomech. 1992;25:297–310.

31. Yazdani SK, Watts B, Machingal M, Jarajapu YP, Van Dyke ME, Christ GJ. Smooth muscle cell seeding of decellularized scaffolds: the importance of bioreactor preconditioning to development of a more native architecture for tissue-engineered blood vessels. Tissue Eng A. 2009;15:827–40.

32. Hopkinson C, Romano V, Kaye R, Steger B, Stewart R, Tsagkataki M, et al. The influence of donor and recipient gender incompatibility on corneal transplant rejection and failure. Am J Transplant. 2017;17:210–7.

33. Ekser B, Cooper DK, Tector AJ. The need for xenotransplantation as a source of organs and cells for clinical transplantation. Int J Surg. 2015;23:199–204.

34. Cooper DK, Ekser B, Ramsoondar J, Phelps C, Ayares D. The role of genetically engineered pigs in xenotransplantation research. J Pathol. 2016; 238:288–99.

4

Emergency transapical mitral valve-in-valve implantation for bioprosthesis failure: transapical implantation of an Edwards Sapien-XT in a dysfunctional mitral bioprosthesis in a critical patient

Marco Zanobini[1], Sabrina Manganiello[1], Giorgia Bonalumi[1], Raoul Biondi[1], Marco Russo[2], Massimo Mapelli[3], Francesco Alamanni[1] and Matteo Saccocci[1,2*] (iD)

Abstract

Background: Valve-in-Valve (VIV) Transcatheter Aortic Valve Replacement (TAVR) is now the treatment of choice in high-surgical-risk patients with failing aortic bioprosthesis. Although less performed, VIV-Transcatheter Mitral Valve Replacement (TMVR) is a valid treatment option for selected high-risk patients with degenerated mitral bioprostheses. Several cases of elective ViV- TAVR and -TMVR have been reported but only few were performed in critical hemodynamic conditions.

Case presentation: We report the case of a patient underwent balloon-expandable transapical mitral valve-in-valve implantation in an emergency setting due to a severe stenosis of a bioprosthesis in mitral position. The procedure was successfully performed, with no residual mitral regurgitation or paravalvular leaks, and uneventful.

Conclusion: Transcatheter transapical mitral valve-in-valve implantation could represent a feasible and effective strategy even in critical setting.

Keywords: Mitral valve stenosis, Bioprosthesis, Transcatheter valve implantation, Valve-in-valve, Transapical, Mitral bioprosthesis, Emergency

Background

Valve-in-Valve (VIV) Transcatheter Aortic Valve Replacement (TAVR) is now the treatment of choice in high-surgical-risk patients with failing aortic bioprosthesis [1]. Although less performed, VIV-Transcatheter Mitral Valve Replacement (TMVR) [2] represents a valid treatment option for selected high-risk patients with degenerated mitral bioprostheses. Several cases of elective ViV-TAVR and -TMVR have been reported, but only a few were performed in critical hemodynamic conditions, especially for dysfunctioning mitral bioprosthesis [3–5].

Over the last decade, the use of bioprosthesis or mitral valve reconstruction, instead of mechanical valves, has shown an important worldwide increase thanks to the improved long-term results and inspired to the desire of avoiding the need of life-long systemic anticoagulation. The durability of bioprostheses, especially in mitral position, can be very variable, depending on patient's and valve characteristics. Although surgical redo operation is often possible, when there are no specific contraindications, it's widely known that is accompanied by an increased mortality depending on age, comorbidities and elective or urgent status of the procedure. In this scenario, the incidence of failing surgical valves in high surgical risk patients will surely increase. Even more important is the choice of the right treatment option in patients with critical conditions with high or

* Correspondence: matteo.saccocci@unimi.it
[1]Department of Cardiac Surgery, IRCCS - Centro Cardiologico Monzino, Università degli Studi di Milano, Via C. Parea 4, 20138 Milano, Italy
[2]Department of CardioVascular Surgery, Heart Center - University Hospital of Zurich, Zurich, Switzerland
Full list of author information is available at the end of the article

unacceptable surgical risks. Usually stented bioprosthesis present a progressive deterioration, evaluable with a correct echocardiographic follow-up, permitting a comfortable planning of the procedure but sometimes patients could be admitted directly to the ER in life-threating conditions without previous important symptoms. We report the case of a patient underwent balloon-expandable transapical mitral valve-in-valve implantation in an emergency setting due to a severe mitral stenosis of a surgical bioprosthesis.

Case presentation

An 82-year-old woman affected by hypertension, grade 1 obesity, severe chronic obstructive pulmonary disease (COPD), atrial fibrillation (AF) and history of previous cardiac surgery was admitted to the emergency room (ER) for acute pulmonary edema and renal insufficiency. Eight years before she underwent aortic and mitral valve replacement (Magna Aortic 23 mm, Magna Mitral 27 mm – Edwards Lifescience, Irvine, CA, US), tricuspid valve repair and atrial fibrillation radiofrequency ablation complicated by complete AV-block and pacemaker implantation. During the years she remained asymptomatic without signs of heart failure. The trans-thoracic echocardiography (TTE) performed at admission showed no signs of endocarditis, no degeneration of the aortic bioprosthesis, good function of the repaired tricuspid valve but a very severe mitral prosthesis stenosis (mean gradient 24 mmHg, PHT 420 msec, area 0,52 cm^2; PAPS 66 mmHg) [Fig. 1; Additional file 1: Video 1]. ECG-gated MDCT (multidetector computed tomography) recorded no significant coronary artery disease, calcified thoracic aorta, a calcified mitral bioprosthesis (outer-diameter 28.9mmx28.6 mm, inner-diameter 24.9 × 24.4 mm) and

bilateral severe pleural effusion. Laboratory testing showed severe anemia. The patient was initially medically treated with endovenous diuretics, blood transfusions, Continous Veno-Venous Hemofiltration (CVVH) and bilateral pleural drainage. Despite medical therapy optimization, the patient 's conditions remained critical with hemodynamic instability, hypotension, initial neurological impairment and acute anuric renal failure. Evaluated morbidity and mortality risk for surgical redo mitral replacement (EuroSCORE II = 19,84; CHA$_2$DS$_2$-VASC Score = 4; HAS BLED score = 4) our multidisciplinary Heart-Team decided for an emergency ViV-TMVR in general anesthesia with TEE-monitoring.

A temporary endocardial pacing leads was introduced in the right ventricle through a 6-F sheath positioned into the left femoral vein. Apex position was optimally detected by TTE evaluation and the pericardium was reached through a left anterolateral thoracotomy. As in our standardized technique for transapical approach, we proceed with the removal of all the adherence and with the positioning of 2 perpendicular "U"-stitches (2/0 polypropylene - Prolene; Ethicon, Inc.), reinforced by pledgets, directly on the myocardial tissue of the apex. Performed the transapical puncture, we positioned a 7-F sheath in order to introduce a 0.035 guide-wire through the ventricle toward the mitral prosthesis reaching the pulmonary vein. Over the guide-wire, we inserted a MultiPurpose catheter to exchange the previous wire with an ExtraStiff .035 in. (Cook Medical). The valve delivery system was introduced through an expandable 21-F E-Sheath (Edwards Lifescience – Irvine, CA, US). Under fluoroscopic and TEE guidance, we proceeded with the deployment of a 29 mm Sapien-3 valve (Edwards Lifescience – Irvine, CA, US) using the

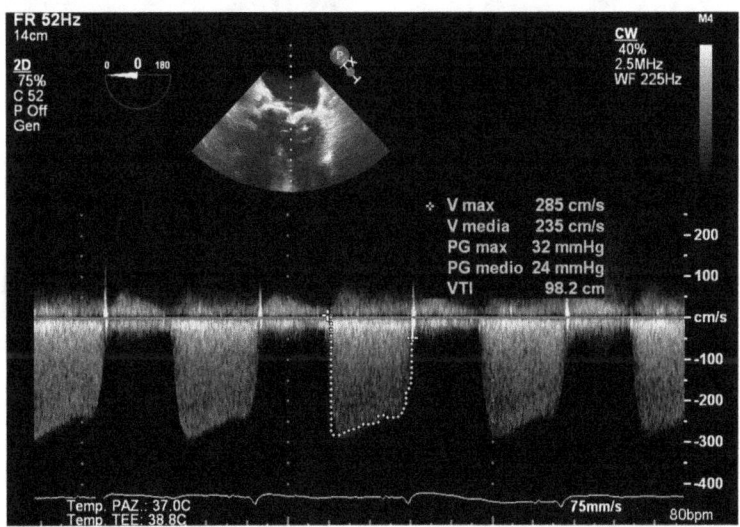

Fig. 1 Preoperative transthoracic echocardiography showing severe mitral stenosis (transvalvular mean gradient 24 mmHg)

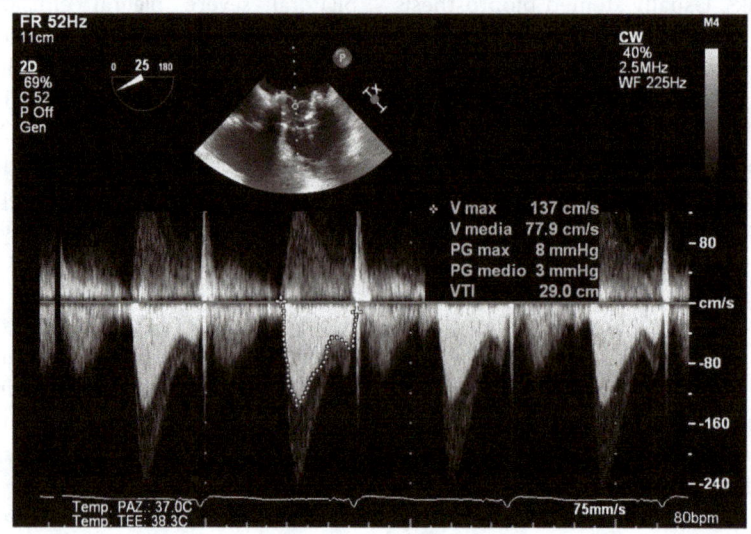

Fig. 2 Valve-in-Valve implantation result

annulus of the surgical bioprosthesis to recognize the correct position (Fig. 2). There were no paravalvular leaks or mitral regurgitation, and we immediately observed a significant improvement in intraprocedural monitoring parameter. The procedure was uneventful, as well as ICU course (no needs of CVVH, inotropes or prolonged mechanical ventilation). The patient was discharged 10 days after ViV-TMVR in good clinical condition (NYHA class I-II). At pre-discharge TTE transvalvular mitral mean gradient was 3 mmHg, PAPS decreased to 29 mmHg and LV Ejection Fraction remained 55% Fig. 3, Additional file 2: Video 2, Additional file 3: Video 3. At 1 month follow-up, the patient was asymptomatic (NYHA class I-II) and the TTE confirmed the absence of valve dysfunction or Paravalvular leak [Fig. 4].

Discussion and conclusions

Degeneration of surgically implanted bioprosthesis in elderly patients is an increasing problem due to the longer life-expectancy. Moreover, this issue is going to interest also a younger population due to the growing percentage of bioprosthesis implantation instead of the

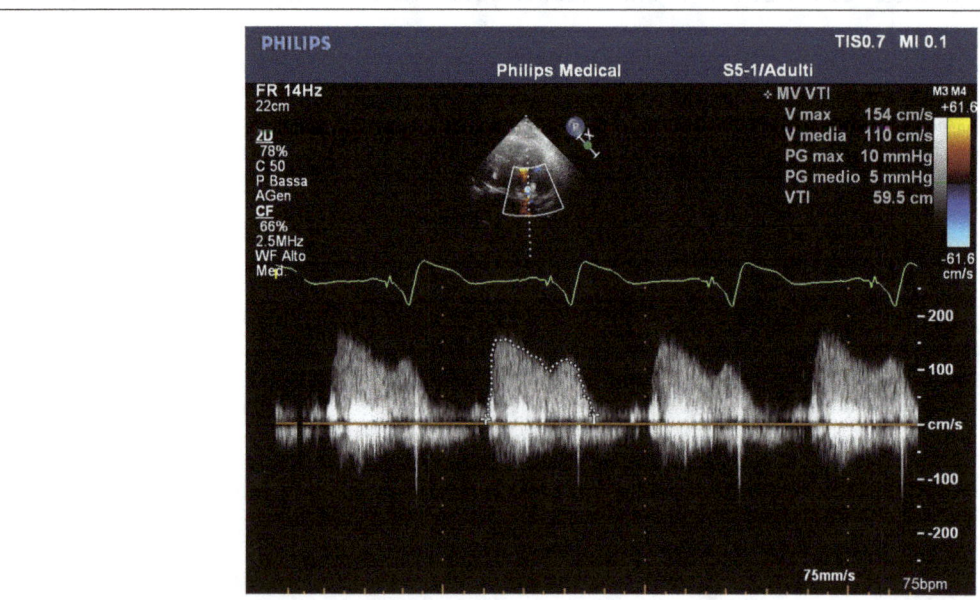

Fig. 3 PreDischarge Trans-Thoracic echocardiography Mitral prosthesis' gradient

Emergency transapical mitral valve-in-valve implantation for bioprosthesis failure: transapical implantation...

25

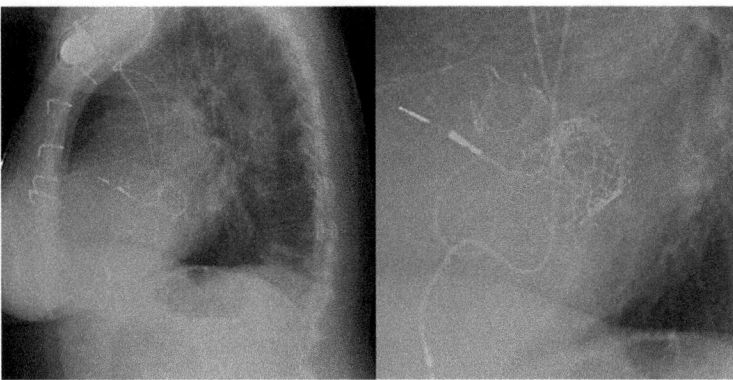

Fig. 4 30-days Trans-Thoracic echocardiography Mitral prosthesis' gradient

mechanical ones. According to the current literature, the perioperative risk of redo surgical intervention may reach high percentage, up to 15% for redo aortic replacement, depending on age, clinical conditions and comorbidities. To this increasing number of patients, we should add the several situations in which surgery can't be performed because of technical contraindications (porcelain aorta, really calcified mitral annulus, multiple redos, frailty, etc.). We are in an era where TAVR is already the therapy of choice for high-risk patients, and in the next year, its indications are moving to the moderate-risk ones. The valve-in-valve concept was developed by Walther et al. in 2007 with the intent of decrease the reoperative risk in patients with a dysfunctional bioprosthesis. ViV-TAVR is nowadays a standard procedure to treat elderly patients with degenerated bioprosthesis, while mitral valve-in-valve implantation is not yet so frequent probably due to the difficulties of reaching the mitral with a peripheral approach. The need of a transapical puncture, as a unique option, is probably going to end with the expanding possibilities linked to transeptal system development. Technically, the deployment of a transcatheter valve into a surgically implanted bioprosthesis is a quite simple procedure for skilled operators thanks to the possibility to use the annulus of the surgical prosthesis as a reference point for the deployment of the new one. Furthermore, using the degenerated valve as a landing zone for the implantation assure a good stability of the transcatheter prosthesis and it's usually not accompanied by significant paravalvular leaks. Transapical approach requests high surgical skills, but with the actual low-profile introducer sheaths the risk of complications is minimized.

According to our experience, transapical valve-in-valve transcatheter mitral implantation can be a feasible and safe way to treat bioprosthesis dysfunc-tion even in urgent and emergency settings, as we have shown in this case.

Abbreviations
AF: Atrial Fibrillation; AV block: atrio-ventricular block; COPD: Chronic Obstructive Pulmonary Disease; CVVH: Continuous Veno-Venous Hemofiltration; ECG-gated MDCT: Electrocardiographic-gated Multiple Detector Computed Tomography; ER: Emrgency Room; LV: Left Ventricle; NYHA: New York Heart Association; PM: Pacemaker; TAVR: Transcatheter Aortic Valve Replacement; TEE: Trans-Esophageal Echocardiography; TMVR: Valve-in-valve Transcatheter Mitral Valve Replacement; TTE: Trans-Thoracic Echocardiography; ViV: Valve-in-Valve

Acknowledgments
All the staff of Centro Cardiologico Monzino.

Funding
Not applicable.

Authors' contributions
First and last authors equally collaborate to the work. Data finding and collecting: MZ, SM, GB, FA, RB. Data analisis: MS, MZ. Paper writing: MS, MZ, MR. All authors read and approved the final manuscript.

Competing interests
The authors have no disclosure.

Author details
[1]Department of Cardiac Surgery, IRCCS - Centro Cardiologico Monzino, Università degli Studi di Milano, Via C. Parea 4, 20138 Milano, Italy. [2]Department of CardioVascular Surgery, Heart Center - University Hospital of Zurich, Zurich, Switzerland. [3]Department of Cardiology -IRCCS - Centro Cardiologico Monzino, Università degli Studi di Milano, Milano, Italy.

References

1. Nishimura RA, Otto CM, Bonow RO, et al. AHA/ACC Focused Update of the 2014 AHA/ACC Guideline for the Management of Patients With Valvular Heart Disease: A Report of the American College of Cardiology/American Heart Association Task Force on Clinical Practice Guidelines. 2017.

2. Condado JF, Kaebnick B, Babaliaros V. Transcatheter mitral valve-in-valve therapy. *Interv*. Cardiol Clin. 2016;5(1):117–23.

3. Summers MR, Mick S, Kapadia SR, et al. Emergency valve-in-valve transcatheter aortic valve replacement in a patient with degenerated bioprosthetic aortic stenosis and cardiogenic shock on veno-arterial extracorporeal membrane oxygenation. Catheter Cardiovasc Interv. 2017;

4. van Garsse LA, Gelsomino S, van Ommen V, et al. Emergency transthoracic transapical mitral valve-in-valve implantation. J Interv Cardiol. 2011;24(5): 474–6.

5. Taramasso M, Maisano F, Michev I, et al. Emergency transfemoral aortic valve-in-valve implantation with the balloon-expandable Edwards-Sapien valve. J Cardiovasc Med (Hagerstown). 2009;10(12):936–9.

5

Abnormal elevation of myocardial necrosis biomarkers after coronary artery bypass grafting without established myocardial infarction assessed by cardiac magnetic resonance

Fernando Teiichi Costa Oikawa, Whady Hueb[*] ⓘ, Cesar Higa Nomura, Alexandre Ciappina Hueb, Alexandre Volney Villa, Leandro Menezes Alves da Costa, Rodrigo Morel Vieira de Melo, Paulo Cury Rezende, Carlos Alexandre Wainrober Segre, Cibele Larrosa Garzillo, Eduardo Gomes Lima, Jose Antonio Franchini Ramires and Roberto Kalil Filho

Abstract

Background: The diagnosis of peri-procedural myocardial infarction is complex, especially after the emergence of high-sensitivity markers of myocardial necrosis.

Methods: In this study, patients with normal baseline cardiac biomarkers and formal indication for elective on-pump coronary bypass surgery were evaluated. Electrocardiograms, cardiac biomarkers, and cardiac magnetic resonance imaging with late gadolinium enhancement were performed before and after procedures. Myocardial infarction was defined as more than ten times the upper reference limit of the 99th percentile for troponin I and for creatine kinase isoform (CK-MB) and by the findings of new late gadolinium enhancement on cardiac magnetic resonance. We assessed the release of cardiac biomarkers in patients with no evidence of myocardial infarction on cardiac magnetic resonance.

Results: Of 75 patients referred for on-pump coronary bypass surgery, 54 (100%) did not have evidence of myocardial infarction on cardiac magnetic resonance. However, all had a peak troponin I above the 99th percentile; 52 (96%) had an elevation 10 times higher than the 99th percentile. Regarding CK-MB, 54 (100%) patients had a peak CK-MB above the 99th percentile limit, and only 13 (24%) had an elevation greater than 10 times the 99th percentile. The median value of troponin I peak was 3.15 (1.2 to 3.9) ng/mL, which represented 78.7 times the 99th percentile.

Conclusion: In this study, different from CK-MB findings, troponin was significantly increased in the absence of myocardial infarction on cardiac magnetic resonance. Thus, CK-MB was more accurate than troponin I for excluding procedure-related myocardial infarction. These data suggest a higher troponin cutoff for the diagnosis of coronary bypass surgery related myocardial infarction.

Keywords: Myocardial infarction, Biomarkers, Coronary bypass surgery, Periprocedural, Troponin

* Correspondence: mass@incor.usp.br
Instituto do Coracao (InCor), Hospital das Clinicas HCFMUSP, Faculdade de Medicina, Universidade de São Paulo, São Paulo, SP, Brazil

Background

Myocardial necrosis biomarkers are frequently elevated after cardiac revascularization procedures. However, the diagnosis of acute myocardial infarction (MI) after a revascularization procedure is still a controversial issue. This inability to diagnose MI makes it more difficult to establish a specific therapeutic strategy. With the appearance of high-sensitivity troponins, a myriad of false-positive diagnoses for myocardial infarction have emerged. In 2000 and 2007 in an attempt to standardize the criteria for diagnosing MI, the European Society of Cardiology, the American College of Cardiology, the American Heart Association, and the World Heart Federation formed a joint task force to address this issue, but the task force was unable to make a satisfactory decision. Therefore, the problem still remained. To reduce diagnostic mistakes, in 2012, this same group arbitrarily raised the cutoff point to 10 times the 99th percentile, but with no solid scientific basis for doing so [1]. Troponin (cTnI) and the creatine kinase isoform (CK-MB) do not reflect, alone, the occurrence of MI related to occlusion of the graft or native artery or varying degrees of myocardial injury. Release of myocardial necrosis markers may be related to incomplete myocardial protection; reperfusion injury; a systemic inflammatory state, including inevitable postsurgical trauma; the handling of intramyocardial vessels; and cardiac defibrillator use [2, 3]. Cardiac troponin may also be increased when nonsurgical damage is present, such as sepsis and thromboembolic phenomena [1]. cTnIs have also been found elevated in athletes after marathons [4]. This makes the identification of small areas of injury very difficult to assess in clinical practice [5].

Parallel to the increased sensitivity of troponin assays, imaging methods have achieved better accuracy for exclusion of the diagnosis of myocardial infarction. Thus, due to the limitations on the interpretation of biomarkers after coronary artery bypass grafting (CABG) and the difficulty of excluding MI, cardiac magnetic resonance imaging (CMR) has enabled a more detailed evaluation of the myocardium.

Therefore, in this study, we aimed to examine the release of biomarkers after CABG in patients with no evidence of late enhancement on CMR.

Patients and methods

Details of the study design, protocol, patient selection, and inclusion criteria have been previously reported [6]. Briefly, patients with preserved left ventricular function and angiographic coronary artery stenosis of more than 70% confirmed by a visually reviewed document, and with multiple-vessel involvement, and documented ischemia were included. Stress testing or evaluation of stable angina according to the Canadian Cardiovascular Society guidelines (Class II or III) established the presence of ischemia.

All patients were candidates for on-pump coronary artery bypass grafting (ONCAB). Patients were excluded if they had undergone any previous mechanical interventions, and had experienced recent thromboembolic events, systemic inflammatory disease, or kidney failure.

Trial outcomes

The primary outcome was the occurrence of MI based on the release of the biomarkers, cTnI and CK-MB, in patients with no late gadolinium enhancement (LGE) assessed by CMR.

Methods
Surgical technique

In accordance with current best practices, the same team of surgeons with experience in ONCAB performed the procedures. Surgical access to the heart was through a standard median sternotomy in all cases. All incisions and closure techniques were performed in the same way in all patients to limit variability among patients.

CMR protocol

CMR was performed before and after the surgical procedure. CMR, considered the gold standard, allows high-precision assessment that is reproducible in the same test. Recent studies indicate that CMR detects MI very accurately and provides results similar or superior to results with radionuclide imaging [7–10].

All patients underwent CMR 2 days before the intervention and 6 days after each invasive procedure during the hospitalization period. A 1.5-T Achieva Magnetic Resonance scanner (Philips Healthcare, Andover, MA) was used. Steady-state free precession cine images were acquired in 2 long-axis (2 and 4 chambers) views and 8 to 10 short-axis views of the left ventricle. Contrast-enhanced images were acquired in long- and short-axis planes identical to the cine images. Typical voxel size was $1.6 \times 2.1 \times 8$ mm, with a reconstruction matrix of 528 and a reconstructed voxel size of 0.6 mm. The method for acquiring and analyzing CMR was standardized in our service and was reproduced according to conventional techniques [11, 12]. Delayed enhancement on CMR was performed with a phase-sensitive inversion recovery (PSIR) sequence (repetition time 6.1 ms echo time 3.0 ms, voxel size $1.6 \times 2.1 \times 8$ mm, flip angle $25°$) following a 5-min time delay after the administration of 0.1 mmol/kg contrast agent (GadoteratemeglumineGd-DOTA™, Guerbet SA, France). Images were acquired in 2 long-axis planes and in a short-axis stack covering the entire left ventricle. The inversion time was meticulously adjusted throughout the acquisition to obtain optimal nulling of remote normal myocardium. The slice thickness at the apex was reduced to 5 mm to avoid a partial volume effect. MI was defined as the identification of

Abnormal elevation of myocardial necrosis biomarkers after coronary artery bypass grafting...

29

hyper-enhancement in the myocardium on CMR. Infarcted regions exhibit this phenomenon, which might be due to an increased volume of distribution of the contrast agent, because of rupture of myocyte membranes and slow contrast washout [10].

CMR analysis

All areas of late gadolinium-diethylene-triamine-pentaacetic acid (DTPA) hyper-enhancement were quantified by 2 experienced observers who interpreted the LGE while blinded to the interventional technique and biochemical data. When measurements differed, a third observer performed a review, and a consensus was obtained. Hyper-enhanced pixels were defined as those with image intensities exceeding 2 standard deviations greater than the mean of image intensities in a remote myocardial region in the same image. Pre-intervention and post-intervention scans were read side by side in both surgical techniques, with and without extracorporeal circulation.

Biochemistry

All blood samples for measurement of cTnI and CK-MB were collected immediately before and 6, 12, 24, 36, 48, and 72 h after on-pump CABG. The surgeon and clinical team were blinded to the CK-MB or cTnI data. All samples were centrifuged at 3000 rpm for 20 min and analyzed within 2 h after collection. Analyses of cTnI and CK-MB were performed using an ADVIA Centaur immunoassay analyzer (Siemens Health Care Diagnostics, Tarrytown, NY). According to the manufacturer, the lower limit of detection of cTnI using the high-sensitivity Ultra kit is 0.006 ng/mL, and the 99th percentile upper reference limit (URL) is 0.04 ng/mL. The assay precision represented by the percentage coefficient of variation is 10% at 0.03 ng/mL. The detection limit of the CK-MB mass kit (Acute Care™ CK-MB assay Siemens™) is 0.18 ng/mL. Cutoff values at the 99th percentile are 3.8 ng/mL for women and 4.4 ng/mL for men. The coefficients of variations for CK-MB mass, as specified by the manufacturer, are 3.91% at 3.55 ng/mL and 3.67% at 80.16 ng/mL.

Definition of CABG-related MI

According to the Third Universal Definition [1], MI type V is defined as an elevation of more than 10 times the 99th percentile during the first 48 h after CABG. Patients with normal baseline cTnI concentrations plus any of the following criteria were considered to have experienced an MI: (1) new pathologic Q waves or new left bundle-branch block (LB-BB), (2) angiographically documented new graft or new native coronary occlusion, or (3) imaging evidence of new loss of viable myocardium or new regional wall motion abnormality.

Electrocardiograms

Twelve-lead electrocardiograms (EKG) were obtained from each patient immediately before and 6, 12, 24, and 36 h after CABG. For the identification of new Q waves, we used the Minnesota code, which is used extensively in epidemiology studies and large-scale clinical trials [13].

Ethics committee approval

All patients provided written informed consent and were assigned to a treatment group. The Ethics Committee of the Heart Institute of the University of São Paulo Medical School, São Paulo, SP, Brazil, approved the trial. All procedures were performed in accordance with the Declaration of Helsinki.

Statistical analysis

Values are expressed as mean and standard deviation or median and interquartile range, as appropriate. The paired-sample t test and the unpaired-sample t test were used to compare means within the study group or between subgroups. The chi-square and the Fisher exact tests were used for comparison of discrete variables. Continuous variables without normal distribution were compared using the Mann-Whitney U test, and correlation between such variables was made with the Spearman rank test. Values of $p < 0.05$ were considered statistically significant.

Results

Between March 2012 and April 2014, 326 consecutive patients who met the inclusion criteria were screened. Of these patients, 107 (32.8%) were excluded (Fig. 1). Of the 219 remaining patients, 148 were referred for CABG (75 ONCAB and 73 OPCAB [off-pump coronary artery bypass]), and 71 patients were referred for PCI (percutaneous coronary intervention). Of the 75 ONCAB patients enrolled in this study, 21 were excluded and 54 completed the study protocol. These 54 patients had no evidence of MI on CMR assessed by LGE. The main reasons for exclusion of the patients are presented in Fig. 1.

The clinical, demographic, and angiographic characteristics are summarized in Table 1. The mean age was 61.3 (± 8.3) years, and 39 (72.2%) were male. In addition, 24 (44.4%) patients had a diagnosis of type 2 diabetes mellitus and 13 (24.1%) had a history of myocardial infarction. Regarding smoking, 18 patients (33.34%) stopped smoking during the inclusion period of the study. The angiographic screening showed that 17 (31.5%) patients had stenosis of the left main coronary artery, 43 (80%) had obstructive lesions in 3 epicardial branches, and 11 (20.4%) had a concomitant bi-arterial obstructive pattern. Additionally, the mean SYNTAX Score was 28. Anginal symptoms were present in 47 (87%) patients, and 15 (27.8%) had grade III angina, according to the

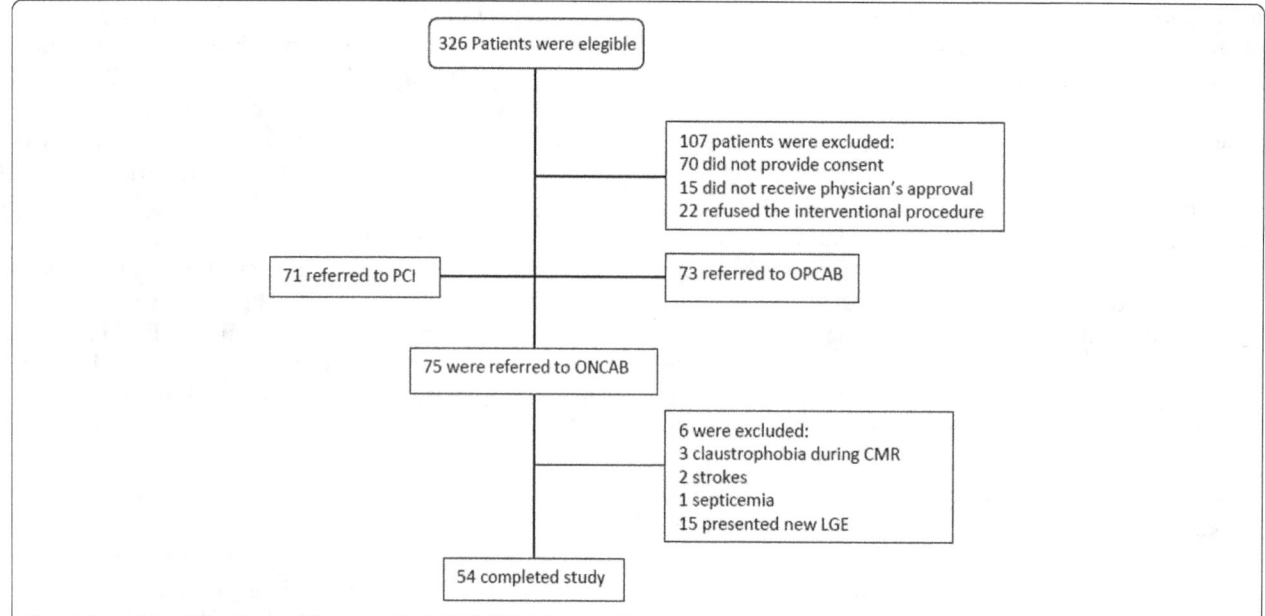

Fig. 1 Consolidated Standards of Reporting Trials (CONSORT) diagram. (CMR = cardiac magnetic resonance; LGE = late gadolinium enhancement; ONCAB = on-pump coronary artery bypass; OPCAB = off-pump coronary artery bypass; PCI = percutaneous coronary intervention)

Table 1 Clinical, demographic and angiographic characteristics of study population

	N = 54
Age, y	61.3 ± 8.3
Male, n %	39 (72.2)
Diabetes mellitus, n (%)	24 (44.4)
Hypertension, n (%)	48 (88.9)
Current smoker, n (%)	6 (11.1)
Former smoker, n (%)	18 (33.3)
Previous myocardial infarction, n (%)	13 (24)
Angina, n (%)	47 (87)
Angina CCS III-IV, n (%)	15 (27.8)
Total cholesterol, mg/dL	161 ± 42.4
LDL cholesterol, mg/dL	93 ± 37
HDL cholesterol, mg/dL	39 ± 13
Triglycerides, mg/dL	160 ± 148
Left main disease, n (%)	17 (31.5)
Double-vessel disease, n (%)	11 (20.4)
Triple-vessel disease, n (%)	43 (80)
SYNTAX Score,	28 ± 10
Ejection fraction, median %	66 ± 8.6

N Number of patients, CCS Canadian Cardiovascular Society, LDL low-density lipoprotein, HDL high-density lipoprotein

Canadian Cardiovascular Society (CCS) scale. Left ventricular ejection fraction was assessed by CRM performed before the procedure and averaged 66 ± 8.6 (Table1).

Cardiac biomarkers

The median value of troponin peak was 3.15 (2.0 to 4.9) ng/mL, which corresponds to 78.7 times the 99th percentile. Two (4%) patients had elevation just above the 99th percentile, and 52 (96%) remaining patients had elevation above 10 times the 99th percentile. There were no patients with a cTnI value below the 99th percentile after the surgical procedure (Fig. 2A).

Regarding CK-MB peak, the median value was 23.0 ng/mL (14.2 to 38.3 ng/mL). Additionally, 41 (76%) patients had elevation above the 99th percentile, and 13 (24%) had an increase higher than 10 times the 99th percentile (Fig. 2B).

The pattern of cTnI elevation in each moment of evaluation after surgery is shown in the chart below (Fig. 3). Values for cTnI above 10 times the 99th percentile are constant over the measurement time in almost the entire sample.

The comparisons of the levels of cTnI in the different periods after the procedure showed a statistically significant difference, $p < 0.001$ in all groups.

The pattern of CK-MB elevation in each moment after surgery is shown in the chart below, respectively (Fig. 4). Only a small part of the sample reached values above the 99th percentile.

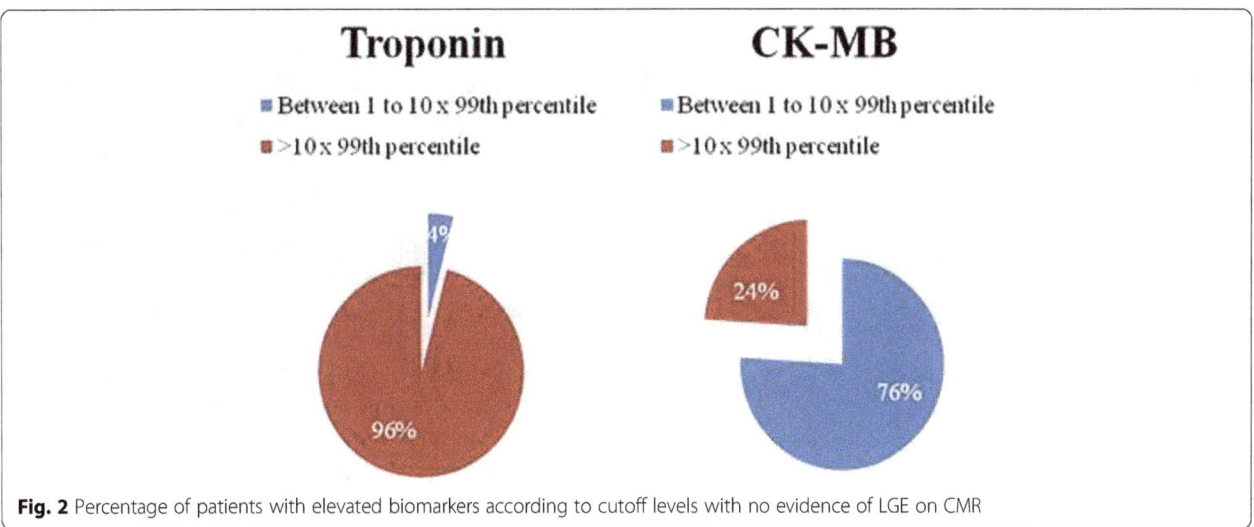

Fig. 2 Percentage of patients with elevated biomarkers according to cutoff levels with no evidence of LGE on CMR

The comparisons of CK-MB values in the different periods after the procedure showed statistically significant differences, $p < 0.001$ in both groups.

Electrocardiogram
All of the 54 patients who were free of late enhancement on the CMR after the procedure and who were selected for this study underwent ECG at entry and sequentially. None of them had a new bundle-branch block, ischemic ST-segment, new pathologic Q wave conduction disorders, or a new Q wave after the procedure.

Renal function
All patients had preserved glomerular filtration rate on admission. Sequential measures of renal function indicated that no loss of this function occurred.

Discussion
In this prospective trial based on current guidelines, we found distinct results when cTnI and CK-MB were simultaneously analyzed in patients after surgical myocardial procedures. All patients had elevated cTnI above the 99th percentile after surgery, with the majority having more than 10 times, reaching an average of 70 times this threshold. Conversely, we found the release of CK-MB predominantly below the recommended threshold of 10 times the 99th percentile. Therefore, our findings conflict with the recommendations of the 2012 European Society of Cardiology/American College of Cardiology/American Heart Association/World Heart Foundation Joint Task Force for the diagnosis of myocardial infarction after surgical revascularization.

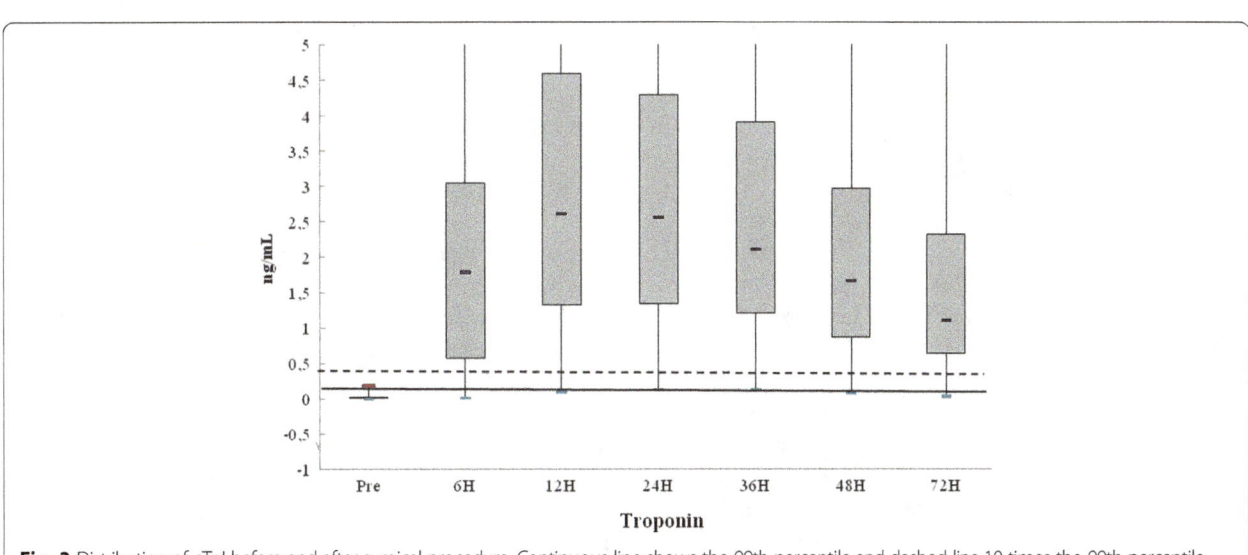

Fig. 3 Distribution of cTnI before and after surgical procedure. Continuous line shows the 99th percentile and dashed line 10 times the 99th percentile

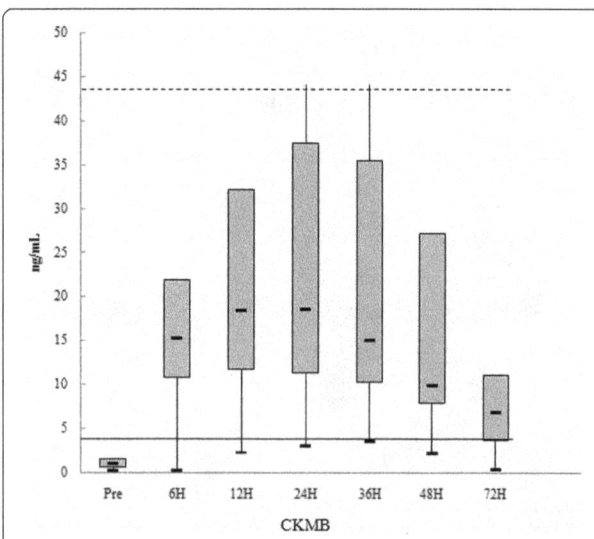

Fig. 4 Distribution of CK-MB before and after surgical procedure. Continuous line shows the 99th percentile and dashed line 10 times the 99th percentile

In this scenario, the EKG remained similar before and after interventions independently of the release of biomarkers. In addition, CMR likewise remained unchanged, without a new delayed enhancement after the procedure.

Over the last decade, elective CABG has progressed to a very standardized and safe surgical procedure with low mortality and low rates of myocardial events [14]. Thus, the present study focused on the possible reasons why our patients, after ONCAB, had elevated troponin above MI levels without the appearance of late enhancement in cardiac magnetic resonance imaging. As we know, perioperative elevation of specific cardiac biomarkers may be due to MI, but may also be associated with routine cardiac surgical procedures.

A study aimed at identifying the release of biomarkers following myocardial revascularization conducted by Pegg et al. [15] identified excessive troponin release in the absence of late enhancement by CMR. On the other hand, they noted that CK-MB behaved as foreseen by the current guideline. Thus, their results confirm the findings of the present study. Likewise, Van Gaal et al. [16], in a study comparing cTnI elevation and appearance of new late enhancement in CMR after CABG, found late enhancement in 28.1% of their patients. However, troponin elevation was found in 100% of patients based on the definition of myocardial infarction by the third Task Force [1]. Similar results were observed by Fellahi et al. [17] who, in an accurate analysis, found 14% troponin elevation in the absence of late enhancement. This lower percentage of discordance was probably due to the use of less-sensitive troponin assays. Wang et al. [18] applying EKG and echocardiography as the gold standard to detect AMI after CABG identified

21% of patients with new regional changes in wall motion on echocardiography without the corresponding change on EKG. The echocardiographic findings were consistent with the Troponin Task Force definition. Conversely, EKG data from our study were consistent with CK-MB release and discordant with troponin release.

The evident release of cTnI in the absence of myocardial necrosis is still questioned in the literature. As a confounding factor, advances in cTnI accuracy after high-sensitivity cTnI onset have been recently observed [18]. It can be postulated that this increase in sensitivity may be related to the power to detect changes in myocyte membrane permeability, which may result from non-physiological intraoperative events, contributing to the increase of cTnI plasma levels in the cytosol even in the absence of necrotic damage (Type 5 troponin elevation) [11, 19]. Therefore, a possible deleterious effect of extracorporeal circulation may contribute to the occurrence of discrete and "diffuse" myocardial damage. This damage can compromise subcellular structures that are difficult to identify, evidencing a clear limitation of CMR analysis.

With the emergence of high-sensitivity troponins, the relationship between the increase in the sensitivity thereof and the increasing rise in false diagnoses has already been described [2]. Currently, there is extensive discussion among manufacturers about the heterogeneity of their troponin kits and the influence of laboratory practices on the use of these kits. The multiplicity of troponin kits, each having different reference values, which use different reagents, different epitopes to bind antibodies, and different incubation times, leads to great difficulty in finding uniformity in the acquired information and studies [20–22]. Unlike that observed with CK-MB, the lack of standardization for calibration of the different tests for assessment of cTnI precludes the establishment of a universal threshold cutoff for the 99th percentile [20].

Clinical implications

Assuming that cardiac biomarkers have limited diagnostic accuracy in myocardial necrosis, the challenges faced for the establishment of definitive values for the diagnosis of myocardial damage include new cutoff values for cTnI. Furthermore, the diagnosis of this condition cannot be exclusively based on cardiac biomarkers or EKG. It is reasonable to include CMR in the set of tools for the accurate diagnosis of procedure-related myocardial injury.

Conclusions

In this study, different from CK-MB findings, troponin was significantly increased in the absence of myocardial infarction on cardiac resonance imaging. Thus, CK-MB was more accurate than cTnI for excluding procedure-related MI. These data suggest a higher troponin cutoff for the diagnosis of CABG-related MI.

Acknowledgments

We would like to thank all members of the MASS-V Trial for hard work in putting together all the forces needed to perform this study. This study has been funded partially by the Zerbini Foundation and Fundação de Amparo á Pesquisa do Estado de São Paulo (FAPESP) Number 2011/20876-2. Medical writing support was provided by Ann Conti Morcos during the preparation of this paper, supported by the Zerbini Foundation.

Funding

Financial support for the present study was provided in part by a research grant from the Zerbini Foundation and also by the FAPESP (2011/20876–2).

Authors' contributions

Contribution of each author: FTCO: concept and design of the manuscript; analysis and interpretation of data; WH; conception and design of this study and final approval of the manuscript; CHN: conception of this trial; ACH: interpretation of data; AVV: acquisition, analysis, and interpretation of data; LMAC: drafting the article or revising it; RMVM: acquisition and analysis of data; PCR: analysis of data; CAWS: drafting the article or revising it; CLG: analysis of data; EGL: interpretation of data, statistical support; JAFR: design of this study and final approval of the submitted manuscript; RKF: final approval of the submitted manuscript. All authors read and approved the final manuscript.

Competing interests

The authors declare that they have no competing interests.

References

1. Thygesen K, Alpert JS, Jaffe AS, et al. Third universal definition of myocardial infarction. J Am Coll Cardiol. 2012;60(16):1581–98.
2. Swaanenburg JC, Loef BG, Volmer M, et al. Creatine kinase MB, troponin I, and troponin T release patterns after coronary artery bypass grafting with or without cardiopulmonary bypass and after aortic and mitral valve surgery. Clinical Chem. 2001;47(3):584–7.
3. Pichon H, Chocron S, Alwan K, et al. Crystalloid versus cold blood cardioplegia and cardiac troponin I release. Circulation. 1997;96(1):316–20.
4. Mingels A, Jacobs L, Michielsen E, Swaanenburg J, Wodzig W, van Dieijen-Visser M. Reference population and marathon runner sera assessed by highly sensitive cardiac troponin T and commercial cardiac troponin T and I assays. Clinical Chem. 2009;55(1):101–8.
5. Testa L, Van Gaal WJ, Biondi Zoccai GG, et al. Myocardial infarction after percutaneous coronary intervention: a meta-analysis of troponin elevation applying the new universal definition. QJM. 2009;102(6):369–78.
6. Hueb W, Gersh BJ, Rezende PC, et al. Hypotheses, rationale, design, and methods for prognostic evaluation of cardiac biomarker elevation after percutaneous and surgical revascularization in the absence of manifest myocardial infarction. A comparative analysis of biomarkers and cardiac magnetic resonance. The MASS-V trial. BMC Cardiovasc Disord. 2012;12:65.
7. Wu E, Judd RM, Vargas JD, Klocke FJ, Bonow RO, Kim RJ. Visualisation of presence, location, and transmural extent of healed Q-wave and non-Q-wave myocardial infarction. Lancet. 2001;357(9249):21–8.
8. KC W, Zerhouni EA, Judd RM, et al. Prognostic significance of microvascular obstruction by magnetic resonance imaging in patients with acute myocardial infarction. Circulation. 1998;97(8):765–72.
9. Selvanayagam JB, Petersen SE, Francis JM, et al. Effects of off-pump versus on-pump coronary surgery on reversible and irreversible myocardial injury: a randomized trial using cardiovascular magnetic resonance imaging and biochemical markers. Circulation. 2004;109(3):345–50.
10. Mahrholdt H, Wagner A, Judd RM, Sechtem U, Kim RJ. Delayed enhancement cardiovascular magnetic resonance assessment of non-ischaemic cardiomyopathies. Eur Heart J. 2005;26(15):1461–74.
11. Porto I, Selvanayagam JB, Van Gaal WJ, et al. Plaque volume and occurrence and location of peri procedural myocardial necrosis after percutaneous coronary intervention: insights from delayed enhancement magnetic resonance imaging, thrombolysis in myocardial infarction myocardial perfusion grade analysis, and intravascular ultrasound. Circulation. 2006;114: 662–9. https://doi.org/10.1161/CIRCULATIONAHA.105.593210.
12. Hudsmith LE, Petersen SE, Francis JM, Robson MD, Neubauer S. Normal human left and right ventricular and left atrial dimensions using steady state free precession magnetic resonance imaging. J Cardiovasc Magn Reson. 2005;7(5):775–82. doi:10.1080/10976640500295516.
13. Mendis S, Thygesen K, Kuulasmaa K, et al. World Health Organization definition of myocardial infarction: 2008-09 revision. Int J Epidemiol. 2001; 40(1):139–46.
14. Gober V, Hohl A, Gahl B, et al. Early troponin T and prediction of potentially correctable in-hospital complications after coronary artery bypass grafting surgery. PLoS One. 2013;8(9):e74241.
15. Pegg TJ, Maunsell Z, Karamitsos TD, et al. Utility of cardiac biomarkers for the diagnosis of type V myocardial infarction after coronary artery bypass grafting: insights from serial cardiac MRI. Heart. 2011;97(10):810–6.
16. van Gaal WJ, Arnold JR, Testa L, et al. Myocardial injury following coronary artery surgery versus angioplasty (MICASA): a randomised trial using biochemical markers and cardiac magnetic resonance imaging. Eur Secur. 2011;6(6):703–10.
17. Fellahi JL, Gue X, Richomme X, et al. Short- and long-term prognostic value of postoperative cardiac troponin I concentration in patients undergoing coronary artery bypass grafting. Anesthesiology. 2003;99(2):270–4.
18. Wang TK, Stewart RA, Ramanathan T, et al. Diagnosis of MI after CABG with high-sensitivity troponin T and new ECG or echocardiogram changes: relationship with mortality and validation of the universal definition of MI. Eur Heart J Acute Cardiovasc Care. 2013;2(4):323–33.
19. White HD. Pathobiology of troponin elevations: do elevations occur with myocardial ischemia as well as necrosis? J Am Coll Cardiol. 2011;57(24):2406–8.
20. Lewandrowski KB. Cardiac markers of myocardial necrosis: a history and discussion of milestones and emerging new trends, Clin Lab Med. 34(1) (2014) 31–41, xi.
21. Araújo MP, Mesquita ET. Avaliação de Marcadores Prognósticos na Síndrome Coronariana Aguda sem Supradesnivelamento do Segmento ST na Sala de Emergência. SOCERJ. 2005:50–6.
22. Ramasamy I. Biochemical markers in acute coronary syndrome. Clin Chim Acta. 2011;412(15–16):1279.

6

A dual therapy of off-pump temporary left ventricular extracorporeal device and amniotic stem cell for cardiogenic shock

Toshinobu Kazui[1,2,6†], Phat L. Tran[2,5†], Tia R. Pilikian[1], Katie M. Marsh[1,2], Raymond Runyan[3], John Konhilas[3], Richard Smith[5] and Zain I. Khalpey[1,2,3,4,5,6*]

Abstract

Background: Temporary mechanical circulatory support device without sternotomy has been highly advocated for severe cardiogenic shock patient but little is known when coupled with amniotic stem cell therapy.

Case presentation: This case reports the first dual therapy of temporary left ventricular extracorporeal device CentriMag with distal banding technique and human amniotic stem cell injection for treating a severe refractory cardiogenic shock of an 68-year-old female patient. A minimally-invasive off-pump LVAD was established by draining from the left ventricle and returning to the right axillary artery with distal arterial banding to prevent right upper extremity hyperperfusion. Amniotic stem cells were injected intramyocardially at the left ventricular apex, lateral wall, inferior wall, and right subclavian vein.

Conclusion: The concomitant use of the temporary minimally-invasive off-pump CentriMag placement and stem cell therapy not only provided an alternative to cardiopulmonary bypass and full-median sternotomy procedures but may have also synergistically enhanced myocardial reperfusion and regeneration.

Keywords: Off-pump, Extracorporeal device, Left Ventricular Assist Device (LVAD), Refractory Cardiogenic Shock (RCS), Amniotic stem cell

Background

Severe refractory cardiogenic shock (RCS) can be defined as significant left or right ventricular dysfunction resulting in sustained hypotension and hypoperfusion of end-organs. Treatment for RCS would include one or more modalities like pharmaco-agents (inotropes and vasopressors), intra-aortic balloon pump (IABP), revascularization in the case of myocardial infarction, and ultimately mechanical circulatory support (MCS) system to hemodynamically unload the heart and restore circulation. One of such MCS system is the centrifugal pumps like CentriMag (Thoratec Corp, Pleasanton, CA), Rotaflow (MAQUET Cardiopulmonary AG, Hirrlingen, Germany), or Sorin Revolution (Sorin Group USA, Inc.,

Arvada, CO). These temporary ventricular assist devices (VAD) have been widely used as bridge-to-decision or bridge-to-recovery in patients with refractory cardiogenic shock [1, 2]. However, cardiac recovery leading to VAD explantation is still observed in a very small population [3].

Most of patients who require this therapy fall into INTERMACS (Interagency Registry for Mechanically Assisted Circulatory Support) profile1. Conventionally, the temporary left VAD implantation has been performed through median sternotomy with or without cardiopulmonary bypass (CPB) support. These critically ill patients tend to bleed more during and after surgery for pre-operative liver dysfunction [4]. Especially for patient with previous sternotomy, the dissection can take longer and bleed more.

Patients with VAD may also be benefited from stem cell therapy (SCT), which has been shown to potentially increase circulatory perfusion [5, 6], promote angiogenesis and reduction of fibrin formation after VAD

* Correspondence: zkhalpey@surgery.arizona.edu
†Equal contributors
¹Department of Surgery, Division of Cardiothoracic Surgery, University of Arizona, Tucson, AZ, USA
²College of Medicine – Tucson, University of Arizona, Tucson, AZ, USA
Full list of author information is available at the end of the article

implantation [7], and improve ejection fraction (EF) [8]. More particularly, Nasseri et al. [5] looked at 10 patients on long-term left ventricular assist device (LVAD) concomitantly injected with bone marrow mononuclear cells. They found one improved cardiac function resulting in LVAD explantation, 2 deaths, and 7 others exhibited increased perfusion. However, these case reports and series are utilizing long-term LVAD support platform with maximal inflammation induction from median sternotomy; therefore creating an unfavorable environment for stem cell engraftment and differentiation that may potentially hinder cardiac recovery.

To recover the heart, a minimally invasive approach with stem cell therapy was applied to reduce surgical insult, avoiding CPB pump and median sternotomy. We cannulated at the apex of the left ventricle and returned through the right axillary artery with distal banding technique to avoid hyperperfusion. We then administered a bimodal delivery of amniotic stem cells with the intention of initiating cellular myocardial recovery.

Case presentation

A 68-year-old female patient with past medical history of, two previous coronary artery bypass grafts, hypertension, chronic kidney disease, and diabetes mellitus, presented to a local hospital with chest pain and shortness of breath following an ST-elevation myocardial infarction. The patient was placed on an IABP and underwent a cardiac catheterization with the placement of five stents in the left anterior descending artery and saphenous vein graft. However she developed postoperative cardiogenic shock and multi-organ hypoperfusion despite her IABP and increased pressor requirements. She was then transferred to our institution for possible ventricular assist device placement.

Preoperative transesophageal echocardiography (TEE) demonstrated EF of 10% with apical akinesis, mild aortic insufficiency, moderate mitral and tricuspid valve regurgitation. Right heart was functional prompting for a CentriMag LVAD placement as Bridge-to-Decision/Recovery.

The patient was placed supine position. The position of Left ventricular (LV) apex was confirmed by transthoracic echocardiography. A 5 cm mini-thoracotomy at 5th intercostal space was made. A pericardial well was created and A Thoratec 34 Fr inflow cannula (Thoratec Corp, Pleasanton, CA) was brought to the field. The Thoratec cuff was sewn into the left ventricular apex using plegetted 3–0 Ethibond sutures followed by a running 3–0 Prolene suture. The right axillary artery was exposed. Activated clotting time guided heparin was confirmed to be more than 200 s. An 8 mm Dacron graft was sewn into the axillary artery in end-to-side fashion using a 4–0 Prolene

running suture. A 20 Fr EOPA cannula was passed through the graft with the tip extending to the level of the anastomosis. Silk ties were used to secure the cannula to the graft. The distal axillary artery was banded with a vessel loop. Banding prevented arterial and right axillary artery distal from over perfusion and ensured adequate cerebral perfusion. Remaining off-pump, the 34 Fr Thoratec inflow cannula was passed into the left ventricle. The position was confirmed by TEE. The cannula was secured to the cuff and was de-aired and connected to the CentriMag device (Fig. 1). The CentriMag was started and flow was established at 4.5 L/min. Human allograft and liquid matrix was inserted into the subclavian vein (2 times of 1cm^3 of PalinGen Kardia Flow, Amnio Technology, Phoenix, AZ, USA) and into the anterior, lateral, and inferior walls of the LV (1cm^3 of PalinGen Kardia Flow each).

Her end organ function recovered during the support. Transthoracic Echocardiography (TTE) was conducted which showed LV recovery, EF 30% with 1.5 LPM of LVAD flow at post op day 13. At post op day 20, fibrin clots developed in both the inflow and outflow cannula connectors prompting for an urgent decannulation at post op day 21. Upon off-pump LVAD removal, a subsequent IABP was placed and inotropic support was started in an effort to increase coronary perfusion. A head CT scan showed evidence of a small right sided ischemic cerebral infarct possibly due to clots dislodgement from the support/plumbing system or thrombotic occlusion of the right brachiocephalic trunk, right common carotid, right internal, and right vertebral arteries resulting in left sided hemiplegia. Extubation, IABP removal, and

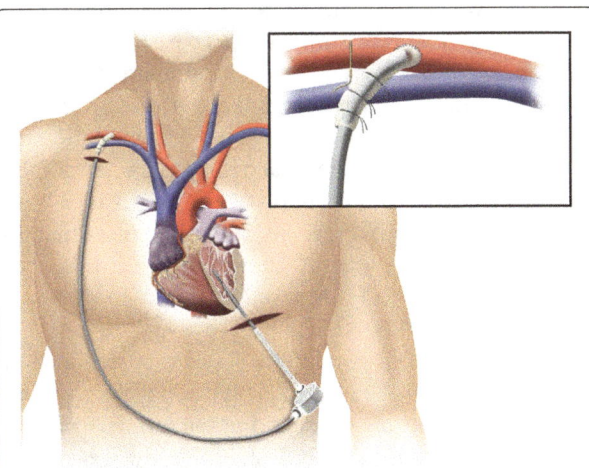

Fig. 1 Application of the Thoratec® CentriMag® LVAD with inflow cannulation from the left ventricular apex, outflow cannulation via 8 mm Dacron graft into the right axillary artery, and arterial banding distal to outflow

BiPAP administration was performed on post-explant day three. The patient was discharge to rehabilitation facility.

Conclusion

With regard to implantable LVAD, off pump placement has been reported [9]. However, to our best knowledge, this is the first dual therapy of using a temporary off-pump implantation of a CentriMag as a left ventricular extracorporeal device with banding technique and human amniotic stem cell. CentriMag LVAD placement was performed in an off-pump fashion with left mini-thoracotomy and adjusted distal arm flow by placing a tourniquet. This is a viable short-term solution as bridge to decision/recovery especially for patients with previous sternotomy. Also, anastomosis of a graft to the right axillary artery can further prevent complications relating to direct axillary artery cannulation. This approach gave us a flexibility to extubate and to mobilize the patient while she was on the support. Avoiding the usage of CPB and full sternotomy can also minimize postoperative inflammation, preserve end organ function, and potentially prevent RV dysfunction [10].

One of the potential disadvantages of this approach was hyperperfusion of the right arm and right carotid artery. We were able to avoid the latter complication by tightening the axillary artery distal to the anastomosed site via a tourniquet such that the right radial pressure matched the left radial pressure upon stable support.

From the hemodynamic point of view, mechanically unloading the heart has been shown to increase survivability and promote differentiation of cardiac stem cells injected in the myocardium of an infarcted animal heart [11]; inhibit apoptotic mechanism and facilitated stem cells engraftment in a mouse model [12]. It appears that our minimally invasive off pump approach minimizes sternotomy-induced myocardial inflammation, reduces myocardial load, improves coronary perfusion such that a favorable environment was created for amniotic stem cell to engraft and resurrect the ailing heart. In fact, our patient's left ventricle EF improved from 10 to 30% by postop day 13. This observed clinical improvement is concurrent to bone marrow stem cell studies reported by Gojo et al. [8] (EF improved from 6.4 to 40%) and Miyagawa et al. [13] (EF improved from 22 to 32%). Aside from safe to use, we think that direct stem cell injection may provide myocardial functional recovery but further study is highly warranted in the future.

The concomitant use of SCT and LVAD have been previously reported by Dib et al. [14] and Pagani et al. [15]. However, they were using skeletal myoblasts, which is less versatile than amniotic stem cells and long term LVAD, which can inflict maximal surgical insults. Our minimally-invasive off-pump CentriMag LVAD placement has the potential to achieve shorter recovery times and improve clinical outcomes in profound RCS and previous cardiac surgery patients. Finally, we further demonstrated that dual therapy of LVAD and SCT is also feasible, safe, and may be efficacious to LVAD explantation; thus moving toward a more prescriptive/individualized medical therapy for early and end stage heart failure patients.

Abbreviations

CPB: CardioPulmonary Bypass; EF: Ejection fraction; IABP: Intra-aortic balloon pump; LV: Left ventricle; LVAD: Left ventricular assist device; MCS: Mechanical circulatory support; RCS: Refractory cardiogenic shock; SCT: Stem cell therapy; TEE: TransEsophageal Echocardiography; TTE: TransThoracic Echocardiography; VAD: Ventricular assist devices

Acknowledgements

The authors thank the OR and ICU staff.

Funding

Authors have no funding to disclose.

Authors' contributions

TK, PLT, KM, RS, and ZK were members of the surgical team. PLT, TRP, RR, and JK were involved in drafting and critical revisions. All authors read and approved the final manuscript.

Consent for publication

Written informed consent was obtained from the patient for publication of this case report and any accompanying images. A copy of the written consent is available for review by the Editor-in-Chief of this journal.

Competing interests

The authors declare that they have no competing interests.

Author details

[1]Department of Surgery, Division of Cardiothoracic Surgery, University of Arizona, Tucson, AZ, USA. [2]College of Medicine – Tucson, University of Arizona, Tucson, AZ, USA. [3]Department of Physiological Sciences, University of Arizona, Tucson, AZ, USA. [4]Department of Biomedical Engineering, University of Arizona, Tucson, AZ, USA. [5]Artificial Heart Program, Banner University Medical Center, Tucson, AZ, USA. [6]Division of Cardiohracic Surgery, Banner University Medical Center Tucson, 1501 N Campbell Ave., Rm 4302A, P.O. Box 245071, Tucson, AZ 85724-5071, USA.

References

1. Takayama H, Soni L, Kalesan B, Truby LK, Ota T, Cedola S, et al. Bridge-to-decision therapy with a continuous-flow external ventricular assist device in refractory Cardiogenic shock of various causes. Circ Hear Fail. 2014;7:799–806.
2. Shuhaiber JH, Jenkins D, Berman M, Parameshwar J, Dhital K, Tsui S, et al. The Papworth experience with the Levitronix CentriMag ventricular assist device. J. Hear. Lung Transplant. 2008;27:158–64.
3. Mancini DM, Beniaminovitz A, Levin H, Catanese K, Flannery M, DiTullio M, et al. Low incidence of myocardial recovery after left ventricular assist device implantation in patients with chronic heart failure. Circulation. 1998;98:2383–9.

4. Bhama JK, Kormos RL, Toyoda Y, Teuteberg JJ, McCurry KR, Siegenthaler MP. Clinical experience using the Levitronix CentriMag system for temporary right ventricular mechanical circulatory support. J. Hear. Lung Transplant. 2009;28:971–6.

5. Nasseri BA, Kukucka M, Dandel M, Knosalla C, Potapov E, Lehmkuhl HB, et al. Intramyocardial delivery of bone marrow mononuclear cells and mechanical assist device implantation in patients with end-stage cardiomyopathy. Cell Transplant. 2007;16:941–9.

6. Anastasiadis K, Antonitsis P, Argiriadou H, Koliakos G, Doumas A, Khayat A, et al. Hybrid approach of ventricular assist device and autologous bone marrow stem cells implantation in end-stage ischemic heart failure enhances myocardial reperfusion. J Transl Med. 2011;9:12.

7. Memon IA, Sawa Y, Miyagawa S, Taketani S, Matsuda H. Combined autologous cellular cardiomyoplasty with skeletal myoblasts and bone marrow cells in canine hearts for ischemic cardiomyopathy. J Thorac Cardiovasc Surg. 2005;130:646–53.

8. Gojo S, Kyo S, Nishimura S, Komiyama N, Kawai N, Bessho M, et al. Cardiac resurrection after bone-marrow-derived mononuclear cell transplantation during left ventricular assist device support. Ann Thorac Surg. 2007;83:661–2.

9. Sileshi B, Haglund NA, Davis ME, Tricarico NM, Stulak JM, Khalpey Z, et al. In-hospital outcomes of a minimally invasive off-pump left thoracotomy approach using a centrifugal continuous-flow left ventricular assist device. J Hear Lung Transplant. 2015;34:107–12.

10. Strueber M, Meyer AL, Feussner M, Ender J, Correia J-C, Mohr F-W. A minimally invasive off-pump implantation technique for continuous-flow left ventricular assist devices: early experience. J Heart Lung Transplant. 2014;33:851–6.

11. Kurazumi H, Li T, Takemoto Y, Suzuki R, Mikamo A. Haemodynamic unloading increases the survival and affects the differentiation of cardiac stem cells after implantation into an infarcted heart. Eur J Cardiothorac Surg. 2014;45:976–82.

12. Suzuki R, Li TS, Mikamo A, Takahashi M, Ohshima M, Kubo M, et al. The reduction of hemodynamic loading assists self-regeneration of the injured heart by increasing cell proliferation, inhibiting cell apoptosis, and inducing stem-cell recruitment. J Thorac Cardiovasc Surg. 2007;133:1051–8.

13. Miyagawa S, Matsumiya G, Funatsu T, Yoshitatsu M, Sekiya N, Fukui S, et al. Combined autologous cellular cardiomyoplasty using skeletal myoblasts and bone marrow cells for human ischemic cardiomyopathy with left ventricular assist system implantation: report of a case. Surg Today. 2009;39:133–6.

14. Dib N, Michler RE, Pagani FD, Wright S, Kereiakes DJ, Lengerich R, et al. Safety and feasibility of autologous myoblast transplantation in patients with ischemic cardiomyopathy: four-year follow-up. Circulation. 2005;112:1748–55.

15. Pagani FD, DerSimonian H, Zawadzka A, Wetzel K, Edge ASB, Jacoby DB, et al. Autologous skeletal myoblasts transplanted to ischemia-damaged myocardium in humans: histological analysis of cell survival and differentiation. J Am Coll Cardiol. 2003;41:879–88.

7

A standardized approach to treat complex aortic valve endocarditis

Anna Gomes[1][*] [iD], Jayant S. Jainandunsing[2], Sander van Assen[3], Peter Paul van Geel[4], Bhanu Sinha[1], Sandro Gelsomino[5], Daniel M. Johnson[5] and Ehsan Natour[5,6]

Abstract

Background: Surgical treatment of complicated aortic valve endocarditis often is challenging, even for experienced surgeons. We aim at demonstrating a standardized surgical approach by stentless bioprostheses for the treatment of aortic valve endocarditis complicated by paravalvular abscess formation.

Methods: Sixteen patients presenting with aortic valve endocarditis (4 native and 12 prosthetic valves) and paravalvular abscess formation at various localizations and to different extents were treated by a standardized approach using stentless bioprostheses. The procedure consisted of thorough debridement, root replacement with reimplantation of the coronary arteries and correction of accompanying pathologies (aortoventricular and aortomitral dehiscence, septum derangements, Gerbode defect, total atrioventricular conduction block, mitral and tricuspid valve involvement).

Results: All highly complex patients included (14 males and 2 females; median age 63 years [range 31–77]) could be successfully treated with stentless bioprostheses as aortic root replacement. Radical surgical debridement of infected tissue with anatomical recontruction was feasible. Although predicted operative mortality was high (median logarithmic EuroSCORE I of 40.7 [range 12.8–68.3]), in-hospital and 30-day mortality rates were favorable (18.8 and 12.5% respectively).

Conclusions: Repair of active aortic valve endocarditis complicated by paravalvular abscess formation and destruction of the left ventricular outflow tract with stentless bioprosthesis is a valuable option for both native and prosthetic valves. It presents a standardized approach with a high success rate for complete debridement, is readily available, and yields comparable clinical outcomes to the historical gold standard, repair by homografts. Additionally, use of one type of prosthesis reduces logistical issues and purchasing costs.

Keywords: Infective endocarditis, Stentless bioprostheses, Abscess, High-risk, Surgery

Background

Infective endocarditis causes in-hospital mortality of 20% and 40% after 1-year, rising further to 79% for aortic valve endocarditis [1, 2]. This high rate is largely due to extended local destruction of heart tissue, e.g. paravalvular abscess formation, with secondary heart failure. Risk factors for endocarditis include rheumatic, congenital, and degenerative valve lesions, intracardiac prosthetic material, intravenous drug use, and healthcare contact [3]. Diagnosis of endocarditis is based on the modified Duke criteria, bearing a sensitivity and specificity of 80% for the total patient population [4]. As this is not optimal, the expert opinion of a multidisciplinairy team is essential for diagnosis. Therapy of endocarditis relies on antimicrobial therapy and surgery for cardiac anatomical damage (vegetation, abscess, fistula, shrunken valve, valve tears or holes, prosthetic valve detachment), as well as uncontrolled infection. In this way, 25–50% of patients are operated upon in the acute phase of infection and an additional 20–40% later in the course due to haemodynamic complications [5].

Paravalvular abscess formation complicates aortic valve endocarditis. Early surgical treatment of complicated endocarditis improves outcome when compared to

* Correspondence: a.gomes@umcg.nl
[1]Department of Medical Microbiology, University of Groningen, University Medical Center Groningen, Groningen, Netherlands
Full list of author information is available at the end of the article

medical therapy alone, reducing 6-month mortality from 33 to 16% [6] and the composite endpoint of death/ embolic events/ recurrence of endocarditis from 28 to 3% [7]. Aortic valve paravalvular abscess formation and root destruction requires radical resection of infected tissue with subsequent reconstruction of the left ventricular outflow tract (LVOT) (modified Bentall procedure) [8]. Therefore, surgical treatment of complicated aortic valve endocarditis is considered challenging, bearing high operative (11–40% in-hospital) and late (60% in 5 years) mortality rates [9].

Various surgical techniques are used to treat complicated aortic valve endocarditis, depending on the surgical preference and with differing results: patch, prosthesis, homograft. Historically, cryopreserved homografts were considered as the gold standard for these patients [10–12]. Homografts offer low recurrence rates, acceptable valve-related morbidity and mortality, and their low transvalvular gradient is associated with improved left ventricular mass regression [13, 14]. Homografts also have disadvantages, including demanding surgical techniques, the need for reoperation due to calcification, limited availability and shelf life [8, 9, 15]. Nowadays, biological stentless valves are more often used in complicated aortic valve endocarditis [8, 9]. Using these prostheses, the surgical versatility of homografts is reached due to their comparable durability, shape and pliability [8]. In addition, stentless bioprostheses have advantages, such as a rather long shelf life and being readily available in various sizes, uniform in quality, technically easier to implant and furnished with anticalcification properties [8, 13, 14, 16–18].

Guidelines support the use of both homografts and stentless bioprostheses in aortic valve endocarditis with paravalvular abscess formation [2, 10, 19]. The choice of prosthesis depends on patient characteristics, technical considerations, and surgeon preferences [8, 14]. In this illustrated series of sixteen patients with aortic valve endocarditis and complicating paravalvular abscess formation, we show that the use of stentless bioprostheses provides a more standardized surgical procedure that consists of thorough debridement, root replacement with reimplantation of the coronary arteries, and treatment of accompanying pathologies.

Methods
Patients
In this case series we aimed at providing evidence for the standardized use of a stentless bioprostheses in complex aortic valve endocarditis. "Standardized use" refers to the use of one type of stentless bioprosthesis for a variety of anatomical problems complicating aortic valve endocarditis. Clinical data and high quality macroscopic pictures from sixteen patients with active aortic valve endocarditis

and paravalvular abscess formation were collected between 2006 and 2015. In this time period, a total of 85 patients underwent aortic valve surgery for endocarditis in our center. Here, we report on those patients treated with stentless bioprostheses. Their endocarditis was not limited to the cusps but also involved the annulus with formation of large paravalvular abscesses at various anatomical locations. Consequently, complications arose, such as root disarrangement with loss of aortaventricular or aortomitral continuity, atrioventricular conduction disturbance, or infection of the septum or the right ventricle. Despite their poor clinical condition, these patients were deemed eligible for surgical valve repair and LVOT reconstruction using stentless bioprostheses.

Definitions
Infective endocarditis was diagnosed based on the modified Duke criteria [4] and expert opinion of a multidisciplinairy team. Prosthetic valve endocarditis was considered early if it occurred during the first year after valve replacement, otherwise it was considered late [2]. Causative microorganisms were identified by culture and molecular testing on peripheral blood and tissue or prosthetic material collected during surgery [2]. Functional cardiac derangements as described by the guidelines were important indications for surgery [2, 19]. Macroscopically visible pathological findings considered an indication for the use of stentless bioprostheses were presence of destructive lesions, including annular abscess, paravalvular leak and cusp perforation. Re-thoracotomy was defined as reopening of the sternum after implantation of the bioprosthesis. Reoperation was defined as any surgical procedure involving the implanted bioprosthesis. Recurrence was used as a combined term for both relapse (repeat episodes of endocarditis caused by the same microorganism) and reinfection (infection caused by a different microorganism) [2].

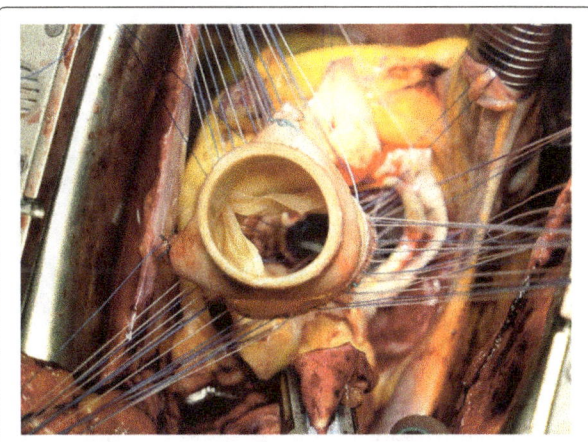

Fig. 1 Stentless bioprosthesis

Prosthesis

The Freestyle® bioprosthesis (Medtronic Inc., Minneapolis, MN, USA) is a stentless porcine aortic root prosthesis with ligated coronary arteries and a thin skirt over the porcine septal myocardium. The bioprosthesis is fixed with low pressure applied to the aortic wall, and zero-net pressure across the leaflets (Fig. 1). Pre-implantation, the bioprosthesis underwent an anticalcification treatment using alpha-amino-oleic acid. The device can be implanted by various techniques: subcoronary valve replacement, root inclusion, or complete aortic root replacement.

Surgical technique

The standard surgical approach was a median (re)sternotomy with mild/moderate hypothermic (32–34 °C) cardiopulmonary bypass and cardioplegic cardiac arrest (retrograde blood cardioplegia). Cardiopulmonary bypass was performed using aortic cannulation and right atrial or bicaval cannulation for venous drainage.

The aorta was transected above the sinotubular junction. After the aortotomy exposure, the abscess regions were inspected (Fig. 2) and infected native cusps or prosthesis as well as any aortic aneurysms were removed with extensive tissue debridement. The aortic sinuses were resected with

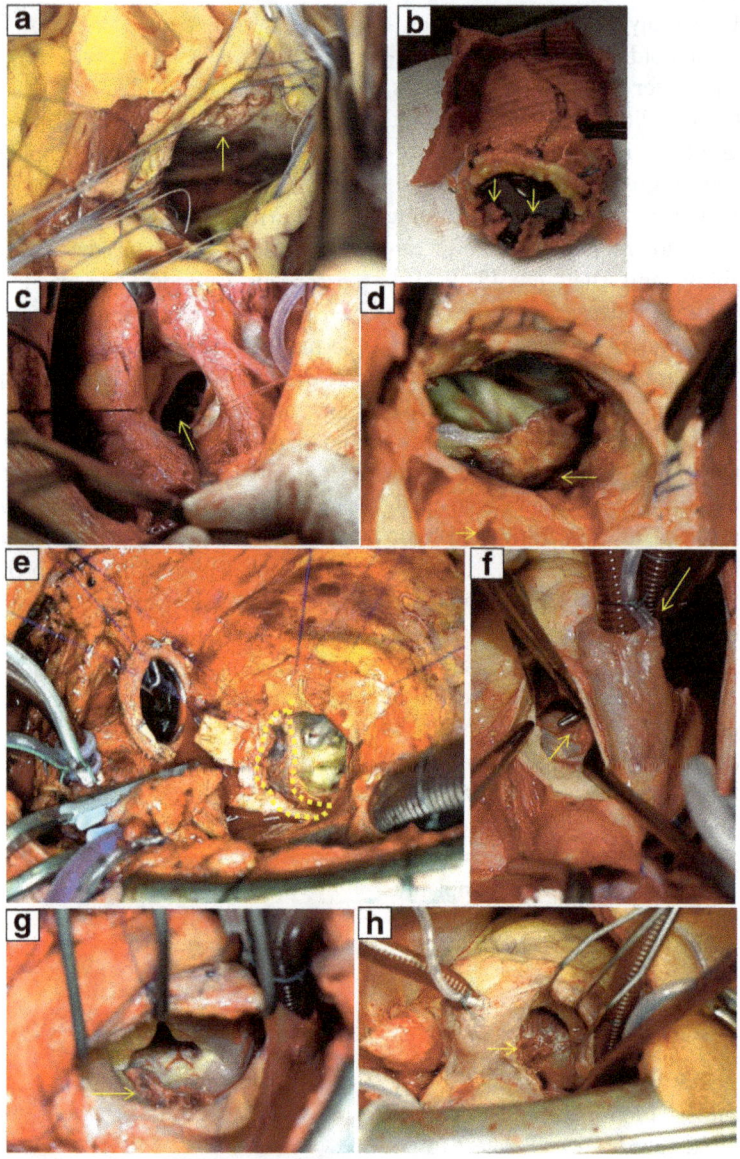

Fig. 2 Aortic valve endocarditis with paravalvular abscess formation, surgical view: **a** view from aortic root, ventricular septal defect, **b** valved conduit with vegetations, **c** total aorto-ventricular dehiscence, with left ventricular outflow tract discontinuity, **d** abscess cavity (large arrow) with left main coronary visible (small arrow), **e** retro-aortal abscess cavity with aorto-mitral involvement and mitral annulus dehiscence, **f** aorto-atrial fistula, Gerbode-like defect, **g** atrial view, tricuspid valve annular abscess with torn septal leaflet and paravalvular leak, **h** tricuspid valve deformity with vegetational mass

trumpet-shaped recesses of the coronary ostia. More specifically, a ventricular septum defect just under the membranous septum was identified in Fig. 2a. In this case a pericardial patch was used, which was distally sutured on the septum covering both the defect and the membranous septum, proximally attached at the level of the aortic annulus. Figure 2b and c depict chronic dehiscence of a mechanical prosthesis (implanted after a Bentall procedure) as a result of abcess formation at the annular level. Interestingly, the prosthesis was found floating above the annulus, only attached by the coronary arteries. Hence, the adhesions surrounding the annulus kept the prosthesis in place. Following resection of the infected prosthesis and clearance of the abcess, the stentless bioprosthesis was sutured on the annulus using a single-stitch technique. Given the chronic nature of disease in this case, the bioprosthesis was parachutted downwards towars the subannular plane to minimize traction of the chronically anchored anterior mitral leaflet (AML). In contrast, Fig. 2d and e illustrate acute subannular abcess formation. In this case, the AML was detached from the annulus while the prosthesis attachment site remained intact. In this case, due to the recent onset of infection, traction of the AML to the annulus plane and a neo-annulus were created after clearance of the abcess and other inflammatory tissue. Afterwards the stentless bioprosthesis was sutured to the annulus. Figure 2f to h depict Gerbode lesions with tricuspid valve involvement. Gerbode(–like) lesions encompass fistulas formed between the left ventricle(aorta) and the right side of the heart, appearing above or below the septal leaflet of the tricuspid valve. Repair of the subvalvular fistula from the right side included temporary resection of the spetal leaflet of the tricupid valve, which was thereafter re-attached.

After debridement, restoration and sizing of the aortic annulus the proximal anastomosis was performed using 20–25 interrupted sutures of Ticron 3–0 in a single plane. If required, the coronary ostia were mobilised using diathermy. After completion of the proximal suture line, the patient's coronary ostia were reimplanted end-to-side to the corresponding sinus of Valsalva of the prosthesis using a continuous 5–0 polyproylene suture. Finally, the bioprosthesis was anastomosed with the aorta using continuous 4–0 polyproylene. If further resection of the ascending aorta was required, a vascular tube graft was interposed.

Ethical considerations

The institutional medical ethical review board of the University Medical Center Groningen approved the use of retrospective patient data for our study and waived informed consent (METc2015/033; February 2015).

Results

Patient characteristics

This series consecutively included 14 males and 2 females with a median age of 63 years (Tables 1 and 2). All patients had an urgent indication for cardiothoracic surgery with implantation of a stentless bioprosthesis as root replacement due to uncontrolled infection and abscess formation (evidence class I and level B [2]). Median New York Heart Association score was III, and median logarithmic EuroSCORE I score was 40.7. Median follow-up for survivors was 4.6 years. All survivors were followed for at least 2 years, 36% were followed for 5 years, and 9% for 10 or more years. In 4 patients (25%) the endocarditis involved native aortic valves, with 2 identified bicuspid valves. In 12 patients (58%) the endocarditis involved prosthetic aortic valves: in 7 patients the aortic valve was replaced once and in 1 patient twice before, in 5 patients a Bentall procedure had been

Table 1 Patient characteristics (n = 16

Characteristic	Value
Age: median [range] (years)	63 [31–77]
Gender: male; female, n (%)	14 (87.5); 2 (12.5)
Reoperation / PVE (%)	75
Follow-up survivors: median [range] (years)	4.6 [2.3–11.7]
NYHA score: median [range]	III [II-IV]
Logarithmic EuroSCORE I: median [range]	40.7 [12.8–68.3]
Microbiology	
PVE	
• *Staphylococcus* spp.: 5 CoNS, 1 *S. aureus*	n = 6 (50%)
• *Streptococcus* spp.: 1 viridans group, 1 *S. bovis*, 1 *S. agalactiae*	n = 3 (25%)
• *Enterococcus* spp.: 2 *E. faecalis*	n = 2 (17%)
• no micro-organism identified	n = 1 (8%)
NVE	
• *Staphylococcus* spp.: *S. aureus*	n = 1 (25%)
• *Streptococcus* spp.: 2 viridans group	n = 2 (50%)
• *Enterococcus* spp.: *E. faecalis*	n = 1 (25%)
Outcome	Value
Cardiopulmonary bypass perfusion time: median [range] (minutes)	358 [186–731]
Aortic cross-clamping time: median [range] (minutes)	266 [107–389]
Intensive care unit stay: median [range] (days)	1.5 [1–21]
Hospital stay: median [range] (days)	55 [29–90]
In-hospital mortality: n (%)	3 (18.8)
30 day mortality: n (%)	2 (12.5)

CoNS coagulase negative staphylococci, *COPD* chronic obstructive pulmonary disease, *e.c.i.* e cause ignota, *NVE* native valve endocarditis, *NYHA* New York Heart Association, *PVE* prosthetic valve endocarditis, *SD* standard deviation

Table 2 Characteristics of included patients

#	Age (yr)	sex	Previous surgery	Micro-organism	Indication for surgery	Euro SCORE	Remarks during stentless bioprosthesis implantation	Outcome			
								rethoracotomy	re-IE	permanent dialysis	PPM
1	66	M	2 yr. bio	*Streptococcus sanguinis*	aortic root abscess	38.92	pericard patch to support MV, 1 RBC	Recovery initially, but death 7.5 months post surgery			
								−	+	−	+
2	70	M	1 yr. bio	*Staphylococcus epidermidis*	aortic root abscess, mycotic aneurysm, loose prosthesis, septic emboli, AV block	65.87	aorta annulus support with pledges and transseptal stiches, CABG, 5 RBC	In-hospital death 40 days post surgery			
								−	−	−	+
3	71	M	1 yr. bio	*Streptococcus agalactiae*	aortic root abscess with Gerbode defect, AV block	47.06	pericard patch reconstruction aorta annulus, atriotomy, TVP and Devega plasty, 14 RBC	Recovery > 6 years post surgery			
								−	−	−	+
4	31	M	–	*Streptococcus mitis*	totally destructed LVOT with Gerbode defect, AV block	42.52	pericard patch reconstruction aorta annulus, TVP, Devega plasty, 0 RBC	Recovery > 4 years post surgery			
								−	−	−	+
5	71	M	29 yr. mech	*Enterococcus faecalis*	aortic root abscess, septic emboli	47.06	3 RBC	Recovery > 3 years post surgery			
								−	−	−	
6	36	M	2 yr. mech	not identified	aortic root abscess, septic emboli	28.55	0 RBC	Recovery > 4 years post surgery			
								−	−	−	−
7	64	M	–	*Staphylococcus aureus*	aortic root abscess, multiple septic emboli, cardiac decompensation	23.42	aorta annulus support with pledges, 2 RBC	Recovery > 2 year (20 months) post surgery			
								−	−	−	+
8	72	M	3mo bio	*Staphylococcus epidermidis*	loose prosthesis, cardiac decompensation	64.48	closure of destructed coronary ostia, CABG, 0 RBC	In-hospital death 14 days post surgery			
9	45	M	12 yr. mech	*Staphylococcus aureus*	aortic root abscess, mycotic aneurysm	28.55	multiple vegetations AV, pericard patch reconstruction aorta annulus, 0 RBC	Recovery initially, but death 13 months post surgery			
								−	+	−	+
10	60	F	4mo bio	*Staphylcoccus epidermidis*	progressive aortic root abscess with Gerbode defect, septic emboli, blood cultures persistantly positive, AV-block	37.28	removal of vegetation from right atrium with affected AML and PPM implantation, 4 RBC	Recovery > 2 years post surgery			
								−	−	−		
11	55	M	–	*Enterococcus faecalis*	aortic root abscess, mycotic aneurysm, conduction disturbance	26.62	pericard patch reconstruction aorta annulus and AML, 1 RBC	Recovery > 4 years post surgery			
								−	−	−	
12	42	M	–	*Streptococcus mutans*	mycotic aneurysm, large vegetation	12.79	MVP, 0 RBC	Recovery > 5 years post surgery			
								−	−	−	
13	75	F	1 yr. bio	*Staphylococcus epidermidis*	aortic wall thickening, septic emboli, AV block	61.76	mobilization of tightly adhered coronary ostia, 2 RBC	Recovery > 8 years post surgery			
								−	−	−	+
14	77	M	2 yr. bio	*Enterococcus faecalis*	septal mycotic aneurysm with fistula and threatened anatomy	52.33	urgent surgery with two times reanimation setting and persistant instability for which	In-hospital death directly post surgery			
								−			

Table 2 Characteristics of included patients *(Continued)*

#	Age (yr)	sex	Previous surgery	Micro-organism	Indication for surgery	Euro SCORE	Remarks during stentless bioprosthesis implantation	Outcome			
								rethoracotomy	re-IE	permanent dialysis	PPM
							sternum left open, 0 RBC				
15	62	M	1 yr. mech	coagulase negative Staphylococci	aortic root abscess, progressive mycotic aneurysm, aortoventricular dehiscence	68.31	4 RBC	Recovery > 11 years post surgery –	–	–	–
16	60	M	7 yr. mech	*Streptococcus bovis*	aortic root abscess, mycotic aneurysm, aortoventricular dehiscence, cardiac decompensation	60.7	drainage of 1 L pleural effusion at both sides, 0 RBC	Recovery > 5 years post surgery –	–	–	–

patient number, *AML* anterior mitral leaflet, *AV* aortic valve, *AV block* atrio-ventricular block, *bio* biological prosthetic valve inplanted, *CABG* coronary artery bypass grafting, *EuroSCORE* logarithimic I, *F* female, *LVOT* left ventricular outflow tract, *M* male, *mech* mechanical prosthetic valve inplanted, *mo* months, *MV* mitral valve, *PPM* placement of permanent pacemaker, *RBC* number of bags with red blood cells given during surgery, *re-IE* recurrence of endocarditis, *rethoracotomy* for bleeding or tamponade, *TVP* tricuspid valve plasty, *yr.* years

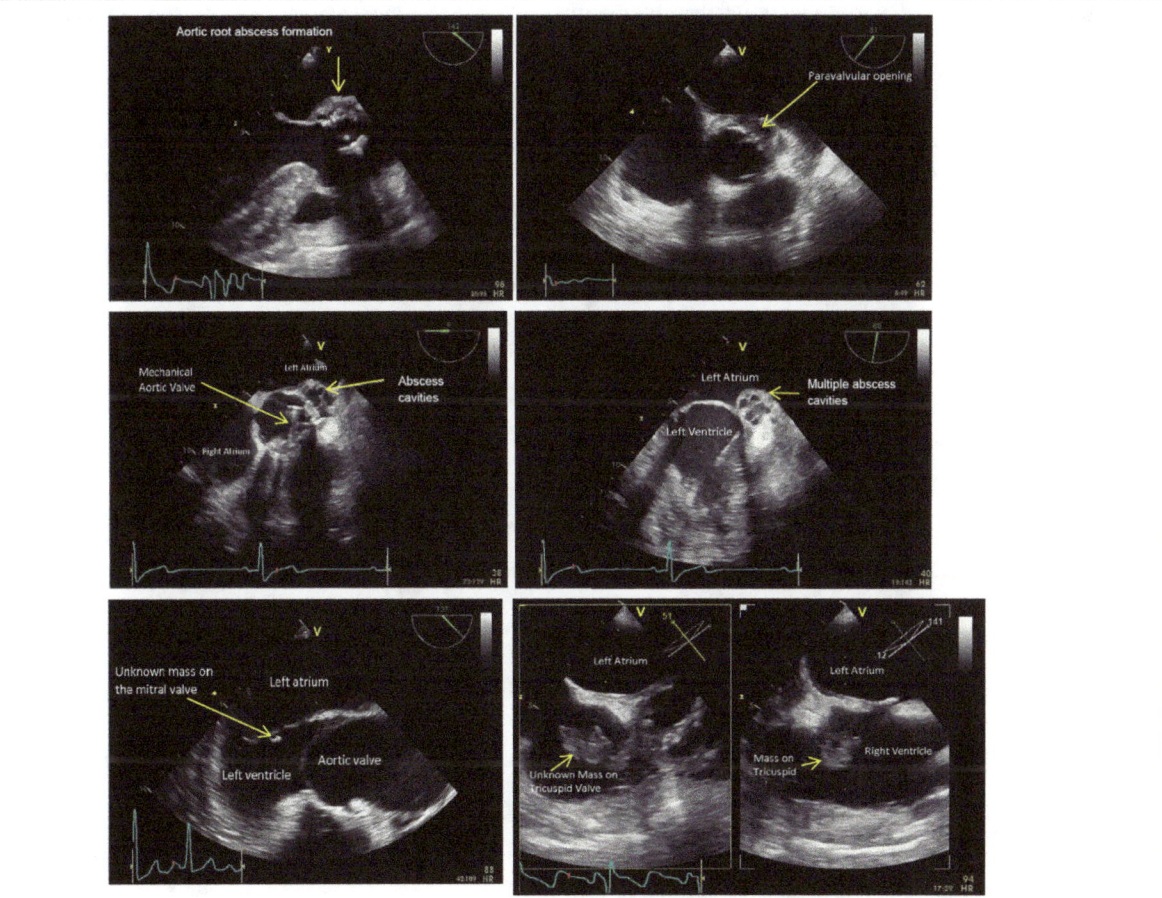

Fig. 3 Aortic valve endocarditis with paravalvular abscess formation, transesophageal echocardiographic view

performed. Of the patients with prosthetic valves, 2 patients had early (3–4 months after surgery) and 10 patients late endocarditis (1–29 years after surgery). In-hospital and 30 day mortality were 18.8% and 12.5%, respectively; 2-year recurrence rate was 14%.

Infectious cardiac anatomical compliations eligible for stentless bioprostheses repair

Several situations of active aortic valve endocarditis with paravalvular abscess formation and accompanying pathologies were deemed eligible for valve repair and LVOT reconstruction with a stentless bioprosthesis (Figs. 2, 3, 4 and 5).

Aortoventricular dehiscence

Seven patients with a prosthetic valve presented with aortoventricular dehiscence. Pathogens included coagulase-negative staphylococci, *Staphylococcus aureus*, *Streptococcus* bovis, *Enterococcus faecalis*. 29% (2/7) of these patients also had extention of infection towards their mitral valve.

Septum derangements

Seven patients presented with infectious derangements of their septum, including vegetations and perforations. Four of these patients had a prosthetic valve. Pathogens included *Staphylococcus epidermidis*, *Staphylococcus aureus*, *Streptococcus agalactiae*, *Streptococcus mitis*, and *Enterococcus faecalis*. 71% (5/7) of these patients had a permanent pacemaker (PPM) implanted and 43%

(3/7) had extention of infection towards the right side of the heart through a Gerbode(–like) defect.

Total atrioventricular conduction block

Six patients presented with a total or third degree atrioventricular conduction block. Five of these patients had a prosthetic valve. Pathogens included *Staphylococcus epidermidis*, *Streptococcus sanguinis*, *Streptococcus agalactiae*, and *Streptococcus mitis*. All these patients had a PPM implanted, 50% had extention of infection towards their right ventricle through a Gerbode(–like) defect, and 50% had extention of infection towards their mitral valve.

Gerbode defect (with tricuspid valve involvement)

Three patients presented with a Gerbode(–like) defect, a left ventricular (aorta) to right atrial shunt [20], causing an infection of their tricuspid valve due to local spread. Two of these patients had a prosthetic valve. Pathogens included *Staphylococcus epidermidis*, *Streptococcus agalactiae* and *Streptococcus mitis*. All patients had a PPM implanted, and needed a tricuspid valve plasty.

Mitral valve involvement (with aortomitral dehiscence)

Seven patients presented with extension of infection towards their mitral valve. Five of these patients had a prosthetic valve. Pathogens included *Staphylococcus epidermidis*, *Streptococcus sanguinis*, *Streptococcus mutans*, and *Enterococcus faecalis*. 57% (4/7) of these patients had septic emboli.

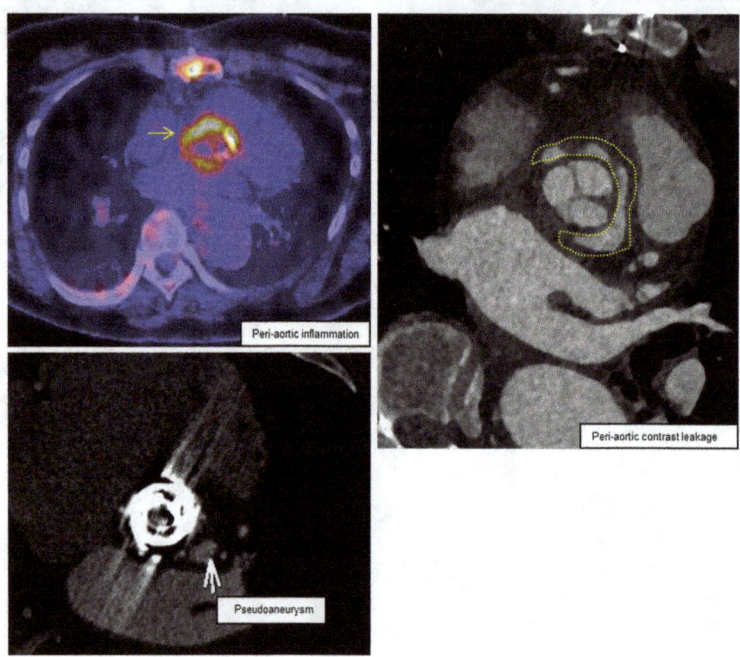

Fig. 4 Aortic valve endocarditis with paravalvular abscess formation, nuclear/radiological view with ^{18}F-fluorodeoxyglucose positron emission tomography/computed tomography

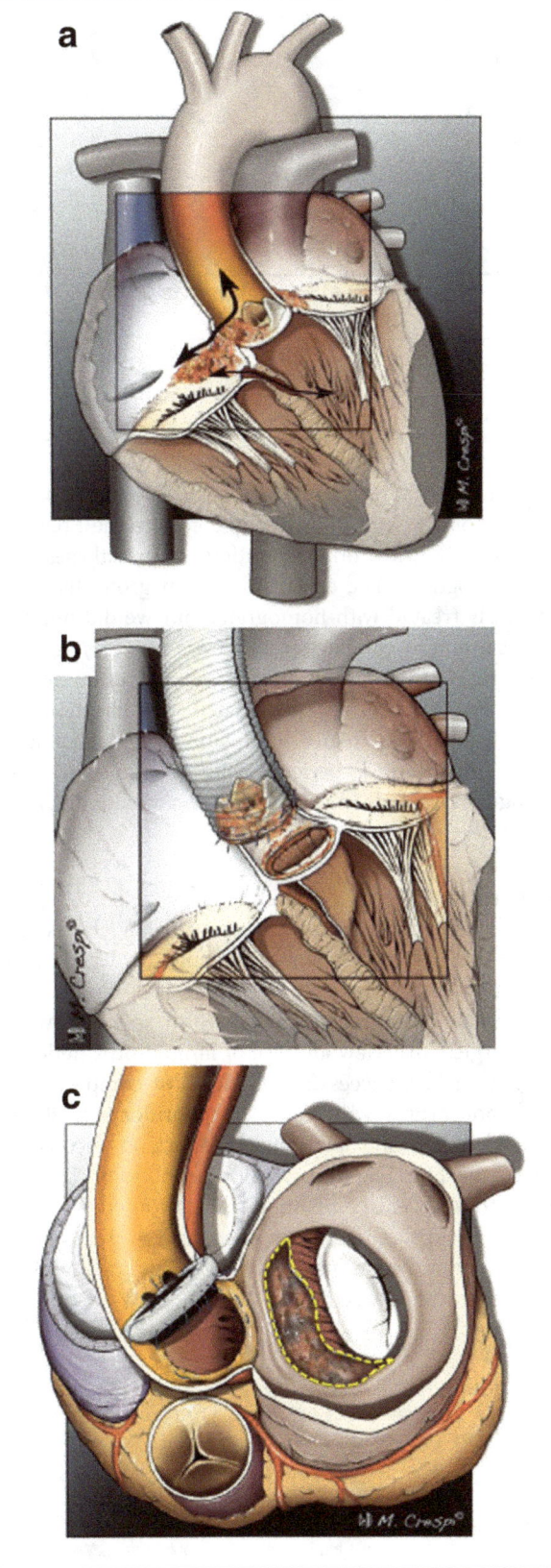

Fig. 5 Aortic valve endocarditis with paravalvular abscess formation, illustrations: **a** coronal view on the heart showing a ventricular septum defect, Gerbode defect (communication between the left ventricle and the right atrium), Gerbode-like defect (communication between the aorta and the right atrium) and tricuspid valve deformity; **b** coronal view on the proximal heart showing total aorto-ventricular dehiscence; **c** horizontal view on the proximal heart showing a retro-aortal abscess cavity with aorto-mitral involvement and mitral annulus dehiscence

Extracardiac complications due to endocarditis

Infective endocarditis is a cardiac disease with extracardiac complications due to hematogenous and embolic spread. In our series, the three most common complications were: mycotic aneurysm ($n = 3$), cerebral emboli ($n = 2$), and vertebral osteomyelitis ($n = 2$).

Patient survival

Figure 6 shows the survival of included patients for 11 years. Five patients died during this period (Table 2), due to: end-stage heart failure 227 days post-surgery; recurrent respiratory insufficiency resulting from sputum retention, encephalopathy and extended postoperative wound infection 40 days post-surgery; active intra-cerebral bleeding without therapeutic options 14 days post-surgery; re-infection of the prosthesis with cerebral embolization, mediastinitis and kidney failure 388 days post-surgery; severe hemodynamic instability immediately post-surgery.

Discussion

We have described and illustrated a series of patients with aortic valve endocarditis, paravalvular abscess formation and accompanying pathologies. All patients underwent cardiothoracic surgery with thorough debridement and restoration of cardiac anatomy using stentless bioprostheses. Patients with native and several types of prosthetic valves were included. Pathogens varied, including staphylococci ($n = 7$), streptococci ($n = 5$) and enterococci ($n = 3$). Predicted mortality was high (median logarithmic EuroSCORE I of 40.7 [range 12.8–68.3]) but actual mortality was relatively low (in-hospital 18.8% [3/16] and 30-day 12.5% [2/16]), showing that the stentless bioprostheses can be successfully used in a variety of surgically challenging situations and allows for a standardized approach. Figures 2, 3 and 4 show the cases of aortic valve endocarditis with various paravalvular abscesses from a surgical (Fig. 2), echocardiographic (Fig. 3) and nuclear/radiological (Fig. 4) view.

Due to its design, it is possible to use the stentless bioprostheses for subcoronary valve replacement, for inclusion of the root, or full root replacement [13, 16]. Using the prostheses for a full root replacement, enables exclusion of abscess cavities and the rebuilding of the LVOT. Furthermore, it maintains root geometry and the integrity of the "leaflet, sinus and root" as a functional entity, both

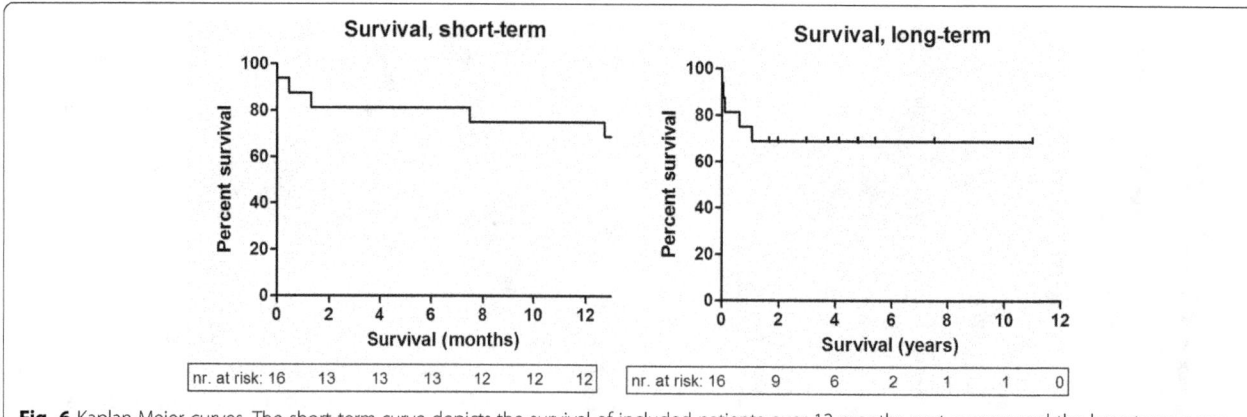

Fig. 6 Kaplan-Meier curves. The short-term curve depicts the survival of included patients over 12 months post surgery and the long-term curve depicts the survival of included patients during the total follow-up time (maximum 11 years)

increasing durability of the bioprostheses [8, 21]. Implantation with the single suture technique is believed to allow placement of the stentless bioprosthesis as full root replacement without narrowing of the LVOT nor obstruction by any rigid structures such as pledgets [21]. Using the stentless bioprothesis as a full root replacement in complex endocarditis was previously reported in 5 patients [22] and now supported with our data of 16 patients with various well described paravalvular abscesses.

Survival rates for the use of stentless bioprostheses when active native or prosthetic aortic valve endocarditis is complicated by extensive destruction of the LVOT have been reported as 81–89%, 76–83%, 62–70%, and 54% at 30 days, 1 year, 5 years, and 10 years, respectively [8, 13, 14, 16, 17]. Although early mortality remains considerably high in the group presented, studies show that stentless bioprostheses yield clinical outcomes, postoperative echocardiographic data, long-term recurrence and survival rates comparable to those of cryopreserved homografts [8, 9, 13, 14, 16, 17]. Indeed, the recurrence rates of homografts (3.8–6.8%) and stentless valves (3.7–8.6%) are similar and lower than that of standard prostheses (33%) [13]. However, as compared with standard aortic valve replacement, the need for re-implantation of coronary arteries conveys an increased risk of atrioventricular conduction block. Also, the use of bioprosthesis conveys an increased risk of reoperation in juvenile patients. Even though stentless and stented valves show equal performance with regard to clinical parameters and valve-related mortality, stentless valves have more favorable hemodynamic and biomechanical characteristics and significantly higher long-term survival rates (78% versus 66% in 8-years) [8, 14, 16]. Compared to homografts, progression of valve dysfunction (37% versus 86%, $p < 0.01$) [23] and need for reoperations are lower for stentless bioprostheses [14, 18, 23]. Furthermore, implantation is less challenging and demanding for stentless bioprostheses and reoperation of a calcified prosthesis may be easier as compared to homografts [9].

A limitation of this study is its retrospective nature. Furthermore, we did not directly compare the Freestyle® bioprosthesis with other stentless bioprostheses, nor with homografts. The described patient group had been previously treated with homografts, but we did not consider it useful to compare results from 10 years ago with recent results. Prospective studies should examine durability and long-term valve-related complication free survival of patients treated with various models of stentless bioprostheses. Experience with reoperation for replacing a bioroot also needs further examination [21].

Conclusion

Aortic valve endocarditis with paravalvular abscess formation remains a therapeutic challenge for which stentless bioprosthesis is a credible surgical option. This prosthesis allows a radical and uniform approach with a good surgical overview and use of limited prosthetic material. It enables successful treatment of complex aortic valve endocarditis with complete debridement, elimination of shunts and anatomical deviations, reconstruction of the LVOT and aortomitral continuity. Stentless bioprostheses yield comparable clinical outcomes as the historical gold standard – the homograft – and are readily available. Of note, use of one type of prosthesis reduces logistical issues and purchasing costs.

Abbreviations
AML: Anterior mitral leaflet; LVOT: Left ventricular outflow tract; PPM: Permanent pacemaker

Acknowledgements
We thank Jakob Wilkens for the high-quality macroscopic pictures. We thank Andor Glaudemans and Niek Prakken for the FDG-PET and CTA images. We thank Massimiliano Crespi for the illustrations of intracardiac pathology. We thank Igor van der Weide for the total number of aortic valve endocarditis surgeries in our center. We thank Sebastian-Patrick Sommer for valuable discussions.

Funding

This work was supported by INTERREG project EurHealth-1Health [grant number 202085]; http://www.eurhealth-1health.eu/nl/home/. INTERREG had not intellectual role.

Authors' contributions

AG composed the report. JJ, SVA, PPVG, BS, SG, DMJ, EN supervised the report. All authors wrote, edited, and reviewed the manuscript. All authors read and approved the final manuscript.

Competing interests

The authors declare that they have no competing interests.

Author details

[1]Department of Medical Microbiology, University of Groningen, University Medical Center Groningen, Groningen, Netherlands. [2]Department of Anesthesiology, University of Groningen, University Medical Center Groningen, Groningen, Netherlands. [3]Department of Internal Medicine, Infectious Diseases, Treant Care Group, Hoogeveen, Netherlands. [4]Department of Cardiology, University of Groningen, University Medical Center Groningen, Groningen, Netherlands. [5]Department of Thoracic Surgery, Maastricht University Medical Center, Maastricht, Netherlands. [6]Department of Cardio-Thoracic Surgery, University of Groningen, University Medical Center Groningen, Groningen, Netherlands.

References

1. Murdoch DR, Corey GR, Hoen B, Miro JM, Fowler VG, Jr BAS, et al. Clinical presentation, etiology, and outcome of infective endocarditis in the 21st century: the international collaboration on endocarditis-prospective cohort study. Arch Intern Med. 2009;169(5):463–73.
2. Habib G, Lancellotti P, Antunes MJ, Bongiorni MG, Casalta JP, Del Zotti F, et al. 2015 ESC guidelines for the management of infective endocarditis: the task force for the management of infective endocarditis of the European Society of Cardiology (ESC). Endorsed by: European Association for Cardio-Thoracic Surgery (EACTS), the European Association of Nuclear Medicine (EANM). Eur Heart J. 2015;36(44):3075–128.
3. Moreillon P, Que YA. Infective endocarditis. Lancet. 2004;363(9403):139–49.
4. Li JS, Sexton DJ, Mick N, Nettles R, Fowler VG, Jr RT, et al. Proposed modifications to the Duke criteria for the diagnosis of infective endocarditis. Clin Infect Dis. 2000;30(4):633–8.
5. Prendergast BD, Tornos P. Surgery for infective endocarditis: who and when? Circulation. 2010;121(9):1141–52.
6. Vikram HR, Buenconsejo J, Hasbun R, Quagliarello VJ. Impact of valve surgery on 6-month mortality in adults with complicated, left-sided native valve endocarditis: a propensity analysis. JAMA. 2003;290(24):3207–14.
7. Kang DH, Kim YJ, Kim SH, Sun BJ, Kim DH, Yun SC, et al. Early surgery versus conventional treatment for infective endocarditis. N Engl J Med. 2012; 366(26):2466–73.
8. Schneider AW, Hazekamp MG, Versteegh MI, Bruggemans EF, Holman ER, Klautz RJ, et al. Stentless bioprostheses: a versatile and durable solution in extensive aortic valve endocarditis. Eur J Cardiothorac Surg. 2016;49(6): 1699–704.
9. Sponga S, Daffarra C, Pavoni D, Vendramin I, Mazzaro E, Piani D, et al. Surgical management of destructive aortic endocarditis: left ventricular outflow reconstruction with the Sorin Pericarbon freedom stentless bioprosthesis dagger. Eur J Cardiothorac Surg. 2016;49(1):242–8.
10. Byrne JG, Rezai K, Sanchez JA, Bernstein RA, Okum E, Leacche M, et al. Surgical management of endocarditis: the society of thoracic surgeons clinical practice guideline. Ann Thorac Surg. 2011;91(6):2012–9.
11. Bonow RO, Carabello BA, Chatterjee K, de Leon AC Jr, Faxon DP, Freed MD, et al. 2008 focused update incorporated into the ACC/AHA 2006 guidelines for the management of patients with valvular heart disease: a report of the American College of Cardiology/American Heart Association task force on practice guidelines (writing committee to revise the 1998 guidelines for the management of patients with valvular heart disease). Endorsed by the Society of Cardiovascular Anesthesiologists, Society for Cardiovascular Angiography and Interventions, and Society of Thoracic Surgeons. J Am Coll Cardiol. 2008;52(13):e1–142.
12. Sabik JF, Lytle BW, Blackstone EH, Marullo AG, Pettersson GB, Cosgrove DM. Aortic root replacement with cryopreserved allograft for prosthetic valve endocarditis. Ann Thorac Surg. 2002;74(3):650–9.
13. Perrotta S, Lentini S. In patients with severe active aortic valve endocarditis, is a stentless valve as good as the homograft? Interact Cardiovasc Thorac Surg. 2010;11(3):309–13.
14. Heinz A, Dumfarth J, Ruttmann-Ulmer E, Grimm M, Muller LC. Freestyle root replacement for complex destructive aortic valve endocarditis. J Thorac Cardiovasc Surg. 2014;147(4):1265–70.
15. Savage EB, Saha-Chaudhuri P, Asher CR, Brennan JM, Gammie JS. Outcomes and prosthesis choice for active aortic valve infective endocarditis: analysis of the Society of Thoracic Surgeons adult cardiac surgery database. Ann Thorac Surg. 2014;98(3):806–14.
16. Miceli A, Croccia M, Simeoni S, Varone E, Murzi M, Farneti PA, et al. Root replacement with stentless freestyle bioprostheses for active endocarditis: a single Centre experience. Interact Cardiovasc Thorac Surg. 2013;16(1):27–30.
17. Edlin P, Sartipy U. Freestyle xenograft for aortic valve endocarditis. J Thorac Cardiovasc Surg. 2014;147(1):542–3.
18. El-Hamamsy I, Clark L, Stevens LM, Sarang Z, Melina G, Takkenberg JJ, et al. Late outcomes following freestyle versus homograft aortic root replacement: results from a prospective randomized trial. J Am Coll Cardiol. 2010;55(4):368–76.
19. Nishimura RA, Otto CM, Bonow RO, Carabello BA, Erwin JP 3rd, Guyton RA, et al. 2014 AHA/ACC guideline for the management of patients with valvular heart disease: a report of the American College of Cardiology/ American Heart Association task force on practice guidelines. J Am Coll Cardiol. 2014;63(22):e57–185.
20. Davies A, Lai K, Bastian B. Acquired Gerbode defects associated with infective endocarditis. Heart Lung Circ. 2016;25(3):e59–61.
21. Dapunt OE, Easo J, Holzl PP, Murin P, Sudkamp M, Horst M, et al. Stentless full root bioprosthesis in surgery for complex aortic valve-ascending aortic disease: a single center experience of over 300 patients. Eur J Cardiothorac Surg. 2008;33(4):554–9.
22. Bozbuga N, Erentug V, Erdogan HB, Kirali K, Ardal H, Tas S, et al. Surgical treatment of aortic abscess and fistula. Tex Heart Inst J. 2004;31(4):382–6.
23. Borger MA, Prasongsukarn K, Armstrong S, Feindel CM, David TE. Stentless aortic valve reoperations: a surgical challenge. Ann Thorac Surg. 2007;84(3): 737–44.

8

Refractory ventricular fibrillations after surgical repair of atrial septal defects in a patient with CACNA1C gene mutation

Ai Kojima[1], Fumiaki Shikata[1,2]* ⓘ, Toru Okamura[1], Takashi Higaki[3], Seiko Ohno[4], Minoru Horie[4], Shunji Uchita[1], Yujiro Kawanishi[1,2], Kenji Namiguchi[1], Takumi Yasugi[1] and Hironori Izutani[1]

Abstract

Background: Congenital long QT syndrome (LQTS) can cause ventricular arrhythmic events with syncope and sudden death resulting from malignant torsades de pointes (TdP) followed by ventricular fibrillations (VFs). However, the syndrome is often overlooked prior to the development of arrhythmic events in patients with congenital heart diseases demonstrating right bundle branch block on electrocardiogram (ECG). We present a case of an adult patient with congenital heart disease who developed VFs postoperatively, potentially due to his mutation in a LQTS related gene, which was not identified on preoperative assessment due to incomplete evaluation of his family history.

Case presentation: A 64-year-old man was diagnosed as having multiple atrial septal defects. He presented with no symptoms of heart failure. His preoperative ECG showed complete right bundle branch block (CRBBB) with a corrected QT interval time of 478 ms. He underwent open-heart surgery to close the defects through median sternotomy access. Three hours after the operation, he developed multiple events of TdP and VFs in the intensive care unit. Cardiopulmonary resuscitation and multiple cardioversions were attempted for his repetitive TdP and VFs. He eventually reverted to sinus rhythm, and intravenous beta-blocker was administered to maintain the sinus rhythm. After this event, his family history was reviewed, and it was confirmed that his daughter and grandson had a medical history of arrhythmia. A genetic test confirmed that he had a missense mutation in CACNA1C, p.K1580 T, which is the cause for type 8.

Conclusions: This case highlights the importance of paying attention to other ECG findings in patients with CRBBB, which can mask prolonged QT intervals.

Keywords: Congenital long QT syndrome, Ventricular fibrillation, Adult congenital heart diseases, Atrial septal defect

Background

Congenital long QT syndrome (LQTS) causes arrhythmic events such as syncope and sudden death due to malignant torsades de pointes (TdP) followed by ventricular fibrillations (VFs). However, in the absence of arrhythmic events, the syndrome can be overlooked, especially in patients with congenital heart diseases, that demonstrate right bundle branch block (RBBB) on electrocardiograms (ECGs) [1, 2]. In addition, QT intervals in ECGs are known to increase for 2 days after open heart surgeries using cardiopulmonary bypasses as a result of electrolyte imbalance and QT prolonging medications. The prolongation of QT interval can trigger arrhythmic events after operations in patients with genetic disorders, such as long QT-related gene mutations or polymorphisms [1, 3]. If the diagnosis of the syndrome is made before open heart surgery, clinicians can avoid factors contributing to the prolongation of QT intervals and, as a result, may be able to prevent ventricular arrhythmias postoperatively [4]. We present an adult patient with congenital heart disease who developed VFs postoperatively,

---

* Correspondence: fumishikata@outlook.com
[1]Department of Cardiovascular Surgery, Ehime University, Shitsukawa, Toon, Ehime 7910295, Japan
[2]Department of Cardiothoracic Surgery, St Vincent's Hospital, Sydney, NSW, Australia
Full list of author information is available at the end of the article

possibly due to his mutation in a LQTS-related gene, which were not identified preoperatively due to incomplete assessment of his family history.

Case presentation

A 64-year-old man with a diagnosis of atrial septal defect (ASD) presented ECG features of incomplete or complete right bundle branch block (CRBBB) during a regular medical check-up. He was asymptomatic, and he had no other significant past medical history. He was referred to our hospital to assess the possibility of catheter device occlusion for ASD, and surgical correction was indicated due to multiple defects and the size of the defects. A chest radiograph showed enlargement of the pulmonary vasculature, indicating pulmonary high flow. An ECG showed CRBBB, and the corrected QT interval (Bazett formula) was 478 ms (Fig. 1). Echocardiography showed preserved left ventricular function, and enlarged right atrium and right ventricle with trivial tricuspid regurgitation and multiple secundum ASDs. The patient was not taking any medications known to prolong the QT interval, and his laboratory data indicated no significant electrolyte disorders. We were informed that he had a child receiving drug treatment for arrhythmia; however, we did not think that this was clinically relevant before the surgery as further information was not provided.

During the operation, anesthetic drugs were used as follows: sevoflurane, remifentanil, dexmedetomidine, propofol, fentanil and rocuronium were administered. Cefazolin was given for the prevention of surgical site infection. After the median sternotomy, an aortic cannula was placed in the ascending aorta, and venous cannulas were inserted into the superior vena cava and the inferior vena cava to establish the cardiopulmonary bypass (CPB). Once the aorta was cross-clamped, cold blood cardioplegic solution was infused through the

cannula in the ascending aorta. The body temperature was cooled down to 33.8° Celsius. Under conditions of cardiac arrest, the right atrium was cut horizontally and opened. Then, three large ASDs were identified at the secundum with thin rims around the holes. The ASDs were closed directly with continuous 4–0 Prolene. After the de-airing, the aorta was de-clamped. The cross-clamp time was 38 min. The patient developed VF. The direct current (DC) cardioversion was successful to convert to sinus rhythm with one attempt of 10 J. The CPB was weaned uneventfully, and its running time was 76 min. The chest was closed using standard techniques, and the patient was sent to the intensive care unit (ICU) with tracheal intubation. In the ICU, dopamine at 4 mcg/kg/min and noradrenaline at 0.05 mcg/kg/min were administered for cardiac support. Propofol and dexmedetomidine were given at the adequate level for sedation. Bipolar temporary pacing wire was placed on the right atrium, and the setting of pacemaker was AAI pacing mode with HR 88 bpm, the sensitivity threshold of 3 mV and the output of 10 mA. The serum level of potassium was 3.8 mEq/l (normal serum potassium value: 3.8–4.8 mmol/l), and that of magnesium was not measured 2 h after the surgery as we do not routinely measure it after low risk operations and the patient was stable. Three hours after the operation, he suddenly presented R on T followed by TdP and Vfs (Fig. 2a). Chest compressions were initiated, and DC cardioversion was attempted. Sinus rhythm was achieved following cardioversion; however, the patient presented repetitive VF (14 times) (Fig. 2b).

Intravenous amiodarone and lidocaine were not effective in managing the arrhythmic storm. After the administration of magnesium and nifecalant, the patient finally recovered to sinus rhythm. Echocardiography revealed normal left ventricular wall motion, which indicated no heart ischemia. After the event, he underwent 24 h of hypothermic treatment to prevent brain damage, and,

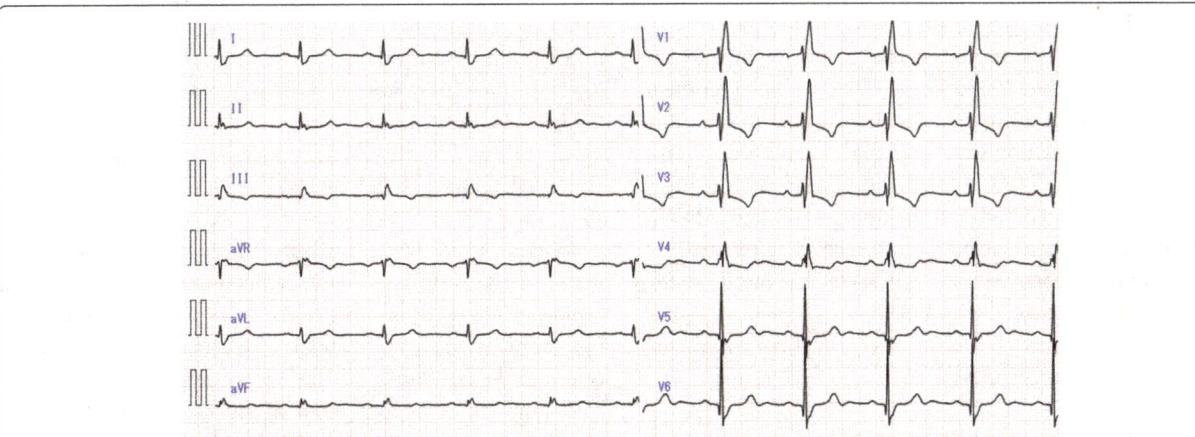

Fig. 1 The preoperative electrocardiogram. The preoperative electrocardiogram showed complete right bundle branch block, and the corrected QT interval time was 478 ms

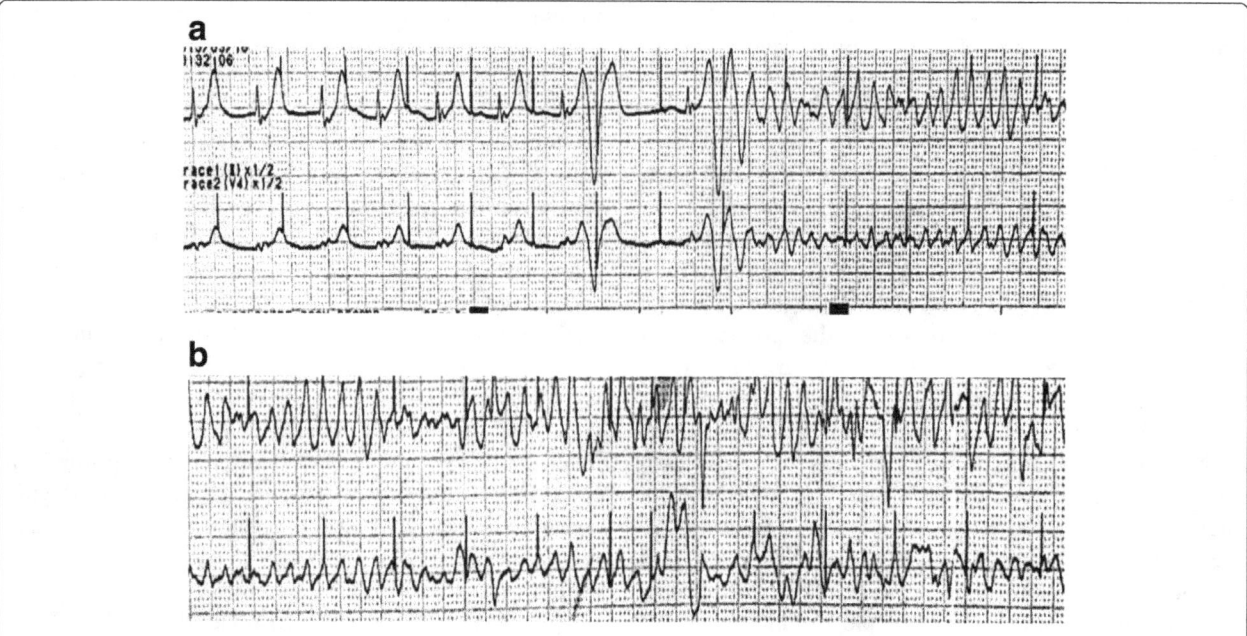

Fig. 2 Refractory ventricular fibrillations after the atrial septal defect repair. **a** Three hours after the surgical correction of multiple atrial septal defects, the patient suddenly presented R on T followed by Torsades de Pointes in the intensive care unit, and eventually, the electrocardiogram shifted to a ventricular fibrillation pattern. **b** The patient presented with repetitive ventricular fibrillations even after he reverted to sinus rhythm with direct current cardioversions

fortunately, there remained no evidence of brain damage on computed tomography. Landiolol had been administered intravenously to maintain sinus rhythm until the patient was able to take bisoprolol tablets orally. Given that his VFs were refractory and the patient had no coronary artery disease and relevant valve disease, we supposed that he might have been a carrier of familial arrhythmic disorders causing repetitive VFs. Therefore, we reviewed his family history and found that his daughter and grandson had congenital LQTS diagnosed at other hospitals, and his grandson was being treated with a beta blocker for this disease.

After obtaining informed consent from the patient, genetic screening for LQTS related genes was conducted to confirm the diagnosis. In the genetic analysis, a CACNA1c missense mutation, c. 4739a > c, p.K1580 T, was identified. CACNA1C is a causative gene for LQTS type 8 (Fig. 3(a)-(c)) [5–7]. The mutation was novel and not reported in the cohort databases; ExAC (http://exac.broadinstitute.org/), gnomAD (http://gnomad.broadinstitute.org/) and HGVD (http://www.hgvd.genome.med.kyoto-u.ac.jp/index.html?). We could not perform genetic analysis for the family members who were diagnosed with LQTS.

He was discharged 2 weeks after the operation with the prescription of bisoprolol.

Discussion

Congenital LQTS is a disease resulting from impaired expression or dysfunctions of cardiac ion channels as a result of their encoding gene variants. It can cause the prolongation of QT intervals and, as a consequence, result in life threatening events such as VFs. Itoh et al. reported that 28% of acquired LQTS patients were actually "congenital" [8]. Moreover, only 60% of patients show symptoms prior to the diagnosis of congenital LQTS [9]. Given that our patient was asymptomatic until the operation, it is presumable that stimulating factors related to perioperative and postoperative procedures or the use of medicines strongly contributed to the event of postoperative TdP followed by VFs. The factors associated with fatal arrhythmias for acquired LQTS are medicines including anesthetic agents, inotropes, hypokalemia, bradycardia, emotional stress, hypothermia and the combinations of these factors [8, 10]. If we had known that the patient had a genetic background of CACNA1C mutations, some of which were reported as cardiac-only Timothy syndrome, we could have avoided potential factors that triggered malignant TdP and VFs [5–7, 10]. In order to prevent malignant arrhythmias postoperatively, some authors have recommended the use of appropriate premedications, avoidance of hypothermia, proper anesthetic agents, adequate pain relief, continuous use of beta blockers during and after operations, avoidance of the excess use of diuretics, and maintenance of proper level of electrolytes such as calcium and magnesium [3, 4, 10, 11]. In our case, sevoflurane, propofol, dopamine and dexmedetomidine were used for anesthesia and postoperative care, and these

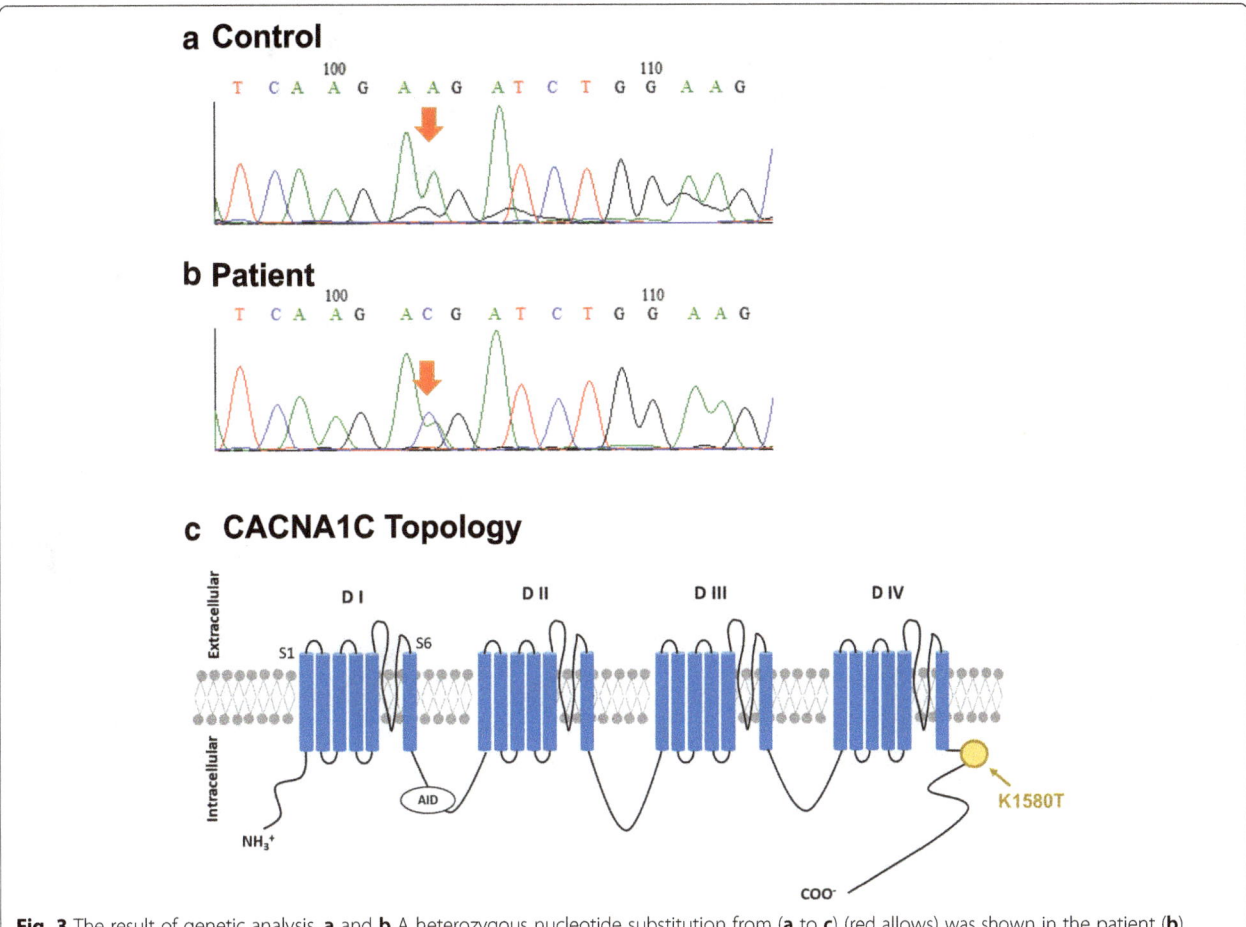

Fig. 3 The result of genetic analysis. **a** and **b** A heterozygous nucleotide substitution from (**a** to **c**) (red allows) was shown in the patient (**b**) compared to control (**a**). **c** The topology of K1580 T mutation in CACNA1C gene

were categorized as possible cause of arrhythmic events or should be avoided in CredibleMeds (https://www.crediblemeds.org/). If the diagnosis was made preoperatively, these possible unsafe drugs could not have been used and, as a result, the patient could not have experienced the refractory VFs in the ICU.

The congenital LQTS is often overlooked and difficult to recognize before the occurrence of arrhythmic events, especially in patients with congenital heart diseases, as in our case. However, preoperative diagnosis of this syndrome is essential as it may help physicians to avoid arrhythmic factors [1, 2, 12]. Diagnostic difficulty is due to the fact that patients with LQTS and ASDs occasionally show a RBBB preoperatively or after surgical correction of tetralogy of Fallot, and this ECG abnormality can mask the prolonged QT time [1]. It has also been reported that QT interval is prolonged after surgical correction of ASD in 42% of patients due to increased coronary flow after the correction [13]. Thus, physicians should carefully evaluate patients' family medical history, especially when they present RBBB and a strong family history of arrhythmias. It is important to note that

Schwartz and Moss score can help medical practitioners to diagnose the LQTS, even in the absence of genetic screening for LQTS [14, 15].

Conclusions

This case highlights the importance of taking a thorough family history in patients due to undergo open heart surgeries. Furthermore, we should pay attention to other ECG findings in patients with CRBBB, which can mask prolonged QT intervals. If preoperative diagnosis of the LQTS is made, we may be able to avoid factors triggering ventricular arrhythmias and prevent arrhythmic events after open heart surgeries.

Abbreviations
ASD: Atrial septal defect; CPB: Cardiopulmonary bypass; CRBBB: Complete right bundle branch block; DC: Direct current; ECG: Electrocardiogram; RBBB: Right bundle branch block; TdP: Torsades de Pointes; Vf: Ventricular fibrillation

Acknowledgements
none.

Funding
none.

Authors' contributions
AI, FS, TO, TH and SU carried out the operation and postoperative care of the patient. NK and TS gathered figures and data to prepare for this manuscript. SO and MH conducted the gene analysis of this case and revised the manuscript. YK, TY and HI supervised and corrected the manuscript. All authors have read and approved the final manuscript.

Competing interests
The authors declare that they have no competing interests.

Author details
[1]Department of Cardiovascular Surgery, Ehime University, Shitsukawa, Toon, Ehime 7910295, Japan. [2]Department of Cardiothoracic Surgery, St Vincent's Hospital, Sydney, NSW, Australia. [3]Department of Pediatric Cardiology, Children's Medical Center, Ehime University, Ehime, Japan. [4]Department of Cardiovascular and Respiratory Medicine, Shiga University of Medical Science, Shiga, Japan.

References
1. Chiu SN, Wu MH, Su MJ, Wang JK, Lin MT, Chang CC, et al. Coexisting mutations/polymorphisms of the long qt syndrome genes in patients with repaired tetralogy of fallot are associated with the risks of life-threatening events. Hum Genet. 2012;131:1295–304.
2. Walls J, Sanatani S, Hamilton R. Post-hoc diagnosis of congenital long qt syndrome in patients with tetralogy of fallot. Pediatr Cardiol. 2005;26:107–10.
3. Krasner BS, Girdwood R, Smith H. The effect of slow releasing oral magnesium chloride on the qtc interval of the electrocardiogram during open heart surgery. Can Anaesth Soc J. 1981;28:329–33.
4. Kim SJ, Pundi KN, Bos JM, Ackerman MJ. Ventricular fibrillation after elective surgery in an adolescent with long qt syndrome. BMJ Case Reports. 2015. doi:10.1136/bcr-2015-212365.
5. Fukuyama M, Wang Q, Kato K, Ohno S, Ding WG, Toyoda F, et al. Long qt syndrome type 8: novel cacna1c mutations causing qt prolongation and variant phenotypes. Europace. 2014;16:1828–37.
6. Boczek NJ, Best JM, Tester DJ, Giudicessi JR, Middha S, Evans JM, et al. Exome sequencing and systems biology converge to identify novel mutations in the l-type calcium channel, cacna1c, linked to autosomal dominant long qt syndrome. Circ Cardiovasc Genet. 2013;6:279–89.
7. Boczek NJ, Ye D, Jin F, Tester DJ, Huseby A, Bos JM, et al. Identification and functional characterization of a novel cacna1c-mediated cardiac disorder characterized by prolonged qt intervals with hypertrophic cardiomyopathy, congenital heart defects, and sudden cardiac death. Circ Arrhythm Electrophysiol. 2015;8:1122–32.
8. Itoh H, Crotti L, Aiba T, Spazzolini C, Denjoy I, Fressart V, et al. The genetics underlying acquired long qt syndrome: impact for genetic screening. Eur Heart J. 2016;37:1456–64.
9. Ackerman MJ. The long qt syndrome: ion channel diseases of the heart. Mayo Clin Proc. 1998;73:250–69.
10. Kies SJ, Pabelick CM, Hurley HA, White RD, Ackerman MJ. Anesthesia for patients with congenital long qt syndrome. Anesthesiology. 2005;102:204–10.
11. Nathan AT, Berkowitz DH, Montenegro LM, Nicolson SC, Vetter VL, Jobes DR. Implications of anesthesia in children with long qt syndrome. Anesth Analg. 2011;112:1163–8.
12. Park YM, Kim SJ, Park CH, Kang WC, Shin MS, Koh KK, et al. Repeated aborted sudden cardiac death with long qt syndrome in a patient with anomalous origin of the right coronary artery from the left coronary cusp. Korean Circ J. 2013;43:830–3.
13. Aburawi EH, Souid AK, Liuba P, Zoubeidi T, Pesonen E. Early changes in myocardial repolarization and coronary perfusion after cardiopulmonary bypass surgery for asd repair in children. BMC Cardiovasc Disord. 2013;13:67.
14. Schwartz PJ, Moss AJ, Vincent GM, Crampton RS. Diagnostic criteria for the long qt syndrome. Circulation. 1993;88:782–4.
15. Tester DJ, Will ML, Haglund CM, Ackerman MJ. Effect of clinical phenotype on yield of long qt syndrome genetic testing. J Am Coll Cardiol. 2006;47:764–8.

9

Porcine pulmonary valve decellularization with NaOH-based vs detergent process: preliminary in vitro and in vivo assessments

Mathieu van Steenberghe[1,2]* ⓘ, Thomas Schubert[3,4], Sébastien Gerelli[5], Caroline Bouzin[6], Yves Guiot[7], Daela Xhema[1], Xavier Bollen[8], Karim Abdelhamid[9] and Pierre Gianello[1]

Abstract

Background: Glutaraldehyde fixed xenogeneic heart valve prosthesis are hindered by calcification and lack of growth potential. The aim of tissue decellularization is to remove tissue antigenicity, avoiding the use of glutaraldehyde and improve valve integration with low inflammation and host cell recolonization. In this preliminary study, we investigated the efficacy of a NaOH-based process for decellularization and biocompatibility improvement of porcine pulmonary heart valves in comparison to a detergent-based process (SDS-SDC0, 5%).

Methods: Native cryopreserved porcine pulmonary heart valves were treated with detergent and NaOH-based processes. Decellularization was assessed by Hematoxylin and eosin/DAPI/alpha-gal/SLA-I staining and DNA quantification of native and processed leaflets, walls and muscles.

Elongation stress test investigated mechanical integrity of leaflets and walls ($n = 3$ tests/valve component) of valves in the native and treated groups ($n = 4$/group).

Biochemical integrity (collagen/elastin/glycosaminoglycans content) of leaflet-wall and muscle of the valves (n = 4/group) was assessed and compared between groups with trichrome staining (Sirius Red/Miller/Alcian blue).

Secondly, a preliminary in vivo study assessed biocompatibility (CD3 and CD68 immunostaining) and remodeling (Hematoxylin and eosin/CD31 and ASMA immunofluorescent staining) of NaOH processed valves implanted in orthotopic position in young Landrace pigs, at 1 ($n = 1$) and 3 months ($n = 2$).

Results: Decellularization was better achieved with the NaOH-based process (92% vs 69% DNA reduction in the wall). Both treatments did not significantly alter mechanical properties. The detergent-based process induced a significant loss of glycosaminoglycans ($p < 0,05$).

In vivo, explanted valves exhibited normal morphology without any sign of graft dilatation, degeneration or rejection. Low inflammation was noticed at one and three months follow-up (1,8 +/− 3,03 and 0,9836 +/− 1,3605 CD3 cells/0,12 mm^2 in the leaflets). In one animal, at three months we documented minimal calcification in the area of sinus leaflet and in one, microthrombi formation on the leaflet surface at 1 month. The endoluminal side of the valves showed partial reendothelialization.

(Continued on next page)

* Correspondence: mathieu.vansteenberghe@uclouvain.be
[1]Pôle de Chirurgie Expérimentale et Transplantation (CHEX), Institut de Recherche Expérimentale et Clinique (IREC), Secteur des Sciences de la Sante, Université Catholique de Louvain, Avenue Hippocrate 55/B1.55.04, B-1200 Brussels, Belgium
[2]Service de chirurgie cardiaque et vasculaire, Clinique Cecil, avenue Louis Ruchonnet 53, 1003 Lausanne, Switzerland
Full list of author information is available at the end of the article

(Continued from previous page)

Conclusions: NaOH-based process offers better porcine pulmonary valve decellularization than the detergent process. In vivo, the NaOH processed valves showed low inflammatory response at 3 months and partial recellularization. Regarding additional property of securing, this treatment should be considered for the new generation of heart valves prosthesis.

Keywords: Cardiovascular engineering, Heart valve, Xenograft, Decellularization, Biocompatibility, Remodeling

Background

Currently, heart valve prostheses are hindered by several limitations. Mechanical valves have excellent long-term durability but require lifelong anticoagulation therapy due to thromboembolic risks. Bioprostheses do not require anticoagulation but show reduced durability and are more prone to degeneration, particularly in younger patients. This phenomenon has been related to a more reactive immunity, higher calcium and phosphate metabolism and physical activity that play a role in prosthesis calcifications [1]. Bioprosthetic valves are usually treated with glutaraldehyde to prevent immune rejection of the xenogeneic scaffold. But it has been early shown that glutaraldehyde modifies mechanical properties of the native tissue, is cytotoxic, does not remove tissue phospholipids, induces a release of cell debris, and does not completely suppress the immune reaction against the graft. These events lead to chronic inflammation and calcifications [1–5].

Finally, cryopreserved homografts with ideal hemodynamic performance but limited availability also show limited durability because of residual tissue immunogenicity [6–9]. Mechanical and bioprosthetic valves share another disadvantage: they cannot grow and remodel, therefore resulting in subsequent revision surgeries in pediatric patients [10].

Decellularization of biological valves is an alternative. This concept involves removing all cellular components that are supposedly immunogenic and may lead to calcifications while minimizing any adverse effect on the composition, biological activity, and mechanical integrity of the matrix. The resulting extracellular matrix (ECM) can be recellularized by the host and functionally and structurally integrated into the body with growth potential [11].

As of today, new products are already commercially available but short term results with some of those implants, essentially those of xenogeneic source, did not demonstrate convincing results in the pediatric population [12, 13], while others, essentially decellularized homografts from allogeneic source seemed to yield better midterm term results [14, 15].

Despite these progresses, no gold standard decellularization process exists. Various decellularization protocols are proposed in the literature and most popular are those using detergents [16, 17].

We previously demonstrated enhanced biocompatibility and vascular remodeling of allogeneic and xenogeneic pericardium with a treatment based on NaOH decellularization in comparison to the glutaraldehyde fixation and detergent process [18, 19].

This NaOH-based process has the particularity of being inactivator for conventional (virus/bacteria) and non-conventional (prion) pathogens and therefore improves the security of those grafts [20–22].

We investigated this treatment as a decellularization process to improve biocompatibility and remodeling of xenogeneic pulmonary heart valves for tissue engineering applications.

In vitro experiments assessed decellularization, antigen removal, mechanical and biochemical integrity of porcine pulmonary heart valves treated with the NaOH-based process (decellularized porcine pulmonary heart valves with NaOH based-process: DPV) as well as porcine pulmonary heart valves treated with a conventional detergent process (decellularized porcine pulmonary heart valves with detergent-based process: DDPV) and native porcine pulmonary heart valves (NPV). Moreover, an in vivo preliminary study was conducted to assess biocompatibility (inflammation and calcifications) and remodeling (endothelialization and recellularization) at 1 and 3 months follow-up of DPV valve in a growing allogeneic/porcine model.

Methods

Sources of matrices

For in vitro study, porcine Landrace hearts were procured from a local slaughterhouse (Eurovlees, Zele, Belgium).

For in vivo study, porcine hearts were procured at our laboratory, from Landrace pigs weighing 20 kg, used for abdominal surgery course/demonstration. Animals were euthanized, and hearts harvested respecting the standards of animal care. The pulmonary valves were then harvested, rinsed with sterile ringer solution and frozen at − 80 °C.

Matrix preparation

Before processing, valves were thawed and washed in sterile ringer solution.

Two treatment protocols were conducted. The detergent-based process was based on a conventional detergent protocol previously published. Briefly, porcine pulmonary valves were incubated for 48 h in an aqueous solution containing 0.5% sodium deoxycholate (SDC) and 0.5% sodium dodecyl sulfate (SDS) under continuous agitation followed by a 72 h rinsing step in a continuous flow of demineralized water [23, 24].

As previously described, the NaOH-based process consists of a succession of baths of acetone, ethanol, NaOH and Hydrogen Peroxyde. This chemical treatment ensures defatting, prions/viruses and bacterial inactivation [18].

Finally, the valves (Fig. 1a) were frozen at − 80 °C without solution and individually packed.

In vitro characterization

Valves were individually characterized for leaflet, pulmonary trunk (wall) and muscle structure.

For histological assessment, the valves were cut longitudinally to explore wall, leaflet and muscle on the same slide (Fig. 1b). The slices were immediately fixed overnight in 4% formaldehyde and embedded in paraffin. Serial sections (thickness of 5 μm) were mounted on glass and dried for 12 h at 37 °C.

Hematoxylin and eosin and DAPI staining

Decellularization was evaluated first by Hematoxylin and eosin (HE) and 40.6-diamidino-2-phenylindole (DAPI; 1 μg/ml/Abbot Molecular Inc-USA) staining. These two methods reveal the nuclei. Sections from 4 different valves per condition (NPV, DPV, DDPV) were stained and slides were then digitalized using a SCN400 slide scanner (Leica Biosystems, Wetzlar, Germany) at

20× magnification for HE. For DAPI assessment, samples were photographed at high definition under structured illumination using a Zeiss AxioImager-Apotome system.

Antigen removal

The presence of residual antigens such as alphagalactosyltransferase antigen (alpha-gal) and swine leucocyte antigen class 1 (SLA-1: the major histocompatibility complex class1 region of pigs) were investigated by immunohistochemistry. Four valves per condition (NPV, DPV, DDPV) were analyzed. After deparaffinization, endogenous peroxidases were inhibited during a 20-min methanol bath with 3% hydrogen peroxide. Primary antibodies (mouse anti-SLA class Ic (1:200; 16.7. E4.2: IgM) [25]); mouse anti-alpha galactose, M86, Enzo Life Sciences®) were revealed with the corresponding Envision HRP-coupled antibodies (Dako) and Diaminobenzidine staining. After counterstaining with hematoxylin, slides were dehydrated and mounted. Stained slices were then digitalized using a SCN400 slide scanner (Leica Biosystems, Wetzlar, Germany) at 20× magnification.

DNA quantification

DNA was extracted with DNeasy® Blood & Tissue Kit (QIAamp DNA Mini Kit, QIAGEN, Hilden, Germany). Three valves per condition were used and one sample per valve region was processed. Extracted DNA was quantified by Quant-it Picrogreen DNA assay kit (Invitrogen, CA, USA), according to manufacturers'

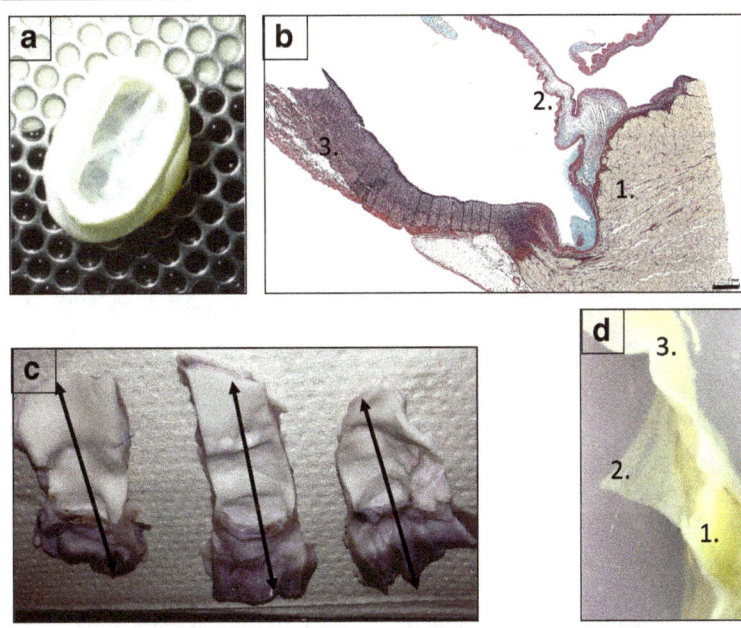

Fig. 1 Valve characterization: methods. **a**: macrophotograph of a DPV. **b**: microphotograph of NPV after trichrome staining illustrating histological assessment of the valves in 3 zones:1: the muscle/2: the leaflet/3: the wall. Scal barr: 1 mm. For histological evaluation, the explanted valves were sectioned in six segments (**c**) to analyze the three zones (**d**)

protocol. Fluorescence was read at 480 nm and 520 nm. Final DNA concentration was expressed in ng/mg dry weight.

Mechanical properties

Uniaxial mechanical resistance tests were performed on a minimum of four valves per condition on the three leaflets and three samples of pulmonary wall per valve. Samples of 15 mm on 15 mm for wall and the whole leaflets were placed between two plastic structure with a central hole of 8,5 mm diameter where a probe comes in contact and applies pressure on the tissue. Mechanical testing was performed, using an Instron traction system with Instron bluehill software (Model 5600, Instron, Canton, MA) with a load-to-failure test set at an elongation rate of 3 mm. min^{-1}. The load to elongation behavior of the matrices and failure modes were recorded. The structural properties of the matrices were represented by stiffness ($Nm.m^{-1}$) and ultimate load (N). Stiffness (k) was calculated as $k = \Delta F/\Delta L$ where, F is the force applied on the body and L is the displacement produced by the force along the same degree of freedom. These parameters were compared between native and treated tissues. Tests were not conducted on muscle.

Biochemical integrity

Longitudinal slices from 4 different valves per condition (NPV, DPV, DDPV) were analyzed. Five micrometer sections were stained using a combined Miller, alcian blue and sirius red trichrome, as described by Sarathchandra P. [26]. The Miller stains elastin in dark blue, the alcian blue colors the glycosaminoglycans (GAGs) in Cyan and the sirius red stains collagen in red.

Quantification was performed individually on leaflet, pulmonary wall and pulmonary trunk using Tissue IA software (Leica Biosystems, Dublin, Ireland). Pixels corresponding to the Miller, Alcian blue and Sirius red staining were selected separately to create three color profiles. Total tissue area was defined by setting an intensity threshold (grey value). Results were expressed as a percentage of stained area and calculated as (stained area/tissue area) × 100.

In vivo study

Surgical procedure

Animals were housed according to the guidelines of the French Ministry of Agriculture and Animal Care. All procedures were approved by the local Ethics Committee for Animal Care of the Ecole de Chirurgie - Université de Lorraine, Nancy (D57–547-5).

Three female Landrace pigs weighting 40 kg were kept unfed for 24 h before the operation. A premedication of ketamine (1000 mg) was administered by IM. The animals were then intubated and kept under general anesthesia throughout the operation. A physiological follow-up (oximetry, pulse, and heart rate) was conducted throughout the entire operating procedure. After longitudinal sternotomy, the heart was exposed. Systemic heparinization was achieved with an activated coagulation time of 400 s. Pediatric cardiopulmonary bypass was then placed and turned on. Then, the native pulmonary artery root was harvested and replaced with DPV with two 5.0 prolene running sutures. After implantation, the pigs were weaned off bypass. The cannulas were removed and the sternum was closed. The pigs received low molecular weight heparin prophylaxis (40 mg/day) for 5 days. The animals did not receive antibiotics. One pig was euthanized at day 30 and 2 pigs were euthanized at day 90. The valves were then removed and cut in order to obtain three parts relating to posterior, right and left leaflets and the corresponding sinus, pulmonary wall and muscular base. Finally, these portions were divided in two parts to obtain six segments (Fig. 1c/d). Tissues were fixed overnight in 4% formaldehyde and embedded in paraffin.

Histological evaluation

Coloration and staining Hematoxylin and eosin, Masson's trichrome and von Kossa stainings assessed remodeling/cell infiltration, structure and calcifications respectively.

Immunohistochemistry for CD3 and CD68 were performed using a Ventana Benchmark XT machine (Roche®, USA) to assess inflammatory reaction. The CD 68 is particularly useful as a marker for the various cells of the macrophage lineage, including monocytes, histiocytes, giant cells, Kupffer cells. CD3 is highly specific of all stages of T-cell development [18]. Slides were digitalized at 20× magnification with a SCN400 slide scanner (Leica, Wetzlar, Germany) and visualized on the Digital Image Hub (Leica Biosystems, Dublin, Ireland).

For immunofluorescent co staining, 5 μm sections were subjected to endogenous peroxidases inhibition for 20 min and then to specific antigen binding sites for 1 h (PBS with 5% BSA and 0.05% Triton). Rabbit anti-CD31 (polyclonal, Abcam, # ab28364, 1/100 dilution for rat, 1/50 dilution for pig) and Mouse anti-ASMA (clone 1A4, Abcam #ab7817, 1/100 dilution, for pig), primary antibodies were incubated overnight at 4 °C in PBS containing 1% BSA and 0.05% Triton X-100. This was followed by an incubation with AlexaFluor 568 anti-rabbit and AlexaFluor647 anti-mouse (Invitrogen) secondary antibodies, incubated at a 1/1000 dilution for 1 h at room temperature. Nuclei were stained with DAPI and labeled sections.

Stained sections were digitized using a Pannoramic P250 FlashIII slide scanner (3DHistech) at 20× magnification and visualized using CaseViewer.

Histomorphometry A minimum of five regions of interest [ROI] in the three parts (wall/leaflet/muscle) of the six segments of the explanted DPV were analyzed at × 20 magnification with a grid representing a surface of 0. 12 mm square. CD3 and CD68 immunohistochemical staining's were assessed by point counting as previously described [18].

Statistical analysis

One-sample Kolmogorov–Smirnov tests and QQ-plots were used to ensure the normal distribution of values. Results were expressed as means ± SD or in ratios. The statistical significance of differences between experimental groups was tested by Student-T or one-way analysis of variance with a Bonferroni's post hoc test. The statistical tests were carried out with PASW 18. Differences were considered to be significant at $p < 0.05$.

Results

In vitro characterization

Decellularization and antigen removal

Staining for HE, DAPI and alpha-gal and SLA-I was positive for controls in the three parts of the valve.

Decellularization and antigen removal were more complete for DPV than for DDPV as well for the muscle, wall or leaflet of treated valves. Positive staining for alpha-gal and SLA-I were still detected for DDPV in the three parts. Cells were also evidenced with hematoxylin and eosin for DDPV muscle and wall (Fig. 2/Table 1).

Mechanical integrity

No differences between NPV, DPV and DDPV regarding elasticity and maximal load of leaflets or pulmonary wall were detected (Fig. 3a).

DNA

Better DNA reduction was achieved with NaOH-based process in comparison with detergent process. The DPV leaflets showed 95% DNA reduction to NPV while DDPV showed 92% DNA reduction. In the wall of DDPV, DNA content was reduced to 69% and in the DPV, the content was reduced to 92%. In the muscle, DNA reduction was quite similar for both treatments: 96% for DDPV vs 97% for DPV (Fig. 3b/Table 2).

Biochemical integrity

Muscle Collagen and elastin staining were maintained in DPV and DDPV in comparison to NPV. However, significant reduction of GAGs staining in DDPV muscle in comparison to NPV occurred ($p = 0.021$) while there was no difference between DPV and NPV (Fig. 4).

Leaflet Histological examination after trichrome staining revealed evidence of GAGs staining reduction after both treatments. Software analysis showed GAGs staining was significantly reduced for both DPV and DDPV to NPV with $p < 0.05$ while elastin staining was significantly reduced for DDPV to NPV (p = 0.021).

Collagen staining was not reduced after both treatments (Fig. 4).

Wall No significant reduction of staining was noticed for DPV and DDPV in comparison to NPV (Fig. 4).

In vivo study

No deaths occurred. The three pigs showed regular growth (to reach 60 kg at 1 month and 120 kg at 3 months).

Macroscopic evaluation

The explanted valves exhibited no signs of graft dilatation, degeneration or rejection. The luminal surface of the arterial wall was similar to the adjacent host artery.

At 1 month, the DPV exhibited two translucent, flexible and mobile leaflets while one small thrombus was detected in the third one (Fig. 5a1).

At 3 months, all leaflets of the two DPVs were translucent, flexible and mobile. We noticed one calcification in one posterior leaflet sinus (Fig. 5a2).

Histological evaluation

Inflammation CD3 infiltration was essentially located in the muscle at 1 month. The CD3 count was significantly the lowest in the leaflets ($p < 0,005$). At 3 months, the CD3 infiltration showed the same repartition than at 1 month with the highest count in the muscle with p < 0,05. At 3 months in comparison to 1 month, infiltration was significantly reduced in the wall and in the muscle with p < 0,005 while leaflet infiltration was still low (0,98 +/− 1,36 cells/0,12 mm^2) (Fig. 5b/c).

At 1 month CD68 infiltration was low in all parts of the valves with the highest count in the muscle part with p < 0,05. The lowest count was in the leaflets (p < 0,05). At 3 months, the CD68 infiltration was still the lowest in the leaflet with $p > 0,05$ but not statistically different than in the wall and in the muscle. The CD68 infiltration significantly decreased at 3 months in the muscle ($p = 0,000$) (Fig. 5c).

Calcifications Von Kossa staining was positive for one sinus at 3 months.

Remodeling HE, AMSA and CD31 staining showed progressive DPV recellularization occurred at one and 3 months (Fig. 6). The interstitial recellularization increased with time and cell colonization, was deeper in the pulmonary trunk at 3 months than at 1 month but was still partial (Fig. 6a). In a similar way,

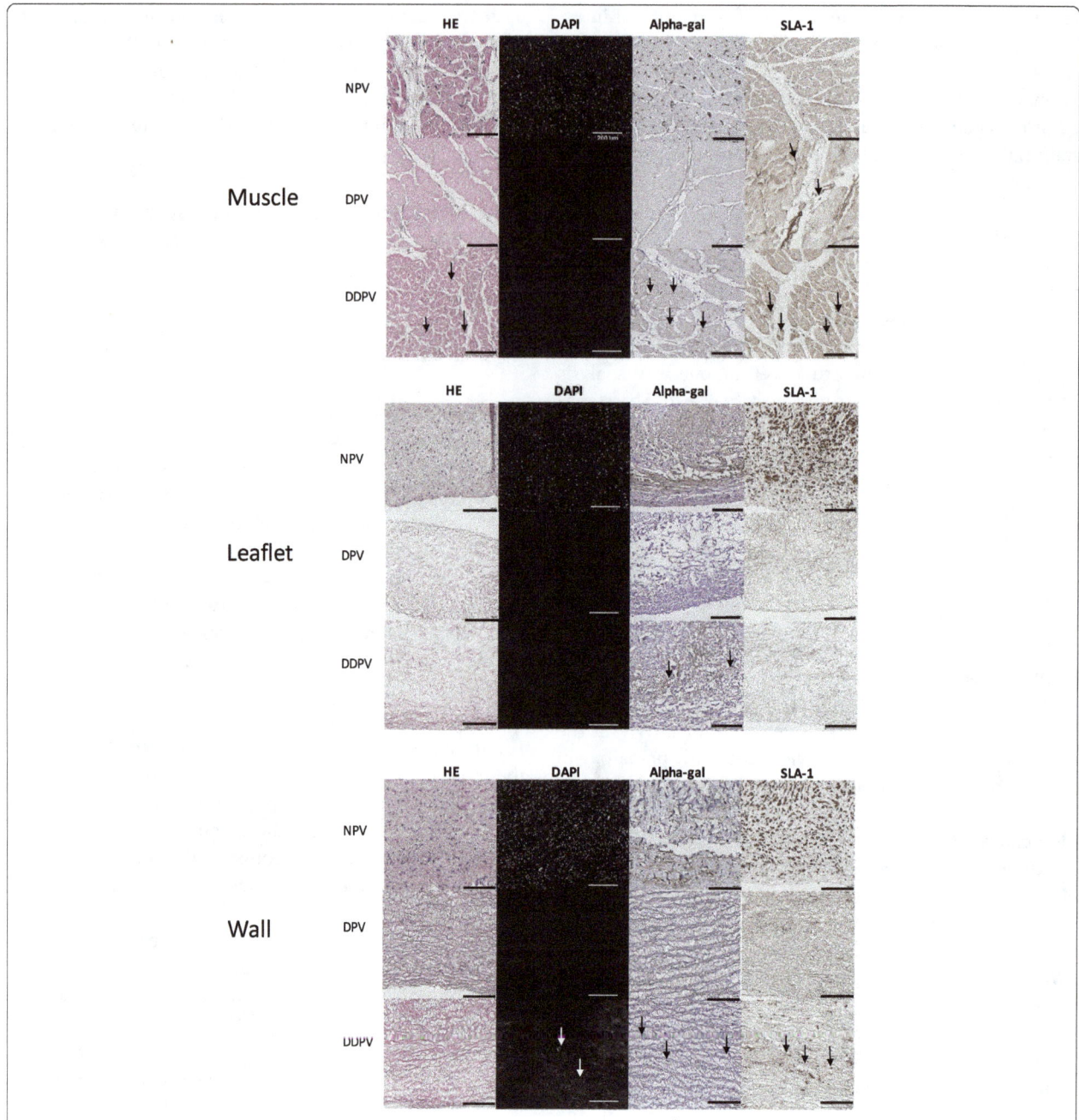

Fig. 2 Histological valves characterization: Hematoxylin and eosin/DAPI/Alpha-gal and SLA-1 staining. Representative histology microphotograph of muscle (first table)/leaflet (second table) and wall (third table) of NPV (first line), DPV (second line) and DDPV (third line) after Hematoxylin and eosin (HE, first column), DAPI (second column) Alpha-gal (third column) and SLA-1 (fourth column) staining. (Black scale bar: 100 μm and white scale bar: 200 μm). The black arrows show positive staining. The staining for NPV (both muscle/leaflet and wall) was positive in all conditions (HE/DAPI/Alpha-gal and SLA-1) and was clear

endothelialisation (endothelial cell monolayer) of DPV was still partial at 1 month and 3 months (Fig. 6b).

Discussion

The aim of the present study was firstly to assess the efficacy of a NaOH-based process to decellularize and

maintain biochemical and mechanical properties of xenogeneic valve in comparison to a standard detergent treatment. This treatment, a combination of 0.5%SDC /0.5%SDS is largely recommended for xenogeneic tissues decellularization as for human valves decellularization with good midterm clinical results in pediatric and adult populations [14, 23, 27–29]. Secondly a preliminary

Table 1 Assessment of HE/DAPI/Alpha-gal and SLA-1 stainings for muscle/leaflet/wall of control (NPV, $n = 4$), DPV($n = 4$) and DDPV($n = 4$)

		H.E.	DAPI	Alpha-gal	SLA-1
Muscle	NPV	+++	+++	+++	+++
	DPV	–	–	–	+
	DDPV	+	–	+	++
Leaflet	NPV	+++	+++	+++	+++
	DPV	–	–	–	–
	DDPV	–	–	+	–
Wall	NPV	+++	+++	+++	+++
	DPV	–	–	–	–
	DDPV	+	+	+	++

Semi-quantitative numerical scale: –: no staining; +: staining traces; ++: moderate staining and +++: intense staining

study investigated in a growing model biocompatibility and remodeling/cell recolonization of NaOH-based processed valve.

The main decellularization agent of our treatment is NaOH. The duration of exposure of the tissue to this agent and the combination with other chemicals offer a supplementary property to inactivate conventional (bacteria and virus) and non-conventional (prion) pathogen agents that a conventional detergent process does not offer, improving grafts security [22]. To our

knowledge, this method for valve decellularization was not yet reported. The NaOH, while known as a decellularization agent, is not commonly used for biological tissue decellularization because it is at risk to denature the tissue. Indeed, decellularization treatments have to respect a perfect balance between decellularization and maintenance of physical properties for optimal in vivo functionality [30, 31]. Our in vitro and in vivo results showed the treatment did not denature the valves and can also ensure this balance for very thin structures such as leaflets.

Moreover, our treatment achieved better results in terms of decellularization and antigen removal than the detergent-based process. The presence of alpha-gal epitope remaining should lead to rapid deterioration of the last in a clinical scenario as it was observed for Synergraft valves [12, 32].

The NaOH-based process led to lower biochemical modifications of the valves in comparison to detergent treatment while mechanical properties of detergent-based processed valves were maintained.

It was shown that SDS might destabilize the triple helical domain of collagen and lead to tissue deterioration [33–35]. We noted the use of SDS lead to extracellular matrix swelling due to destruction of extracellular glycosaminoglycans as in our study while we did not observe direct consequences on mechanical tests not altered in comparison to native valves.

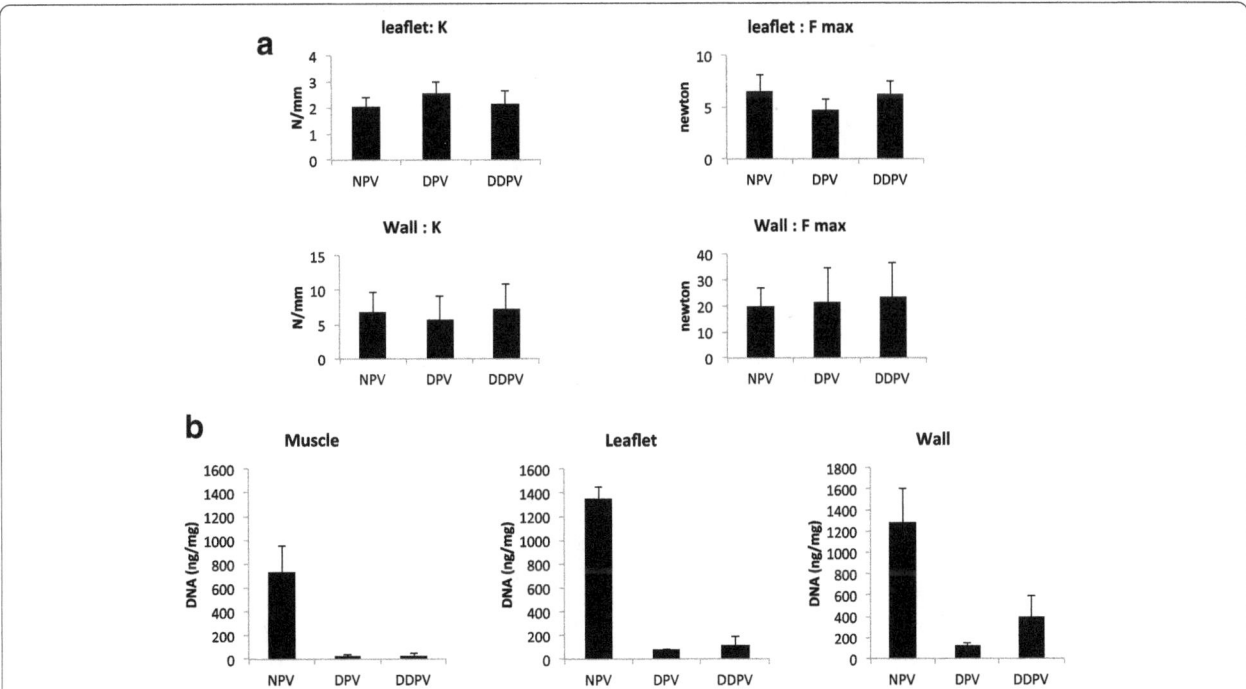

Fig. 3 Valves characteristics: Mechanical properties and DNA content. **a**: Stiffness (K: N/mm) and maximal load before rupture (F max: Newton) of leaflet and wall of NPV, DDPV and DPV. No significant differences were observed between groups. **b**: DNA content (ng/mg) in muscle, leaflet and wall of NPV, DDPV and DPV

Table 2 DNA content (ng/mg) in NPV, DDPV, DPV and DNA reduction in DDPV and DPV

	Native (n = 3)	DDPV (n = 3)		DPV (n = 3)	
	Total DNA (ng/mg)	Total DNA (ng/mg)	% reduction	Total DNA (ng/mg)	% reduction
Muscle	730,58+/−223,20	31,02+/− 20,07	96%	23,35+/− 18,92	97%
Leaflet	1345,65+/−100,64	110,3231+/−85,27	92%	77,16+/−7,94	95%
Wall	1278,85+/− 332,05	396,60+/−196,30	69%	122,34+/−23,52	92%

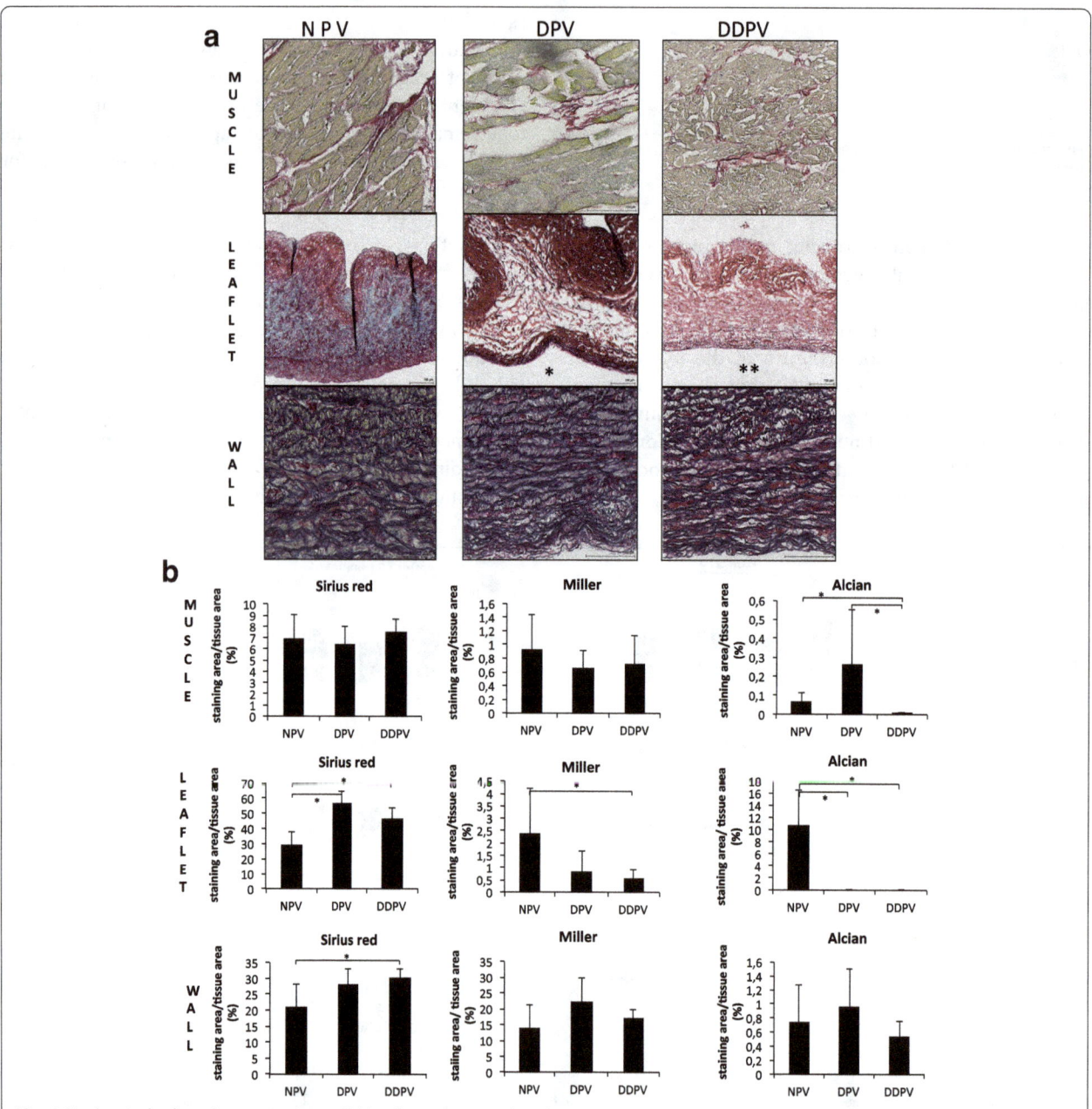

Fig. 4 Biochemical valves characterization. **a**: Table of representative histologic microphotographs of the three parts (muscle/leaflet and wall) of NPV (first column), DPV (second column) and DDPV (third column) after trichrome staining. Scale bar: 100 μm. Note reduction of blue staining (GAGs) in treated leaflets (*: DPV leaflet and **: DDPV leaflet) while coloration of wall in the different conditions are quite similar. **b**: Quantification of staining area for Sirius red (collagen), Miller (elastin) and Alcian blue (GAGs) /analyzed tissue area in muscle (first line) /leaflet (second line) and wall (third line) of NPV, DPV and DDPV after trichrome staining. *: $p < 0.05$

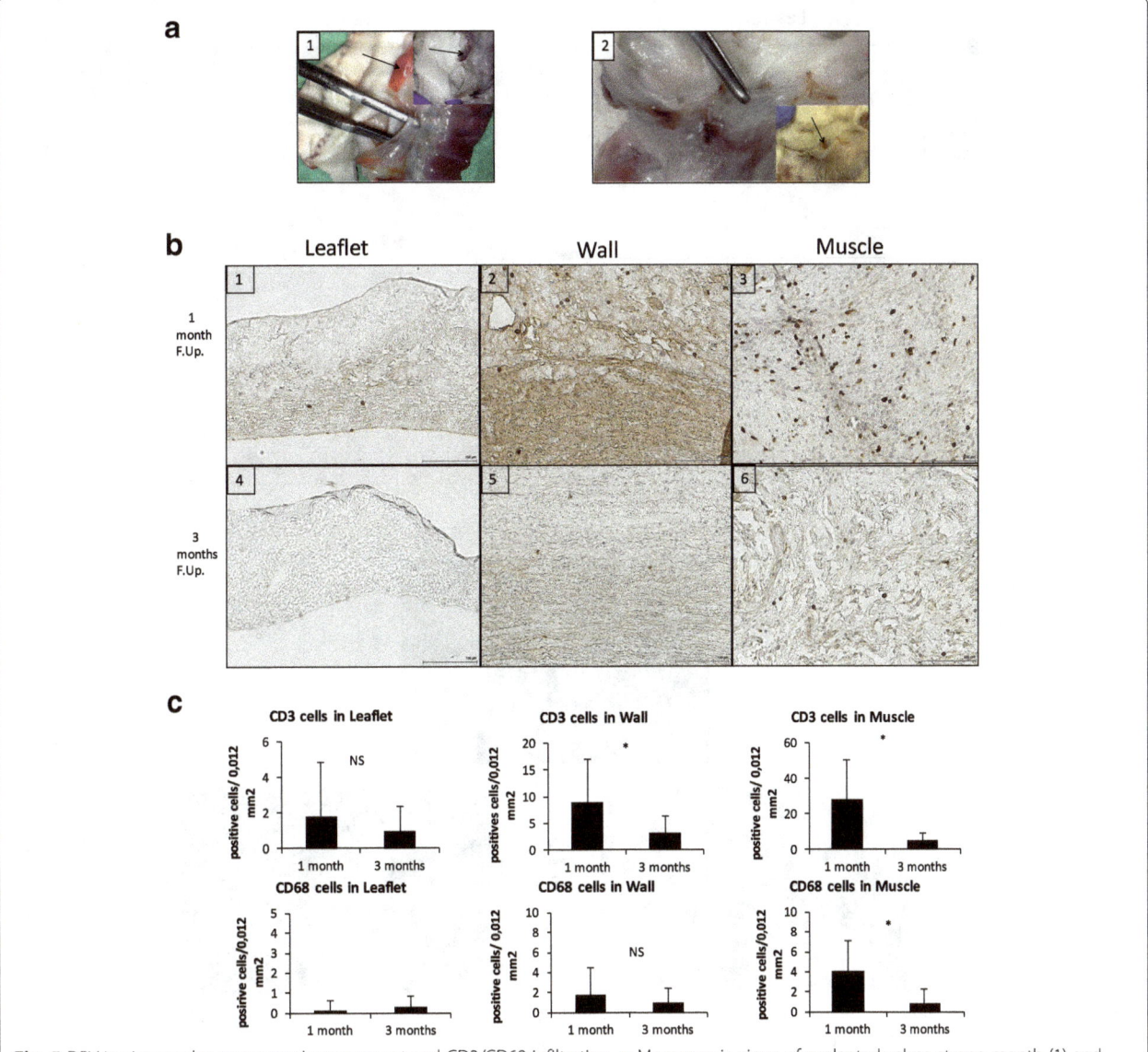

Fig. 5 DPV in vivo results: macroscopic assessment and CD3/CD68 infiltration. **a**: Macroscopic views of explanted valves at one month (1) and three months (2) follow-up. The forceps indicate translucent and flexible leaflets. The black arrow in 1 shows thrombi formation and in 2, a micro calcification in the posterior sinus. **b**: Representative histological findings of CD3 staining of DPV at one month (first line) and three months (second line) of follow-up in leaflet (1;4), wall (2;5) and muscle (3;6). Note staining was the highest in muscle at one month (3) and reduction of staining at three months in comparison to one month (1->4 for leaflets/2->5 for wall and 3->6 in muscle). Scale bar: 100 μm. **c**: Results of histomorphometry for CD3 (first line) and CD68 (second line) staining in the three portions of DPV at one month and three months showing a decrease of inflammatory reaction at three months in all portions of the valve and significantly (*: p < 0,05) in wall and muscle portions for CD3 infiltration and in wall portion for CD68 infiltration. Low inflammation in the leaflet, the wall and muscle portions was found at 3 month: for CD3 infiltration: respectively 0,98 +/− 1,36; 3,1+/− 3,28 and 5,08 +/− 4,35 cells/0,12 mm^2 and for CD68 infiltration: respectively CD68: 0,32 +/− 0,69; 0,93 +/− 1,44 and 0,87 +/− 1,34 cells/0,12mm^2)

Additional studies also showed that the cytotoxicity of SDS can have an influence on the ingrowth of host valvular endothelial and interstitial cells [6, 36].

On the contrary, the NaOH-based process showed previously good clinical results regarding biocompatibility and cytotoxicity for other allogeneic biological tissues in different implantation sites with good host cell incorporation and remodeling [18, 19, 37, 38].

Our in vivo study confirmed this aspect. The in vivo results showed very low inflammation while the leaflets were thin and translucent at 3 months. Moreover, a recellularization, which is also of major concern for decellularized scaffolds integration and function,

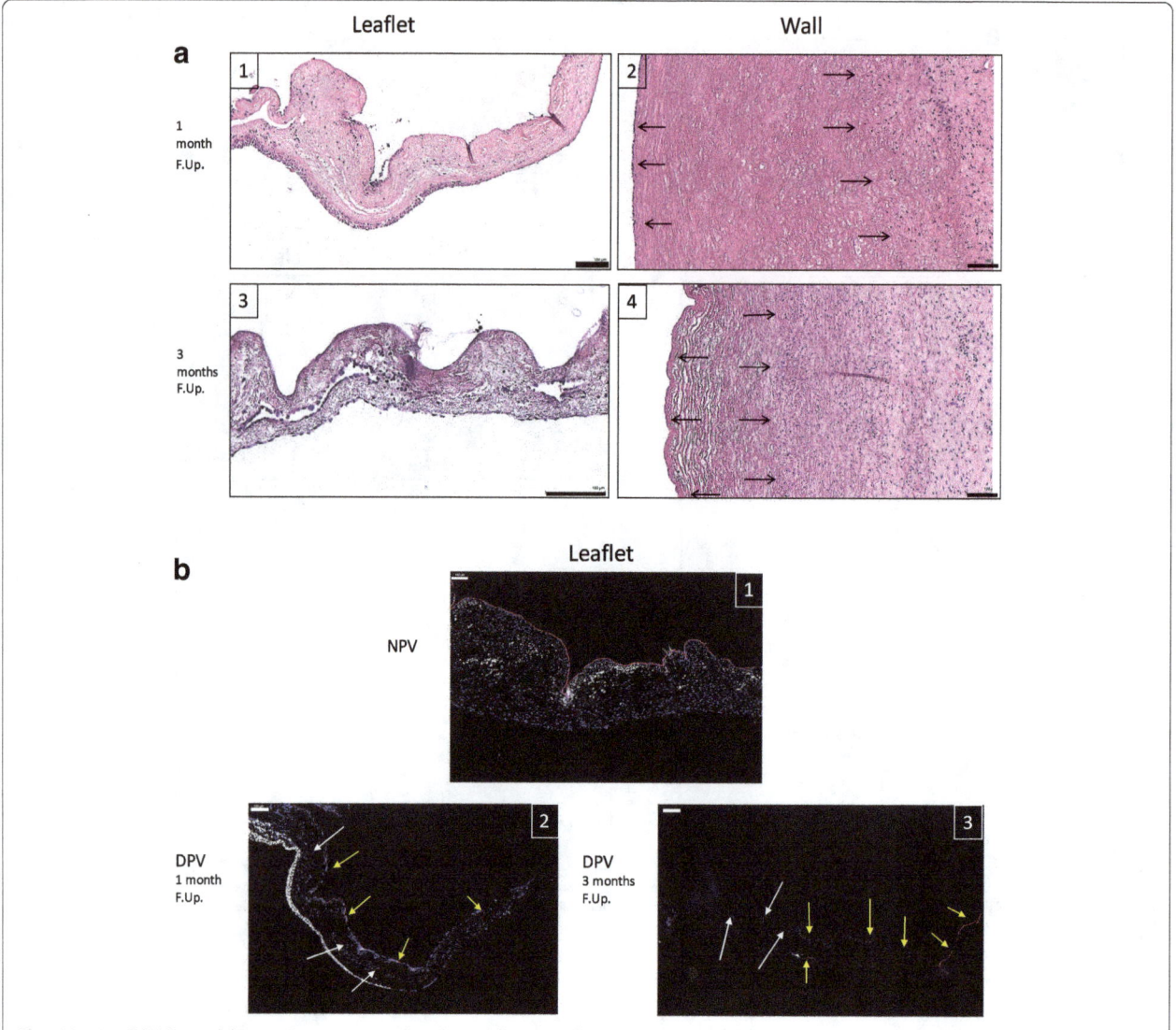

Fig. 6 In vivo DPV Remodeling. **a**: Representative histological findings of Hematoxylin and eosin staining of DPV Leaflet (1,3) and Wall (2,4) of at one month (1;2) and three months (3;4) of follow-up illustrating the recellularization process. The black arrows indicate cell nuclei. Scale bar: 100 μm. **b**: Representative histological findings of CD31 (red) and ASMA (white) IHF stainings counterstained with DAPI (blue) of NPV leaflet (1), DPV leaflet at one month (2) and DPV leaflet at three months (3). Scale bar: 100 μm. The yellow arrows indicate CD31 + cells and white arrows DAPI + cells

occurred and was progressive but still partial at 3 months. This phenomenon was also observed by others and a longer follow-up will investigate if complete recellularization can be achieved [39].

Another crucial point for cardiovascular prosthesis assessment is calcification occurrence. In this aspect, of the three implanted valves, in this growing model we observed one calcification focus in a sinus at 3 months. One explanation is although histologic examinations showed adequate decellularization and antigen removal, DNA quantification revealed only 92% DNA reduction in comparison to native in this region. This is less than the recommended threshold of 95% DNA reduction as nulceic acid can act as nucleation sites for calcifications [1, 16]. Unfortunately, a link is difficult to establish due to the small sample which constitutes a limit in our study.

Additionally, acetone and ethanol are part of the process. As detergents, these chemicals are recognized as antimineralization agents in heart valve substitutes by removal of phospholipids and cholesterol [1, 40–42].

Alcohols also aid in tissue decellularization by dehydrating and lysing cells. However, alcohol and acetone as tissue fixatives can damage ECM ultrastructure. In comparison to detergent treatments, acetone and alcohol crosslink ECM can produce stiffer scaffolds with mechanical properties further removed from those of native tissue [16]. We did not observe this phenomenon and conclude the proposed dilutions and duration of tissue exposure are not deleterious.

Last, the preservation method that we used is simple, cost effective, and the valve can be easily stored and banked for a long time as musculo-skeletal tissues in a tissue bank [18].

The results of this preliminary study are encouraging to consider this NaOH-based process for xenogeneic valve decellularization. In the clinical setup, xenogeneic source is advantageous regarding availability. But xenogeneic tissue transplantation to humans imposes high caution in view of controversial results with xenogeneic decellularized gafts [12]. We investigated only alpaha gal epitope removal. Others xeno non alpha-gal antigens exist and especially a recently highlighted, highly immunogenic xenoantigen, N-glycolylneuraminic acid antigen. This should be also investigated. The new genetically modified pigs for these major xenoantigens (alphagalactosyltransferase KO N-glycolylneuraminic acid KO pigs) offer new possibilities in this direction [43]. On the other hand, it would be impossible and inappropriate to check the disappearance of all xeno antigens [44] and, as suggested by G Gerosa, a step back to the preclinical evaluation in human-like models (non-human primates) is mandatory to assess effective biocompatibility [17].

Moreover, larger samples with a longer follow-up and echocardiographic data are prerequisite before considering clinical translation.

Conclusions

The NaOH-based process does not alter biomechanical valve properties and can be used for xenogeneic heart valve decellularization. It ensures better decellularization and antigen removal than detregent-based process. In a preliminary in vivo study, the NaOH-based processed valve showed recellularization, low inflammation, and absence of structural deterioration. Regarding additional property of graft securing, this treatment should be considered for the new generation valves.

Abbreviations

alpha-gal: Alphagalactosyltransferase antigen; ASMA: Alpha smooth muscle cells actin; BSA: Bovine serum albumin; DAPI: 40.6-diamidino-2-phenylindole; DDPV: Decellularized porcine pulmonary heart valves with detergent-based process; DNA: Desoxyribonucleic acid; DPV: Decellularized porcine pulmonary heart valves with NaOH-based process; HE: Hematoxylin and eosin; MHC-1: Major histocompatibility complex class 1; NPV: Native porcine pulmonary heart valves; PBS: Phosphate buffered saline; SD: Standard deviation; SDC: Sodium deoxycholate; SDS: Sodium dodecyl sulfate; SLA-1: Swine leucocyte antigen: MHC class 1 region of pigs

Acknowledgements
We thank Ecole de chirurgie de Nancy for technical assistance, Pascale Segers and Eric Legrand (CHEX) for writing and administrative assistance.
We thank Prof. P. Astarci (cardiac surgery department, Cliniques universitaires Saint-Luc) for having made possible the realization of the in vitro tests.

Funding
This research did not receive any specific grant from funding agencies in the public, commercial or not-for-profit sectors.
The content of the work is solely the responsibility of the authors.

Authors' contributions
MvanS, PG, and TS contributed for study conception and design. Data acquisition was carried out by MvanS, DX, SG, CB, YG, XB and KA. Analysis and data interpretation were carried out by MvanS, PG, TS, DX, and CB. The authors MvanS drafted the manuscript, PG, DX, CB, critically revised the article. All authors read and approved the final manuscript.

Competing interests
The authors declare that they have no competing interests.

Author details
[1]Pôle de Chirurgie Expérimentale et Transplantation (CHEX), Institut de Recherche Expérimentale et Clinique (IREC), Secteur des Sciences de la Sante, Université Catholique de Louvain, Avenue Hippocrate 55/B1.55.04, B-1200 Brussels, Belgium. [2]Service de chirurgie cardiaque et vasculaire, Clinique Cecil, avenue Louis Ruchonnet 53, 1003 Lausanne, Switzerland. [3]Service d'orthopédie et de traumatologie de l'appareil locomoteur, Cliniques universitaires Saint-Luc, Avenue Hippocrate 10, B-1200 Brussels, Belgium. [4]Unité de thérapie tissulaire et cellulaire de l'appareil locomoteur, Cliniques universitaires Saint Luc, Avenue Hippocrate 10, B-1200 Brussels, Belgium. [5]Service de chirurgie cardiaque, Centre hospitalier Annecy-Genevois, site Annecy, 1 Avenue de l'Hopital, F-74370 Pringy, France. [6]Institut de Recherche Expérimentale et Clinique (IREC), IREC Imaging Platform (2IP), Université catholique de Louvain, Avenue Hippocrate 55/B1.55.20, B-1200 Brussels, Belgium. [7]Service d'anatomie pathologique, Cliniques universitaires Saint Luc, Avenue Hippocrate 10, B-1200 Brussels, Belgium. [8]Institute of Mechanics, Materials and Civil Engineering, Mechatronic, Electrical Energy, and Dynamic Systems (MEED), Secteur des Sciences et Technologies, Université Catholique de Louvain, Place du Levant 2/L5.04.02, B-1348 Louvain-la-Neuve, Belgium. [9]Service d'oncologie, Centre hospitalier universitaire vaudois, Rue du Bugnon 46, CH-1011 Lausanne, Vaud, Switzerland.

References
1. Schoen FJ, Levy RJ. Calcification of tissue heart valve substitutes: progress toward understanding and prevention. Ann Thorac Surg. 2005;79:1072–80.
2. Umashankar PR, Mohanan PV, Kumari TV. Glutaraldehyde treatment elicits toxic response compared to decellularization in bovine pericardium. Toxicol Int. 2012;19:51–8.
3. Manji RA, Zhu LF, Nijjar NK, Rayner DC, Korbutt GS, Churchill TA, Rajotte RV, Koshal A, Ross DB. Glutaraldehyde-fixed bioprosthetic heart valve conduits calcify and fail from xenograft rejection. Circulation. 2006;114:318–27.
4. Choi SY, Jeong HJ, Lim HG, Park SS, Kim SH, Kim YJ. Elimination of alpha-gal xenoreactive epitope: alpha-galactosidase treatment of porcine heart valves. J Heart Valve Dis. 2012;21:387–97.
5. Hu XJ, Dong NG, Shi JW, Deng C, Li HD, Lu CF. Evaluation of a novel tetrafunctional branched poly(ethylene glycol) crosslinker for manufacture of crosslinked, decellularized, porcine aortic valve leaflets. J Biomed Mater Res B Appl Biomater. 2014;102:322–36.
6. Dohmen PM. Clinical results of implanted tissue engineered heart valves. HSR Proc Intensive Care Cardiovasc Anesth. 2012;4:225–31.
7. Shaddy RE, Hawkins JA. Immunology and failure of valved allografts in children. Ann Thorac Surg. 2002;74:1271–5.
8. Carpentier A, Lemaigre G, Robert L, Carpentier S, Dubost C. Biological factors affecting long-term results of valvular heterografts. J Thorac Cardiovasc Surg. 1969;58:467–83.
9. Rajani B, Mee RB, Ratliff NB. Evidence for rejection of homograft cardiac valves in infants. J Thorac Cardiovasc Surg. 1998;115:111–7.
10. Ruel M, Chan V, Bedard P, Kulik A, Ressler L, Lam BK, Rubens FD, Goldstein W, Hendry PJ, Masters RG, Mesana TG. Very long-term survival implications of heart valve replacement with tissue versus mechanical prostheses in adults <60 years of age. Circulation. 2007;116:1294–300.

11. Keane TJ, Swinehart IT, Badylak SF. Methods of tissue decellularization used for preparation of biologic scaffolds and in vivo relevance. Methods. 2015;84:25–34.

12. Simon P, Kasimir MT, Seebacher G, Weigel G, Ullrich R, Salzer-Muhar U, Rieder E, Wolner E. Early failure of the tissue engineered porcine heart valve SYNERGRAFT in pediatric patients. Eur J Cardiothorac Surg. 2003;23:1002–6.

13. Ruffer A, Purbojo A, Cicha I, Glockler M, Potapov S, Dittrich S, Cesnjevar RA. Early failure of xenogenous de-cellularised pulmonary valve conduits–a word of caution! Eur J Cardiothorac Surg. 2010;38:78–85.

14. Sarikouch S, Horke A, Tudorache I, Beerbaum P, Westhoff-Bleck M, Boethig D, Repin O, Maniuc L, Ciubotaru A, Haverich A, Cebotari S. Decellularized fresh homografts for pulmonary valve replacement: a decade of clinical experience. Eur J Cardiothorac Surg. 2016;50:281–90.

15. Brown JW, Elkins RC, Clarke DR, Tweddell JS, Huddleston CB, Doty JR, Fehrenbacher JW, Takkenberg JJ. Performance of the CryoValve SG human decellularized pulmonary valve in 342 patients relative to the conventional CryoValve at a mean follow-up of four years. J Thorac Cardiovasc Surg. 2010;139:339–48.

16. Crapo PM, Gilbert TW, Badylak SF. An overview of tissue and whole organ decellularization processes. Biomaterials. 2011;32:3233–43.

17. Iop L, Gerosa G. Guided tissue regeneration in heart valve replacement: from preclinical research to first-in-human trials. Biomed Res Int. 2015;2015:432901.

18. van Steenberghe M, Schubert T, Guiot Y, Bouzin C, Bollen X, Gianello P. Enhanced vascular biocompatibility of decellularized xeno–/allogeneic matrices in a rodent model. Cell Tissue Bank. 2017;18:249–62.

19. van Steenberghe M, Schubert T, Xhema D, Bouzin C, Guiot Y, Duisit J, Abdelhamid K, Gianello P. Enhanced vascular regeneration with chemically/physically treated bovine/human pericardium in rodent. J Surg Res. 2018;222:167–79.

20. Cornu O, Schubert T, Libouton X, Manil O, Godts B, Van Tomme J, Banse X, Delloye C. Particle size influence in an impaction bone grafting model. Comparison of fresh-frozen and freeze-dried allografts. J Biomech. 2009;42:2238–42.

21. Fawzi-Grancher S, Goebbels RM, Bigare E, Cornu O, Gianello P, Delloye C, Dufrane D. Human tissue allograft processing: impact on in vitro and in vivo biocompatibility. J Mater Sci Mater Med. 2009;20:1709–20.

22. WHO. Decontamination methods for transmissible spongiform encephalopathies. Report of a WHO consultation, Geneva, Switzerland, 23-26 march 1999. In: WHO infection control guidelines for transmissible spongiform encephalopathies. WHO/CDS/CSR/APH/2000.3; 2009. p. 29–32.

23. Hulsmann J, Grun K, El Amouri S, Barth M, Hornung K, Holzfuss C, Lichtenberg A, Akhyari P. Transplantation material bovine pericardium: biomechanical and immunogenic characteristics after decellularization vs. glutaraldehyde-fixing. Xenotransplantation. 2012;19:286–97.

24. Cebotari S, Tudorache I, Ciubotaru A, Boethig D, Sarikouch S, Goerler A, Lichtenberg A, Cheptanaru E, Barnaciuc S, Cazacu A, Maliga O, Repin O, Maniuc L, Breymann T, Haverich A. Use of fresh decellularized allografts for pulmonary valve replacement may reduce the reoperation rate in children and young adults: early report. Circulation. 2011;124:S115–23.

25. Duisit J, Orlando G, Debluts D, Maistriaux L, Xhema D, de Bisthoven YJ, Galli C, Peloso A, Behets C, Lengele B, Gianello P. Decellularization of the porcine ear generates a biocompatible, nonimmunogenic extracellular matrix platform for face subunit bioengineering. Ann Surg. 2017; Epub ahead of print

26. Sarathchandra P, Smolenski RT, Yuen AH, Chester AH, Goldstein S, Heacox AE, Yacoub MH, Taylor PM. Impact of gamma-irradiation on extracellular matrix of porcine pulmonary valves. J Surg Res. 2012;176:376–85.

27. Theodoridis K, Muller J, Ramm R, Findeisen K, Andree B, Korossis S, Haverich A, Hilfiker A. Effects of combined cryopreservation and decellularization on the biomechanical, structural and biochemical properties of porcine pulmonary heart valves. Acta Biomater. 2016;43:71–7.

28. Booth C, Korossis SA, Wilcox HE, Watterson KG, Kearney JN, Fisher J, Ingham E. Tissue engineering of cardiac valve prostheses I: development and histological characterization of an acellular porcine scaffold. J Heart Valve Dis. 2002;11:457–62.

29. Pu L, Wu J, Pan X, Hou Z, Zhang J, Chen W, Na Z, Meng M, Ni H, Wang L, Li Y, Jiang L. Determining the optimal protocol for preparing an acellular scaffold of tissue engineered small-diameter blood vessels. J Biomed Mater Res B Appl Biomater. 2017; Epub ahead of print

30. Badylak SF, Freytes DO, Gilbert TW. Extracellular matrix as a biological scaffold material: structure and function. Acta Biomater. 2009;5:1–13.

31. Wong ML, Wong JL, Vapniarsky N, Griffiths LG. In vivo xenogeneic scaffold fate is determined by residual antigenicity and extracellular matrix preservation. Biomaterials. 2016;92:1–12.

32. Kasimir MT, Rieder E, Seebacher G, Wolner E, Weigel G, Simon P. Presence and elimination of the xenoantigen gal (alpha1, 3) gal in tissue-engineered heart valves. Tissue Eng. 2005;11:1274–80.

33. Rieder E, Kasimir MT, Silberhumer G, Seebacher G, Wolner E, Simon P, Weigel G. Decellularization protocols of porcine heart valves differ importantly in efficiency of cell removal and susceptibility of the matrix to recellularization with human vascular cells. J Thorac Cardiovasc Surg. 2004;127:399–405.

34. Kasimir MT, Rieder E, Seebacher G, Silberhumer G, Wolner E, Weigel G, Simon P. Comparison of different decellularization procedures of porcine heart valves. Int J Artif Organs. 2003;26:421–7.

35. Bodnar E, Olsen EG, Florio R, Dobrin J. Damage of porcine aortic valve tissue caused by the surfactant sodiumdodecylsulphate. Thorac Cardiovasc Surg. 1986;34:82–5.

36. Caamano S, Shiori A, Strauss SH, Orton EC. Does sodium dodecyl sulfate wash out of detergent-treated bovine pericardium at cytotoxic concentrations? J Heart Valve Dis. 2009;18:101–5.

37. Dufrane D, Marchal C, Cornu O, Raftopoulos C, Delloye C. Clinical application of a physically and chemically processed human substitute for dura mater. J Neurosurg. 2003;98:1198–202.

38. Dufrane D, Mourad M, van Steenberghe M, Goebbels RM, Gianello P. Regeneration of abdominal wall musculofascial defects by a human acellular collagen matrix. Biomaterials. 2008;29:2237–48.

39. Navarro FB, Costa FD, Mulinari LA, Pimentel GK, Roderjan JG, Vieira ED, Noronha L, Miyague NI. Evaluation of the biological behavior of decellularized pulmonary homografts: an experimental sheep model. Rev Bras Cir Cardiovasc. 2010;25:377–87.

40. Jorge-Herrero E, Fernandez P, de la Torre N, Escudero C, Garcia-Paez JM, Bujan J, Castillo-Olivares JL. Inhibition of the calcification of porcine valve tissue by selective lipid removal. Biomaterials. 1994;15:815–20.

41. Schmidt CE, Baier JM. Acellular vascular tissues: natural biomaterials for tissue repair and tissue engineering. Biomaterials. 2000;21:2215–31.

42. Mendoza-Novelo B, Cauich-Rodriguez JV. Decellularization, stabilization and functionalization of collagenous tissues used as cardiovascular biomaterials. In: Pignatello R, editor. Biomaterials - physics and chemistry. InTech; 2011. p. 159–82.

43. Lee W, Long C, Ramsoondar J, Ayares D, Cooper DK, Manji RA, Hara H. Human antibody recognition of xenogeneic antigens (NeuGc and gal) on porcine heart valves: could genetically modified pig heart valves reduce structural valve deterioration? Xenotransplantation. 2016;23:370–80.

44. Griffiths LG, Choe LH, Reardon KF, Dow SW, Christopher OE. Immunoproteomic identification of bovine pericardium xenoantigens. Biomaterials. 2008;29:3514–20.

10

Impact of connective tissue disease on the surgical outcomes of aortic dissection in patients with cystic medial necrosis

Toshiki Fujiyoshi[4*], Kenji Minatoya[1], Yoshihiko Ikeda[2], Hatsue Ishibashi-Ueda[2], Takayuki Morisaki[3], Hiroko Morisaki[3] and Hitoshi Ogino[4]

Abstract

Background: A retrospective analysis was performed to determine the impact of genetically diagnosed connective tissue disease (CTD) on the early and late outcomes of surgical treatment for aortic dissection in patients having aortic pathology associated with cystic medial necrosis (CMN).

Methods: Between 2003 and 2013, a total of 43 patients (37 ± 12.8 years old, 23 men, 20 women) who had undergone surgery for aortic dissection associated with CMN in the aortic wall underwent genetic examinations. Subsequently, there were 30 patients with CTD (CTD group) and 13 without CTD (non-CTD group).

Results: There were no early or late deaths (the follow-up rate was 100% for 57.1 ± 43.0 months). The median age was significantly lower in the CTD group ($p = 0.030$). The rate of elastic fiber loss was significantly higher in the CTD group ($p = 0.014$). In the long-term follow-up, there were no significant differences in the incidences of re-dissection ($p = 0.332$). However, re-operations were required more frequently in the CTD group ($p = 0.037$).

Conclusions: In patients with CTD as well as CMN, the onset of aortic dissection tends to be earlier, which would result in higher rates of re-operation, compared with the non-CTD group. Closer and stricter follow-up with medication and adequate surgical treatments with appropriate timing are mandatory for such high-risk patients.

Keywords: Aortic dissection, Surgery, Genetically diagnosed connective tissue disease, Cystic medial necrosis

Background

Cystic medial necrosis (CMN) or degeneration is found in surgical specimens of aortic dissection, and tends to be associated with higher risks of various aortic complications including aortic dissection and dilatation [1–3]. In addition, CMN is also considered as one of the histological markers for connective tissue diseases (CTD), including Marfan syndrome, Loeys-Dietz syndrome, and Ehlers-Danlos syndrome. Although some differences are found in the degree of loss of elastic fibers, there are no significant differences in the histopathological patterns within the aortic wall between CTD and non-CTD patients, especially in patients who are of advanced age and have systemic hypertension for a long time [4, 5].

Further genetic examinations are then highly recommended to diagnose CTD more precisely. However, for every patient with aortic dissection, there are difficulties in performing routine genetic examinations which are generally carried out when association with CTD is suspected, based on bodily features and family histories. On the other hand, there have been few published studies looking at the adverse effects and relationships of CTD and CMN to the surgical outcomes of aortic dissection. Under these circumstances, we wanted to determine the impact of genetically diagnosed CTD on the early and late outcomes of surgical treatment for aortic dissection in patients having pathologies associated with CMN.

Methods

Patient profiles

We reviewed our institutional database to identify patients who underwent initial surgery for aortic dissection

* Correspondence: fff.toshiki@gmail.com
[4]Cardiovascular Surgery, Tokyo Medical University, 6-7-1 Nishishinjuku Shinjuku-ku Tokyo, 160, Tokyo –0023, Japan
Full list of author information is available at the end of the article

between April 2003 and March 2013 at the National Cerebral and Cardiovascular Center, Osaka, Japan. A total of 321 patients underwent initial surgery for aortic dissection and 298 patients (64.0 ± 15.7 years old, 56% male) underwent postoperative pathological examinations of the surgical specimen during this period, in which CMN was present in 141 patients (47.3%). Of them, 43 patients (37.0 ± 12.8 years old, 53% male) subsequently underwent genetic examinations. Our criteria for genetic examination were as follows: (1) patients with bodily features consistent with the current Ghent criteria, (2) young patients under 50 years of age, and (3) patients with family history of aortic diseases. This study was approved by the National Cerebral and Cardiovascular Center of Japan Institutional Review Board waived the need for individual patient consent under the provisions for deidentified human subject and quality improvement research.

The patient characteristics are shown in Table 1. Thirty patients (69.8%, CTD group) were diagnosed genetically as having CTD, whereas the remaining 13 patients (30.2%, non-CTD group) did not have any genetic disorders. The details of genetic disorders are shown in Table 2. Preoperative variables were compared between the CTD and non-CTD groups (Table 3). The median age at the onset of aortic dissection was significantly lower in the CTD group, namely 33.5 years in the CTD group vs. 42.0 years in the non-CTD (p = 0.030). In addition, there were differences in the Stanford classification of aortic dissection (p = 0.015) and the stages of aortic dissection (p = 0.009) between the two patient groups. In the CTD group, there were type A aortic dissections in 11 patients (37%, 7 acute and 4 chronic) and type B aortic dissections in 19 patients (63%, 1 acute and 18 chronic). In the non-CTD group, there were type A aortic dissections in 10 patients (77%, 9 acute and 1 chronic) and type B in 3 patients (23%, 3 chronic). The incidence of type B aortic dissection was higher in the CTD group. Two patients in the CTD group developed

Table 1 Patient characteristics

Patient characteristics (n = 43)	
Male: Female	23: 20
Mean age at AD (years)	37.0 ± 12.8
Stanford AD classification	
Type A	21 (48.8%)
Type B	22 (51.2%)
Stage of aortic dissection	
Acute	17 (39.5%)
Chronic	26 (60.5%)
Connective tissue disorder[a]	30 (69.8%)

AD aortic dissection
[a]genetically diagnosed

Table 2 Genetic disorders in CTD

Genetic disorders in CTD	Number
FBN1	19
TGFBR2	4
ACTA2	3
MYH11	1
SMAD3	1
TGFB2	1
COLIAI	1

CTD genetically diagnosed connective tissue disease

three-channel aortic dissection, although it was not found in the non-CTD group. The incidence of family history of aortic dissection was significantly higher in the CTD group (57% vs. 23%, p = 0.043). The rate of preoperative renal dysfunction (serum creatinine ≥2.0) was significantly higher in the non-CTD group (p = 0.028).

In these series, the surgical treatments were performed according to the same indication criteria at the single center with the same surgical team staff. In the acute phase, emergent or urgent surgeries were carried out, in cases with acute type A aortic dissection with patent false channels excluding intramural hematoma, and with complicated acute type B aortic dissection. In patients with chronic aortic dissection or with residual aortic dissection in the long term after the initial surgical replacement, surgical interventions were indicated when the

Table 3 Preoperative variables

Preoperative variables (n = 43)	CTD (n = 30)	non-CTD (n = 13)	p value
Male	14 (46.7%)	9 (69.2%)	0.303
Median age at AD (years [range])	33.5 [19–65]	42.0 [28–71]	0.030
Stanford AD classification			
Type A	11 (36.7%)	10 (76.9%)	0.015
Type B	19 (63.3%)	3 (23.1%)	
Aortic pathology			
Acute	8 (26.7%)	9 (69.2%)	0.009
Chronic	22 (73.3%)	4 (30.8%)	
Three-channel AD	2 (6.7%)	none	0.518
Family history of AD	17 (56.7%)	3 (23.1%)	0.043
Other coexisting conditions			
Hypertension	16 (53.3%)	8 (61.5%)	0.870
Hyperlipidemia	1 (3.3%)	2 (15.4%)	0.440
Diabetes mellitus	none	1 (7.7%)	0.677
CKD (Cr ≥ 2.0)	none	2 (15.4%)	0.028
Smoker	9 (30.0%)	5 (38.5%)	0.850

CTD genetically diagnosed connective tissue disease, AD aortic dissection, CKD chronic kidney disease, Cr creatinine value, NS no significant difference

aortic maximum diameter exceeded 50 to 55 mm. Root repairs such as aortic valve-sparing surgery or composite valve-graft root replacement were carried out with the site of the root over 40 to 45 mm, predominantly for the CTD patients [6]. In 2 patients described above, surgical treatments were indicated for 3-channel dissection, even though the diameter was less than 50 mm.

Histopathological examination

The samples were surgically resected from the dissecting aortic wall. Histopathological examination consisted of light microscopy on the surgical specimen stained with hematoxylin-eosin stain, Masson's trichrome stain, elastica van Gieson stain, and toluidine blue stain. CMN was diagnosed if the aorta displayed fragmentation of elastic fibers associated with cystic accumulation of the extracellular matrix. The degree of loss of elastic fibers was defined as elastin fragmentation in the media stained with elastica van Gieson using a diagram of the grading system. Three grades were recognized as follows: grade 0 or 1+ (no loss or minimal loss or mild fragmentation of elastic fibers), grade 2+ (intermediate change), and grade 3+ (complete loss of elastic fibers in some full-thickness portions of the media) (Fig. 1) [5]. Afterwards,

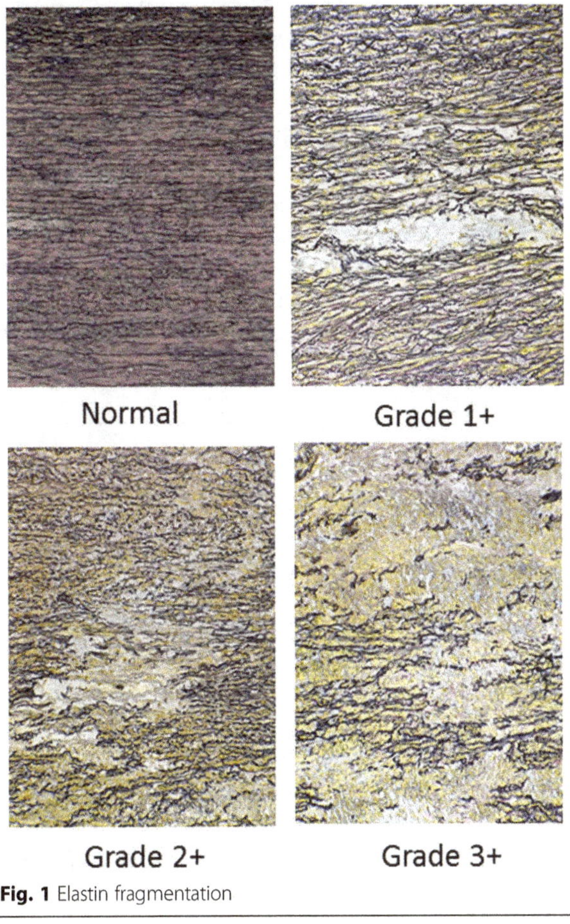

Fig. 1 Elastin fragmentation

loss of elastic fibers was combined into two clinically relevant categories, namely, (1) no or minimal loss of elastic fibers (grade 0 or 1+ representing no loss or minimal loss or mild fragmentation of elastic fibers), and (2) loss of elastic fibers (grade 2+ or 3+ representing a significant loss of elastic fibers in some portion of the media) [5, 7].

Genetic examination (sequencing and mutation analysis)

Mutation analyses were performed by bidirectional Sanger sequencing of exons and exon-intron boundaries of FBN1, TGFBR1, and TGFBR2 genes first [8–11]. PCR products were purified and sequenced using BigDye Terminator chemistry v.1.1 on an ABI Prism3130xl or 3730xl (Applied Biosystems). In cases in which mutations of FBN1 gene were not found, mutations were further examined with the multiple ligation probe amplification method on an ABI Prism3130xl (Applied Biosystems). In cases in which these two methods failed to find mutations in patients, SMAD3, ACTA2, and TGFB2 genes were additionally analyzed by bidirectional Sanger sequencing of exons and exon-intron boundaries. For patients without mutations in FBN1, TGFBR1, TGFBR2, SMAD3, ACTA2, or TGFB2 genes, exome sequencing was performed after TruSeq Exome enrichment on HiSeq1000 (Illumina) for searching mutations in MYH11, COL3A1, COLIAI (COL1A1), and COL1A2 genes [12–16]. Nonsense, missense, or splicing variations in these genes were further analyzed by Sanger sequencing if they were not present in SNP databases, predicted to be damaging by PolyPhen-2, or the SIFT program, or previously reported to be a pathogenic mutation.

Follow-up

Data were collected from hospital admission and out-patient medical records. All patients were regularly followed, either at our center or at other local hospitals. All of them underwent strict blood pressure control before leaving the hospital, with β-blockers in all cases and angiotensin II receptor blockers in some cases. The follow-up rate was 100% and the duration was 57.1 ± 43.0 (range, 6–132) months.

Statistical analysis

Two-tailed Student's t tests for continuous variables and chi-square tests for categorical variables were used to make univariate comparisons between the two groups. The long-term outcomes including re-dissection and re-operation were analyzed using Kaplan-Meier methods and compared with log-rank tests. The risk factors (see Appendix) for mortality and late aortic re-operations were estimated using a multivariate proportional hazard regression analysis (Cox model). A p value of <0.05 was considered statistically significant. SPSS software, version

22.0 for Windows (IBM SPSS Inc., Chicago, IL) was used for all calculations.

In this study, between the CTD and the non-CTD groups, the early and late outcomes of the initial aortic surgery for aortic dissection were compared to demonstrate the impact of CTD on the surgical outcomes in the patients with aortic dissection associated with CMN.

Results

Initial surgeries for aortic dissection

As shown in Table 4, in the CTD group, there were initial surgical repairs of the ascending aorta in 5 patients and the aortic arch in 9 patients. Simultaneous aortic root repairs were performed in 11 of these 14 patients. The others underwent repairs of the descending aorta (in 10 patients), the thoracoabdominal aorta (in 2 patients), and the abdominal aorta (in 4 patients). In the non-CTD group, the surgical repairs were for the ascending aorta in 3 patients and the aortic arch in 7 patients. Simultaneous aortic root repair was carried out in 1 patient. The other 3 patients underwent repairs of the descending aorta (in 1 patient) and the thoracoabdominal aorta (in 2 patients). There were concomitant mitral valve surgeries in 2 patients in the CTD group.

Histopathological findings

CMN classification showed minimal or no loss of elastic fibers in 3 patients (10%) and loss of elastic fibers in 27 patients (90%) of 30 CTD patients, whereas minimal or no loss of elastic fibers was found in 6 patients (46.2%) and loss of elastic fibers in 7 patients (53.8%) of 13 non-

CTD patients. The rate of loss of elastic fibers was significantly higher in the CTD group ($p = 0.014$).

Postoperative data

There were no early deaths. In the long term, despite of there being no late deaths, new aortic dissection occurred at the same sites (three-channel aortic dissection) in 3 patients or at different sites in 3 patients (a total of 6 patients [20.0%] of the CTD group), whereas only 1 patient (7.7%) in the non-CTD group developed it at a different site ($p = 0.310$). The absence of re-dissection was not significantly different between the two groups (log-rank, $p = 0.380$) (Fig. 2), that is, 83.2% in the CTD group and 85.7% in the non-CTD at 5 years.

In contrast, in all, there were no significant differences in the incidences of re-dissection and re-operation, when all of the patients were divided into the two patient groups according to the grade of CMN. Of 43 patients, 9 patients had no or minimal loss of elastic fibers (Grade 1+) and 34 patients had loss of elastic fibers (Grade 2+ or 3+). There were no occurrences of re-dissection and 5 (55.6%) patients required re-operation in the former group, whereas 7 patients (20.6%) developed re-dissection and 25 patients (73.5%) required re-operation in the latter group. However, interestingly, all 7 patients who suffered from aortic re-dissection had high-grade CMN, that is, loss of elastic fibers (Grade 2+ or 3+); these 7 patients consisted of 6 (22.2%) of 27 CTD patients and 1 (14.7%) of 7 non-CTD patients ($p = 0.951$).

There were no significant differences in the re-operation rates between the Stanford aortic dissection classification groups ($p = 0.332$), that is, 13 of 21 with type A (62.0%) and 17 of 22 with type B (77.3%). There were also no significant differences in the absence of aortic re-operation (log-rank, $p = 0.404$), that is, 13.8% with type A and 14.5% with type B at 5 years. In contrast, re-operations were required more frequently ($p = 0.037$); there were 24

Table 4 Initial surgery

Initial surgery (n = 43)	CTD (n = 30)	non-CTD (n = 13)	p value
Surgical site of aorta			
Ascending aorta	5 (16.7%)	3 (23.1%)	0.944
Aortic arch	9 (30.0%)	7 (53.8%)	0.253
Descending aorta	10 (33.3%)	1 (7.7%)	0.164
Thoraco-abdominal aorta	2 (6.7%)	2 (15.4%)	0.740
Abdominal aorta	4 (13.3%)	none	0.417
Simultaneous aortic root	11 (36.7%)	1 (7.7%)	0.115
Concomitant mitral valve surgery	2 (6.7%)	none	0.869
Conditions of false channel after the initial surgery			
Double barrel	23 (76.7%)	8 (61.5%)	0.519
Partial thrombosed	2 (6.7%)	2 (15.4%)	0.740
Thrombosed (IMH)	5 (16.7%)	3 (23.1%)	0.945

CTD genetically diagnosed connective tissue disease, *NS* no significant difference, *IMH* intramural hematoma

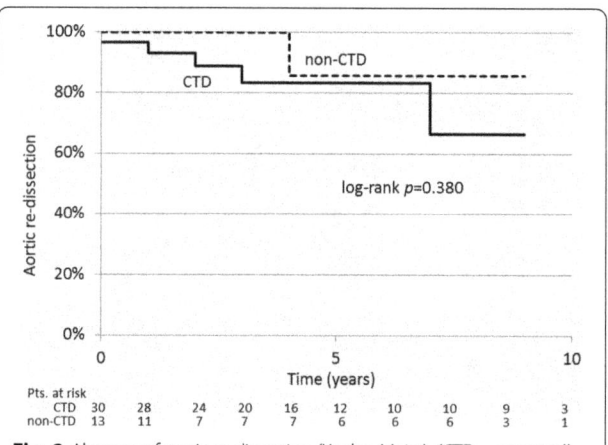

Fig. 2 Absence of aortic re-dissection (Kaplan-Meier). (CTD = genetically diagnosed connective tissue disease)

(80.0%) patients in the CTD group versus 6 patients (46.0%) in the non-CTD group. *The absence of aortic reoperation tended to be worse* (log-rank, $p = 0.052$), that is, 7.9% in the CTD group and 31.0% in the non-CTD group at 5 years (Fig. 3). *Twelve of 24 CTD patients (50.0%) and 3 of 6 non-CTD patients (50.0%) required thirdly surgical interventions.* Despite no substantial differences in the initial and following surgical procedures between the two patient groups, the rate of surgical interventions to the descending aorta was significantly higher in the CTD group ($p = 0.021$), that is, 16 patients (53.3%) versus 2 patients (15.4%). The rate of surgical interventions to the aortic root was also significantly higher in the CTD group ($p = 0.037$), that is, 15 patients (50.0%) versus 2 patients (15.4%). Regarding the time frame for aortic re-interventions, 15 of 24 patients (62.5%) in the CTD group underwent re-operations during the two years of follow-up after the initial surgery, compared with 3 of 6 patients (50.0%) in the non-CTD group. Univariate analysis revealed that patent false channel ($p = 0.019$), and simultaneous aortic root repair ($p = 0.024$) were significant risk factors for re-operation. In the multivariate analysis of risk factors for re-operation, patent false channel, simultaneous aortic root repair, and preoperative systemic hypertension were independent risk factors (Table 5).

Discussion

CMN is often observed in the resected aorta in patients with CTD and tends to be associated with the worst long-term prognoses; this also causes aortic dilatation and dissection in non-CTD patients as well as in CTD patients [1, 17, 18]. However, it is difficult to demonstrate pathologically remarkable differences in the fragmentation of elastic fibers and accumulation of extracellular matrix in the formation of the cystic structures between CTD and non-CTD patients, especially in elderly patients with systemic hypertension [4, 5]. In this study, we hypothesized

Table 5 Multivariate analysis of risk foctors for re-operation

Variables	HR	95% CI	p value
Patient-related risk factors			
Hypertension	3.45	1.12–10.63	0.031
Dissection-related risk factor			
Patent false channel	5.22	1.37–19.89	0.016
Procedure-related risk factor			
Simultaneous aortic root repair	4.31	1.37–13.60	0.013

HR hazard ratio, *CI* confidence i

that coexistence of genetically identified CTD would be associated with worse postoperative prognoses after surgeries for aortic dissection in patients with CMN. To elucidate it, we compared early and late outcomes, including occurrence of new aortic events after the initial surgeries for aortic dissection of CMN-positive patients, between the CTD and non-CTD groups.

CMN might be due to long-term hemodynamic forces (hypertension) and age [4, 5]. It was demonstrated that patients with CMN have increased risks of serious vascular complications [19, 20]. However, few studies have seemed to look at adverse effects of CMN on the surgical outcomes of aortic dissection, as far as we investigated. With regard to findings of histological examinations, Trotter and Olsen reported that the degrees of elastic fragmentation were variable in Marfan patients, and can also be found even in non-Marfan subjects [4]. Nakajima et al. pointed out a higher degree of elastic fiber loss or fragmentation in Marfan patients, compared with non-Marfan patients having CMN [21]. Similarly, in our study, the grade of loss or fragmentation of elastic fibers was higher in the CTD patients than that of the non-CTD patients. Clinically, in this study, the age of the onset of initial aortic dissection was also significantly younger in the CTD patients, and aortic re-dissection occurred only in the patients with high-grade CMN, that is, loss of elastic fibers. Such clinical phenomena may be affected directly by such fragility of the aortic walls due to higher degree of loss or fragmentation of elastic fibers in the aortic wall. Consequently, the presence of coexisting CTD should be suspected or examined genetically in relatively young patients with higher grades of loss or fragmentation of elastic fibers in the aortic wall.

With regard to occurrence of re-dissection in the long term after the initial aortic dissection, the incidence was higher in CTD patients, despite no significant statistical differences. Interestingly, in the CTD group, 2 patients had suffered from three-channel dissection before the initial surgery and another 3 patients developed it in the long term after surgery; this may show a more severe fragility of the degenerative aortic wall in CTD patients. In the histopathological examinations, the grades of loss or fragmentation of elastic fibers were higher in CTD

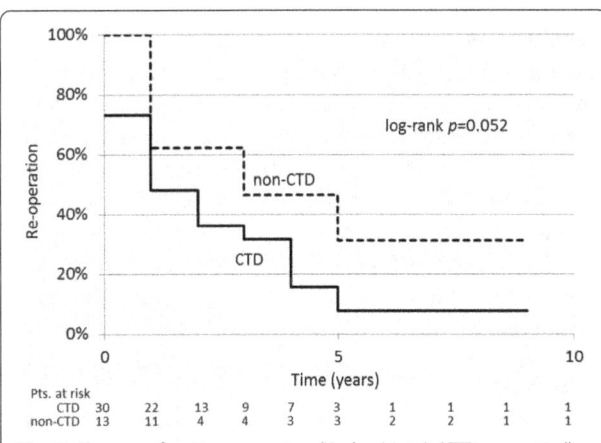

Fig. 3 Absence of aortic re-operation (Kaplan-Meier). (CTD = genetically diagnosed connective tissue disease)

patients than in those of the non-CTD group. Looking at the relationship between the histopathological findings and the re-dissection rate, there were no significant differences between patients with no or minimal loss of elastic fibers and those with loss of elastic fibers. However, interestingly, all of the CTD and non-CTD patients suffering from aortic re-dissection had high-grade CMN, that is, loss of elastic fibers in the histopathological examinations. Consequently, it is important to estimate the long-term outcome after initial surgery for aortic dissection according to the results of genetic examinations as well as the histopathological findings.

In contrast, regarding re-operations, in CTD patients, higher rates of redo surgery were reported than in non-CTD patients [22, 23]. In our study, redo surgeries were also required more frequently in CTD patients. In particular, the rate of descending aortic repairs was significantly higher, compared with non-CTD patients. In patients with CMN combined with CTD, higher onset rates of type B aortic dissection were demonstrated than the others [24]. Our study also demonstrated the higher rate of type B aortic dissection in CTD patients. Related to this issue, Schoenhoff et al. reported that 86% of Marfan patients with type B aortic dissection required redo surgery for residual aortic enlargement [25]. In our study, similar findings were revealed. In the CTD group, 80.0% of the patients required re-operations after the initial surgical repairs in the long term, 72.7% in type A and 84.2% in type B.

The rate of surgical interventions to the aortic root was also significantly higher in the CTD group. Progressive enlargement of the aortic root is one of the characteristics of CTD patients, which is related directly to the early onset of type A aortic dissection. In cases with aortic root enlargement of 40 to 50 mm in diameter, prophylactic root repairs such as aortic valve-sparing surgery or composite valve-graft root replacement are recommended in the guidelines to eliminate risks of ruptured type A aortic dissection [26]. Progressive aortic root enlargement also should be one of the reasons for redo surgery after various surgical repairs for type A or B aortic dissection, whether it is associated with aortic dissection or not. In our study, a total of 39.5% of all patients underwent aortic root repairs; this included 63.6% of CTD patients and 20.0% of non-CTD patients with type A aortic dissection, and 42.1% of CTD patients with type B aortic dissection. Moreover, simultaneous aortic root repair was a significant risk factor for re-operation in the univariate and multivariate analyses. Consequently, these circumstances resulted in the higher rates of redo surgeries in the CTD patients.

Obviously, there are some limitations to this study. First, this is a retrospective study dealing with a small number of enrolled patients. In particular, the number of the patients undergoing genetic examinations was too small to elucidate exactly the impact of CTD on the outcomes of surgeries for aortic dissection. Aortic dissection was also variable, such as acute or chronic, and type A or B. Apart from the histological aortic pathologies, there are other factors or requirements for redo surgeries after initial surgeries for aortic dissection, relating to types of aortic dissection, conditions of the false channels, surgical techniques, extent of repairs, and so on. The surgical procedures of the initial operations for aortic dissection were variable, which depended on a variety of conditions, including the stages of aortic dissection, such as acute and chronic, and the settings of the surgery, such as emergent/urgent and elective. Theoretically, the re-operation rates become significantly higher in cases with no tear resection and patent false channel [27, 28]. Actually, there may be some differences in the incidences of re-operation between limited ascending/hemiarch replacement and entire arch replacement. The rates should also be different after the total arch replacement between with or without elephant trunk procedures on the distal anastomosis site [29]. The conditions of aortic dissection, including the patency of the false channel, were also variable. More detailed studies dealing with a larger number of patients is required to elucidate precisely the impact of genetically identified CTD on the surgical outcomes of aortic dissection in patients with CMN.

Finally, most (90.0%) of the CTD patients showed high-grade CMN, that is, loss of elastic fibers. However, similar findings were also found in a half (53.8%) of non-CTD patients. The genetic examinations are still limited by the issue of availability. There might be other different CTDs with unknown genetic characteristics. Consequently, in case of high-grade CMN, it is necessary to recognize, even without genetically diagnosed CTD at present, potentially high-risk subjects who would develop re-dissection and require re-operations at relatively shorter intervals after surgery for aortic dissection.

Conclusions

Patients with CTD as well as CMN in the aortic wall tend to develop aortic dissection, particularly of type B, at an earlier age. They require re-operation more frequently due to enlargement of the residual dissecting aorta and/or the aortic root, compared with non-CTD patients. Therefore, closer and stricter follow-up with medication and with earlier and more adequate surgical treatments including more extended repairs should be considered for such high-risk patients having CTD and CMN, and for some non-CTD patients having high-grade CMN.

Abbreviations

CMN: Cystic medial necrosis; CTD: Connective tissue disease

Acknowledgements
Not applicable.

Funding
None.

Authors' contributions
TF carried out the molecular genetic studies, participated in the sequence alignment and drafted the manuscript. TM and HM carried out the genetic examinations. YI and HIU carried out the histopathological examination. TF participated in the design of the study and performed the statistical analysis. HO and KM conceived of the study, and participated in its design and coordination and helped to draft the manuscript. All authors read and approved the final manuscript.

Competing interests
The authors declare that they have no competing interests.

Author details
[1]Departments of Cardiovascular Surgery, National Cerebral and Cardiovascular Center, Osaka, Japan. [2]Departments of Pathology, National Cerebral and Cardiovascular Center, Osaka, Japan. [3]Departments of Bioscience and Genetics, National Cerebral and Cardiovascular Center, Osaka, Japan. [4]Cardiovascular Surgery, Tokyo Medical University, 6-7-1 Nishishinjuku Shinjuku-ku Tokyo, 160, Tokyo –0023, Japan.

References

1. Girdauskas E, Kuntze T, Borger MA, Doenst T, Mochalski M, Walther T, et al. Long-term prognosis of type a aortic dissection in non-Marfan patients with histologic pattern of cystic medial necrosis. Ann Thorac Surg. 2008;85(3):972–7.
2. Marsalese DL, Moodie DS, Lytle BW, Cosgrove DM, Ratliff NB, Goormastic M, et al. Cystic medial necrosis of the aorta in patients without Marfan's syndrome: surgical outcome and long-term follow-up. J Am Coll Cardiol. 1990;16(1):68–73.
3. Larson EW, Edwards WD. Risk factors for aortic dissection: a necropsy study of 161 cases. Am J Cardiol. 1984;53(6):849–55.
4. Trotter SE, Olsen EG. Marfan's disease and Erdheim's cystic medionecrosis. A study of their pathology. Eur Heart J. 1991;12(1):83–7.
5. Schlatmann TJ, Becker AE. Histologic changes in the normal aging aorta: implications for dissecting aortic aneurysm. Am J Cardiol. 1977;39(1):13–20.
6. Tanaka H, Ogino H, Matsuda H, Minatoya K, Sasaki H, Iba Y. Midterm outcome of valve-sparing aortic root replacement in inherited connective tissue disorders. Ann Thorac Surg. 2011;92(5):1646–9.
7. Roberts WC, Vowels TJ, Ko JM, Filardo G, Hebeler RF Jr, Henry AC, et al. Comparison of the structure of the aortic valve and ascending aorta in adults having aortic valve replacement for aortic stenosis versus for pure aortic regurgitation and resection of the ascending aorta for aneurysm. Circulation. 2011;123(8):896–903.
8. Morisaki H, Akutsu K, Ogino H, Kondo N, Yamanaka I, Tsutsumi Y, et al. Mutation of ACTA2 gene as an important cause of familial and nonfamilial nonsyndromatic thoracic aortic aneurysm and/or dissection (TAAD). Hum Mutat. 2009;30(10):1406–11.
9. Dietz HC, Cutting GR, Pyeritz RE, Maslen CL, Sakai LY, Corson GM, et al. Marfan syndrome caused by a recurrent de novo missense mutation in the fibrillin gene. Nature. 1991;352(6333):337–9.
10. Mizuguchi T, Collod-Beroud G, Akiyama T, Abifadel M, Harada N, Morisaki T, et al. Heterozygous TGFBR2 mutations in Marfan syndrome. Nat Genet. 2004;36(8):855–60.
11. Loeys BL, Chen J, Neptune ER, Judge DP, Podowski M, Holm T, et al. A syndrome of altered cardiovascular, craniofacial, neurocognitive and skeletal development caused by mutations in TGFBR1 or TGFBR2. Nat Genet. 2005; 37(3):275–81.
12. De Paepe A, Devereux RB, Dietz HC, Hennekam RC, Pyeritz RE. Revised diagnostic criteria for the Marfan syndrome. Am J Med Genet. 1996; 62(4):417–26.
13. Guo DC, Papke CL, Tran-Fadulu V, Regalado ES, Avidan N, Johnson RJ, et al. Mutations in smooth muscle alpha-actin (ACTA2) cause coronary artery disease, stroke, and Moyamoya disease, along with thoracic aortic disease. Am J Hum Genet. 2009;84(5):617–27.
14. Superti-Furga A, Gugler E, Gitzelmann R, Steinmann B. Ehlers-Danlos syndrome type IV: a multi-exon deletion in one of the two COL3A1 alleles affecting structure, stability, and processing of type III procollagen. J Biol Chem. 1988;263(13):6226–32.
15. Zhu L, Vranckx R, Khau Van Kien P, Lalande A, Boisset N, et al. Mutations in myosin heavy chain 11 cause a syndrome associating thoracic aortic aneurysm/aortic dissection and patent ductus arteriosus. Nat Genet. 2006; 38(3):343–9.
16. Pannu H, Tran-Fadulu V, Papke CL, Scherer S, Liu Y, Presley C, et al. MYH11 mutations result in a distinct vascular pathology driven by insulin-like growth factor 1 and angiotensin II. Hum Mol Genet. 2007;16(20):2453–62.
17. Bähr M, Postler E, Meyermann R. Fatal stroke in a patient with carotid and middle cerebral artery dissection associated with cystic medial necrosis. J Neurol. 1996;243(10):722–3.
18. Takeda K, Matsumiya G, Nishimura M, Matsue H, Tomita Y, Sawa Y. Giant circumflex coronary artery aneurysm associated with cystic medial necrosis in a non-Marfan patient. Ann Thorac Surg. 2007;83(2):668–70.
19. Pande AK, Gosselin G, Leclerc Y, Leung TK. Aortic dissection complicating coronary angioplasty in cystic medial necrosis. Am Heart J. 1996;131:1221–3.
20. Isner JM, Donaldson RF, Fulton D, Bhan I, Payne DD, Cleveland RJ. Cystic medial necrosis in coarctation of the aorta: a potential factor contributing to adverse consequences observed after percutaneous balloon angioplasty of coarctation sites. Circulation. 1987;75:689–95.
21. Nakashima Y, Kurozumi T, Sueishi K, Tanaka K. Dissecting aneurysm: a clinicopathologic and histopathologic study of 111 autopsied cases. Hum Pathol. 1990;21(3):291–6.
22. Finkbohner R, Johnston D, Crawford ES, Coselli J, Milewicz DM. Marfan syndrome long-term survival and complications after aortic aneurysm repair. Circulation. 1995;91:728–33.
23. Iba Y, Minatoya K, Matsuda H, Sasaki H, Tanaka H, Ogino H, et al. Surgical experience with aggressive aortic pathologic process in Loeys-Dietz syndrome. Ann Thorac Surg. 2012;94(5):1413–7.
24. Cameron DE, Alejo DE, Patel ND, Nwakanma LU, Weiss ES, Vricella LA, et al. Aortic root replacement in 372 Marfan patients: evolution of operative repair over 30 years. Ann Thorac Surg. 2009;87:1344–9.
25. Scharfschwerdt M, Sievers HH, Greggersen J, Hanke T, Misfeld M. Prosthetic replacement of the ascending aorta increases wall tension in the residual aorta. Ann Thorac Surg. 2007;83(3):954–7.
26. Judge DP, Dietz HC. Marfan's syndrome. Lancet. 2005;366(9501):1965–76.
27. Heinemann M, Laas J, Borst HG, et al. Surgery extended into the aortic arch in acute type a dissection. Indications, techniques, and results. Circulation. 1991;84(5 Suppl):III25–30.
28. Girdauskas E, Kuntze T, Borger MA, Falk V, Mohr FW. Distal aortic reinterventions after root surgery in Marfan patients. Ann Thorac Surg. 2008; 86(6):1815–9.
29. Watanuki H, Ogino H, Minatoya K, Matsuda H, Sasaki H, Ando M, et al. Is emergency total arch replacement with a modified elephant trunk techniquejustified for acute type a aortic dissection? Ann Thorac Surg. 2007; 84(5):1585–91.

11

Modified 'candy-plug' technique for chronic type B aortic dissection with aneurysmal dilatation

Sohsyu Kotani[1][*] (iD), Yoshito Inoue[1], Mio Kasai[1], Satoru Suzuki[1] and Takashi Hachiya[2]

Abstract

Background: The original 'candy-plug' technique has been reported to be beneficial for the treatment of residual perfused false lumen in patients with aortic dissection. However, this technique is also associated with several problems, such as narrowing of the true lumen and damage to the flap or vessel wall. Therefore, we modified the procedure to overcome these problems. Here we report a case in which the patient was successfully treated using the modified procedure.

Case presentation: A 59-year-old man presented with chronic type B aortic dissection with aneurysmal dilatation. The patient had undergone prosthetic graft replacement of the ascending aorta for acute type A aortic dissection 3 years previously and replacement of the descending aorta for residual type B aortic dissection with aneurysmal dilatation 1 year previously. After these procedures, the residual false lumen aneurysm of the distal descending aorta expanded to 57-mm in diameter. Endovascular stent grafting was successfully performed using the modified 'candy-plug' technique with relining of the true lumen and occlusion of the false lumen. The patient was discharged 10 days after the procedure. Follow-up imaging at 1 year showed a completely thrombosed false lumen aneurysm.

Conclusion: The modified 'candy-plug' technique is useful for treatment of residual type B aortic dissection with aneurysmal dilatation.

Keywords: Candy-plug technique, Residual type B aortic dissection with aneurysmal dilatation, Endovascular repair

Background

Recently, thoracic endovascular aortic repair (TEVAR) has become a useful operative treatment for complicated chronic type B aortic dissection by covering the primary entry. However, retrograde flow through distal entries or branch vessels makes complete false lumen thrombosis difficult.

Successful exclusion of the false lumen in chronic dissection remains a challenge. Survival is associated with aortic remodelling, which is related to persistence of flow in the false lumen [1].

The original 'candy-plug' technique was described for occlusion of a large false lumen aneurysm of the descending aorta using a 'candy-shaped' stent-graft [2]. However, endovascular intervention with this technique alone still has two major problems: 1. the possibility of narrowing the true lumen by compression of the 'candy-plug' stent [3] and 2. The possibility of flap or vessel wall injury by the stent [3]. To avoid these complications, we designed an efficient modification of the 'candy-plug' device, which is deployed adjacent to the distal end of the stent-graft in the true lumen at the same distal end.

Here, we report a case of residual type B chronic aortic dissection with aneurysmal dilatation that was successfully treated using the modified 'candy-plug' technique with an Excluder aortic extender after a staged operation for type A aortic dissection.

Case presentation

A 59-year-old man with a medical history of hypertension and smoking was diagnosed with acute type A aortic dissection in 2012. The patient underwent emergency surgery, and prosthetic graft replacement of the ascending aorta was performed. Residual type B aortic dissection

---
* Correspondence: sohsyu_k@yahoo.co.jp
[1]Department of Cardiovascular Surgery, Hiratsuka City Hospital, Kanagawa, Japan
Full list of author information is available at the end of the article

with a perfused false lumen aneurysm from the proximal aortic arch to the right iliac artery was followed up by periodic computed tomography angiography (CTA) every 6 months. In 2015, the patient underwent prosthetic graft replacement using a 28-mm Dacron graft (J-Graft SHIELD NEO; Japan Lifeline Co., Ltd., Tokyo, Japan) from the hemi-arch to the descending aorta due to false lumen aneurysm dilatation. Six months after the second procedure, retrograde blood flow persisted through the distal entry in the false lumen, and the dissection with false lumen aneurysm expanded from 47 to 57-mm at its maximum diameter (Fig. 1). It also exhibited a 28-mm false lumen aneurysm and an 8-mm true lumen immediately above the celiac trunk. To dilate the true lumen and occlude the large false lumen, TEVAR was performed using the modified 'candy-plug' technique.

Two Conformable TAG stent-grafts (TGU282820J, TGU343420J; W. L. Gore & Associates, Flagstaff, AZ, USA) were selected to deploy in the true lumen. Since proximal diameter was the same as a 28-mm prosthetic graft, a 34*200-mm aortic stent-graft was chosen for proximal true lumen to achieve oversizing by just 20%. The dissection with false lumen aneurysm tapered toward the celiac trunk (8-mm true lumen and 28-mm false lumen), therefore a 28*200-mm aortic stent-graft (two sizes smaller than the proximal device in diameter) was chosen for distal true lumen. Length of thoracic coverage from a 28-mm prosthetic graft to the level of celiac trunk was 168-mm. To keep adequate landing zone, two different size of stent-grafts were required. A 36*45-mm Excluder aortic extender (PLA360400J; W. L.

Gore & Associates, Flagstaff, AZ, USA) was chosen for placement of the 'candy-plug' in the distal false lumen based on the preoperative CTA results.

This procedure was performed under general anesthesia. To prepare the 'candy-plug' device, a 36*45-mm Excluder aortic extender was partially unloaded from the delivery system. To restrict opening of the stent-graft, a 2–0 Ethibond (Ethicon, Somerville, NJ, USA) suture was placed at the middle of the stent-graft, also using a 22-Fr DrySeal Sheath (DSL2228; W. L. Gore & Associates, Flagstaff, AZ, USA) to limit its maximum diameter to 10-mm, producing a shape similar to a wrapped candy (Fig. 2). Then, the stent-graft was reloaded and prepared in a standard manner.

The patient had a false lumen of the left femoral artery and a true lumen of the right femoral artery. First, a Radifocus guidewire (RF-GA35183; Terumo Medical, NJ, USA) was placed through the false lumen via an 8-Fr left femoral sheath, and then a double curve Lunderquist guidewire (TSCMG-35-300-LESDC-JP; Cook Medical, Bloomington, IN, USA) was positioned carefully in exchange for the Radifocus guidewire. Second, a Radifocus guidewire and a double curve Lunderquist guidewire were placed through the true lumen via the right femoral artery in a similar manner. Third, TEVAR was performed via a 24-Fr right femoral sheath. A 28*200-mm Conformable TAG stent-graft was placed in the small true lumen of the descending aorta immediately above the celiac trunk, and then a 34*200-mm Conformable TAG stent-graft was placed at the mid-portion of the 28-mm prosthetic graft of the descending aorta. Next, a customized 36*45-mm Excluder aortic extender was deployed in the large false lumen at the

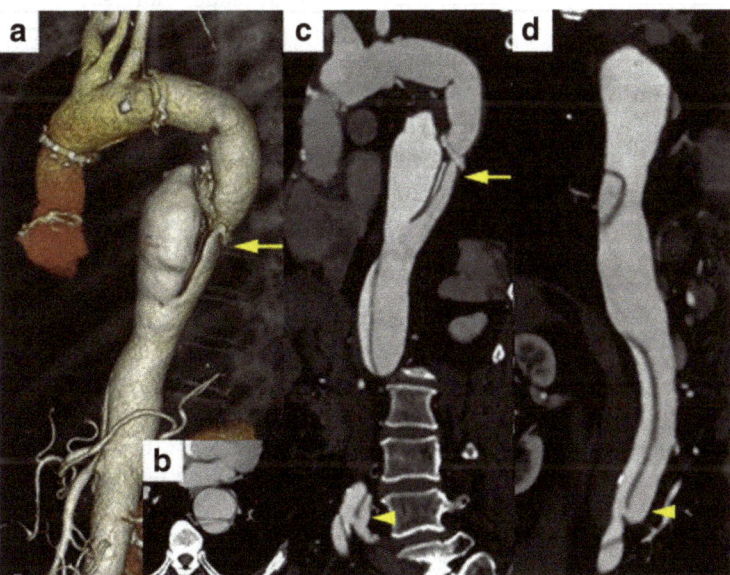

Fig. 1 a Preoperative 3D–CTA imaging of a 59-year-old patient showing an aortic dissection with a 28-mm false lumen aneurysm and an 8-mm true lumen immediately above the celiac trunk. **b** An axial slice at the level of the arrow showing the aortic dissection with a 57-mm triple lumen aneurysm. **c, d** A saggital slice showing a major distal entry just above the aortic bifurcation (arrowhead)

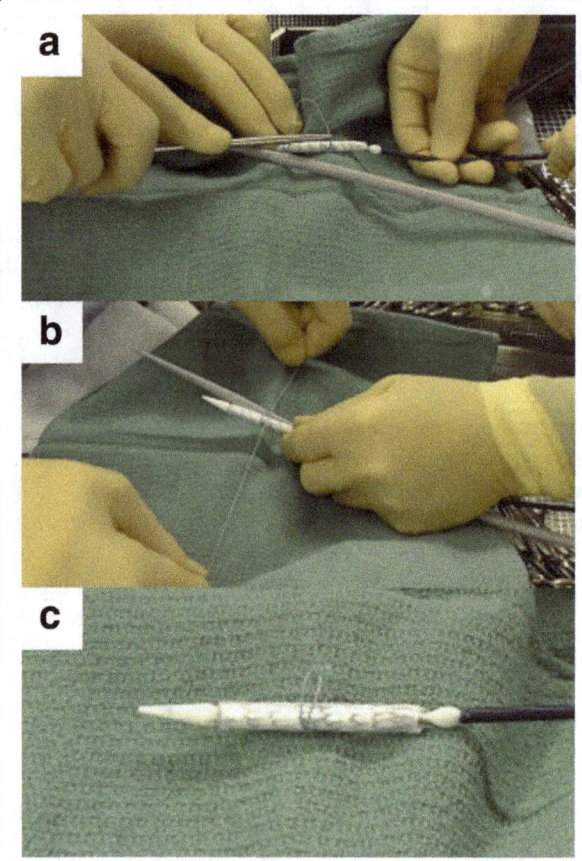

Fig. 2 How to prepare the 'candy-plug' device. **a** A 2–0 polyester suture placed at the middle of the stent-graft to restrict opening of the stent-graft. **b** Using a 22-Fr sheath to limits its maximum diameter of its waist to 10-mm. **c** After customization of the stent-graft. Then the stent-graft was reloaded and prepared in a standard fashion

dissection. Kölbel et al. originally described this technique using a Zenith TX-2 ProForm stent-graft (Cook Medical, Bloomington, IN, USA) [2]. In this report, the plug was placed in a false lumen in which the true lumen is guarded by a stent-graft. Rholffs et al. reported early results of 18 patients using this 'candy-plug' technique for endovascular false lumen occlusion in chronic aortic dissection [4]. They said their technique was feasible and associated with low morbidity and mortality due to its minimal invasiveness [4].

Ogawa et al. recommended using an Excluder aortic extender for the 'candy-plug' device instead of the Zenith TX-2 due to the ease of modification [3]. However, they placed it at an unprotected level without a stent-graft in the true lumen. They were also concerned about the possibility of complications caused by the 'candy-plug' device. One of the technical problems of the 'candy-plug' is the possibility of narrowing the true lumen as the result of expanding the 'candy-plug' within the false lumen [3]. This possibility presents the risk of thrombosis of the branch vessels, which are located near the distal entries. Another concern is the possibility of flap or vessel wall injury due to continuous shear stress from the 'candy-plug' device [3].

Disproportionate stress from the 'candy-plug' device edge has the risk of intimal injury [5]. According to this previous report, the intimal flap is barely stabilized by being sandwiched the embolized false lumen and stented true lumen. We think that a stent-graft in the true lumen should be deployed at the level of distal end of the occluder device in the false lumen.

Our modified 'candy-plug' technique with an Excluder aortic extender can reduce the risk of these complications by deploying it adjacent to the distal end of the stent-graft in the true lumen. A stent-graft in the true lumen can avoid narrowing the true lumen and will thus protect the flap from damage by the 'candy-plug' device.

We chose 34-mm and 28-mm aortic stent grafts for the true lumen and a 'candy-shaped' 36*45-mm Excluder aortic extender for the false lumen while using a 28-mm prosthetic graft in the descending aorta; the 28-mm false lumen aneurysm and the 8-mm true lumen were located immediately above the celiac trunk. In TEVAR for aortic dissection, the size of stent-graft is determined by the diameter of the proximal landing zone. Generally, 10–20% oversizing of the stent-graft based on the proximal landing zone diameter is recommended. In this case, since proximal diameter was the same as a 28-mm prosthetic graft, a 34*200-mm stent-graft was chosen for proximal true lumen to achieve oversizing by just 20%. The dissection with false lumen aneurysm tapered toward the celiac trunk, therefore a two sizes smaller diameter stent-graft was chosen for distal true lumen. A 36*45-mm Excluder aortic extender was selected because of the easy modification and based on the mean

distal end of the 28*200-mm Conformable TAG stent-graft via a 24-Fr left femoral sheath. Finally, a 16-mm Amplatzer Vascular Plug II (9-AVP2–016; AGA Medical Corp., North Plymouth, MN, USA) was placed into the center of the 'candy-plug' of the Excluder extender to complete the occlusion. Postprocedural angiography demonstrated no major complications and no residual retrograde flow into the false lumen aneurysm.

The patient was discharged on the 10th postoperative day without any complications.

Follow-up CTA at 1 month post-TEVAR showed no endoleak and almost complete thrombosis of the false lumen above the 'candy-plug' device. CTA at 1 year also showed decreased maximum aneurysm diameter (47-mm), greater expansion of the true lumen, and volume reduction of the thrombosed false lumen (Fig. 3).

Discussion

The 'candy-plug' technique is a useful treatment option for occlusion of the false lumen in chronic type B aortic

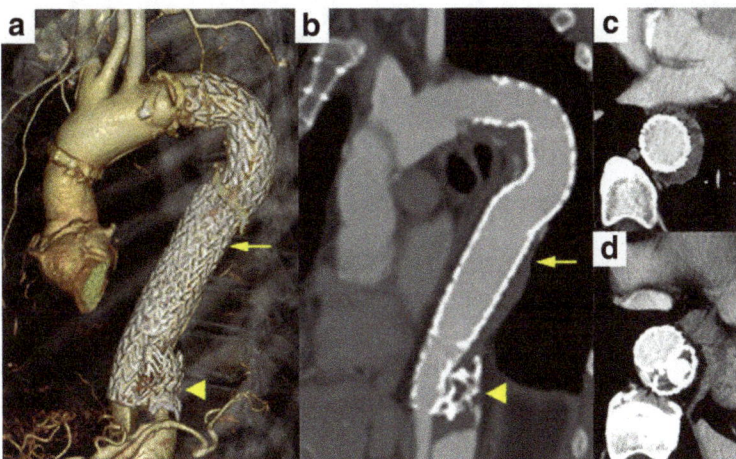

Fig. 3 a Postoperative 3D–CTA imaging 1 year after TEVAR with implantation of a 'candy-plug'. **b** A saggital slice showing the 'candy-plug' device with the Amplatzer vascular plug. **c** Decreased aneurysm diameter and false lumen thrombus formation (at the level of the arrow). **d** The 'candy-plug' with the Amplatzer vascular plug filling the central lumen (at the level of arrowhead)

diameter of false lumen which was 31.3-mm. It is difficult to determine the appropriate size of stent-grafts because the thrombosed false lumen will become smaller after 'candy-plug' deployment, and the radial force of its frame may increase. Kölbel et al. selected their customized 42-mm TX-2 ProForm stent-graft based on preoperative CTA results, which identified a false lumen diameter < 36-mm. Ogawa et al. based the diameter of their Excluder extender on the mean diameter of the false lumen observed on axial CTA images.

This case had the risk of paraplegia due to long coverage with total false lumen thrombosis. The incidence of symptomatic spinal cord ischemia after TEVAR is ranging between 1 and 5% [6]. Some patients with occluded lower thoracic levels may not suffer from paraplegia whereas others with these segments preserved may well show symptomatic spinal cord ischemia. There are 4 vascular territories supplying the spinal cord (left subclavian, intercostal, lumbar, and hypogastric arteries) and simultaneous closure of some of these vascular territories has association with symptomatic spinal cord injury [6]. We could keep these arteries except intercostal arteries in this case. In addition, we always avoid intraoperative prolonged hypotension. This case didn't show no sign of paraplegia in the perioperative period.

Conclusion

We performed a successful endovascular repair using the modified 'candy-plug' technique for a residual large false lumen aneurysm in the descending aorta. This technique has the potential to effectively occlude large distal false lumen aneurysms within chronic aortic dissection with aneurysmal dilatation.

Abbreviations

CTA: Computed tomography angiography; TEVAR: Thoracic endovascular aortic repair

Acknowledgements

Not applicable.

Funding

The authors declare no funding for this publication.

Authors' contributions

SK was a major contributor in writing the manuscript. YI and TH performed described surgery, interpreted data, and revised manuscript. MK and SS conceived of the study and participated in its design and coordination. All authors read and approved the final manuscript.

Competing interests

The authors declare that they have no competing interests.

Author details

[1]Department of Cardiovascular Surgery, Hiratsuka City Hospital, Kanagawa, Japan. [2]Department of Cardiovascular Surgery, Kawasaki City Hospital, Kanagawa, Japan.

References

1. Mani K, Clough RE, OTA L, et al. Predictors of outcome after endovascular repair for chronic type B dissection. Eur J Vasc Endovasc Surg. 2012;43:386–91.
2. Kölbel T, Lohrenz C, Kieback A, et al. Distal false lumen occlusion in aortic dissection with a homemade extra-large vascular plug: the candy-plug technique. J Endovasc Ther. 2013;10:484–9.
3. Ogawa Y, Nishimaki H, Chiba K, et al. Candy-plug technique using an excluder aortic extender for distal occlusion of a large false lumen aneurysm in chronic aortic dissection. J Endovasc Ther. 2016;23:483–6.

4. Rohlffs F, Tsilimparis N, Fiorucci B, et al. The candy-plug technique: technical aspects and early results of a new endovascular method for false lumen occulusion in chronic aortic dissection. J Endovasc Ther. 2017;24:549–55.
5. Furukawa T, Uchida N, Yamane Y, et al. A pitfall of false lumen embolization in chronic aortic dissection: intimal injury caused by the embolization device edge. Interact Cardiovasc Thorac Surg. 2017;24:153–5.
6. Czerny M, Eggebrecht H, Sodeck G, et al. Mechanisms of symptomatic spinal cord ischemia after TEVAR. J Endovasc Ther. 2012;19:37–43.

12

Retrograde type a dissection in a 24th gestational week pregnant patient – the importance of interdisciplinary interaction to a successful outcome

Jerry Easo[1]*[iD], Michael Horst[1], Bernhard Schmuck[2], Rohit Philip Thomas[2], Steffen Saupe[3], Malte Book[4] and Alexander Weymann[1]

Abstract

Background: Type A Dissection in pregnancy is a devastating medical condition with 2 lives at stake and unclear strategy at early gestational stages. We describe a successful outcome, clearly dependent on the coordination of all involved disciplines.

Case presentation: This case history describes a 28 year old female with a 24th week pregnancy gravida 2 para 0 with a DeBakey Type I aortic dissection, diagnosed via ultrasound. Surgery was perfomed on the day of diagnosis. After conferral with the mother, caesarean section was performed and a 690 g fetus could be delivered and was immediately transferred to the neonatal unit. Subsequent aortic repair was performed after hysterectomy, with replacement of the ascending aorta and hemiarch treatment. Intraoperatively no entry in the ascending aorta or transverse arch could be demonstrated, so that a retrograde Type A with entry distal to the left subclavian had to be postulated. We decided to perform subsequent computer tomography, demonstrating multiple entry sites in the descending aorta distal to the left subclavian artery. Successful endovascular treatment could be performed with a Medtronic Valiant Stent via a transfemoral approach. The further hospital stay was uneventful and the patient could be discharged on the 18th postoperative day. The baby demonstrated fighter qualities and could be discharged home after a 3 month hospital stay to be reunited with his mother.

Conclusion: Prompt diagnosis, precise coordination between all involved subspecialties and ultimately, as in this case, definitive treatment in consensus with operative and interventional departments have led to a successful outcome and encourages us in our daily struggle in this often demanding surgery.

Keywords: Aortic dissection, Pregnancy, Stent-grafting

Background

Aortic dissection remains a devastating medical condition with a prevalence of estimated 2.9 per 100,000 person years [1], associated mainly with arterial hypertension and often related to connective tissue disorders such as Marfan's Syndrome or Ehlers Danlos Syndrome. In pregnancy, acute aortic type A dissection has an overall incidence of 0.4 per 100,000 person years, often presenting in the third trimester attributed to hemodynamic alterations taking place in late pregnancy. In woman under 40 years of age half of all aortic dissections occur during pregnancy or during the peri-partum period [2]. Gestational hypertension, pre-eclampsia and hormonal changes during pregnancy may predispose to aortic dissection, in addition high levels of oestrogen and progesterone may cause degeneration of the aortic wall, similar to cystic medial necrosis [3–8]. Early diagnosis and successful coordination of care between the cardiothoracic surgeon, anaesthesiology, interventional radiologist, obstetrician and paediatrician is mandatory for successful outcome of such complex patients.

* Correspondence: easo.jerry@klinikum-oldenburg.de
[1]Department of Cardiac Surgery, European Medical School Oldenburg-Groningen, University Hospital Oldenburg, Carl von Ossietzky University Oldenburg, Rahel Straus Str. 10, 26133 Oldenburg, Germany
Full list of author information is available at the end of the article

Case presentation

A 28 year old woman with a 24th -week intrauterine pregnancy gravida 2 para 0 was admitted to the emergency department of the referring hospital with chest and back pain. Ultrasound diagnostic demonstrated pericardial effusion and a dissection membrane in the ascending and descending aorta (Fig. 1). The patient was immediately transferred with the diagnosis of a DeBakey Type I Aortic dissection. Further comorbidities included arterial hypertension, renal insufficiency stage 4 with a history of kidney transplant 2014 after preeclampsia after childbirth 2007, among others.. Initial consensus was found to minimise the operative risk for the mother and to perform surgery leaving the fetus in vivo and choosing an optimal operative strategy with a mild hypothermia and arch inspection to limit the period of circulatory arrest to an absolute minimum. After conferring with the pregnant mother however, she decided to deliver the baby via caesarean section despite the early phase of prior to aortic repair. To minimise the perioperative risk of bleeding the patient consented to an operative hysterectomy before heparinisation for the establishment of extracorporal circulation.

Surgery was performed on the day of diagnosis in a collaborative manner, with induction of general anaesthesia immediately prior to caesarean section performed via a Misgav Ladach operative technique and subsequent supracervical hysterectomy. The fetus was immediately transferred to the neonatal paediatricians, the initial body weight was 690 g with an APGAR 2/4/6 and a naval pH of 7.19.. After semi-closure of the abdomen we proceeded with the surgical treatment of the aortic dissection. Arterial cannulation was established via the right subclavian artery, mild hypothermia was targeted and exposition of the aorta and supraaortic vessels was achieved. Aortotomy demonstrated the dissection reaching into the acoronary sinus, the right and left coronary sinus showed no signs of dissection. After resection of the dissected aorta to the sinotubular ridge and application of Bioglue® (Cryolife Inc. Kennesaw, U.S.A) for stabilisation of the dissected noncoronary Sinus a pledget strip stabilised supracoronary ascending aortic replacement using a 28 mm Vascutek Gelweave vascular prosthesis was performed. After reaching the aimed 28 °C temperature, circulatory arrest was established and selective antegrade cerebral perfusion was administered over the brachiocephalic trunk and the left common carotid artery. The left subclavian artery was snared down by tape to reduce subclavian steal. Inspection of the aortic arch showed however no entry site in the ascending aorta or the transverse arch, even distal to the left subclavian artery as far as visible. A possible retrograde type A dissection had to be postulated as possible cause of the aortic pathology. A rapid decision had to be made as to whether to extensify the procedure in form of a frozen elephant trunk procedure to occlude possible entry sites in the descending aorta, or to secondarily visualise the tears of the descending aorta via computed tomography and secondary treatment of the underlying pathology. The less radical approach was chosen and a hemi-arch replacement was performed in a circulatory arrest of 21 min using SACP for 12 min, INVOS® (Somanetics, U.S.A) monitoring showed no hemispheral differences in saturation. Postoperative echocardiographic examination demonstrated trivial aortic regurgitation. After adequate haemostasis was achieved the gynaecologists were contacted for definitive closure of the abdomen.

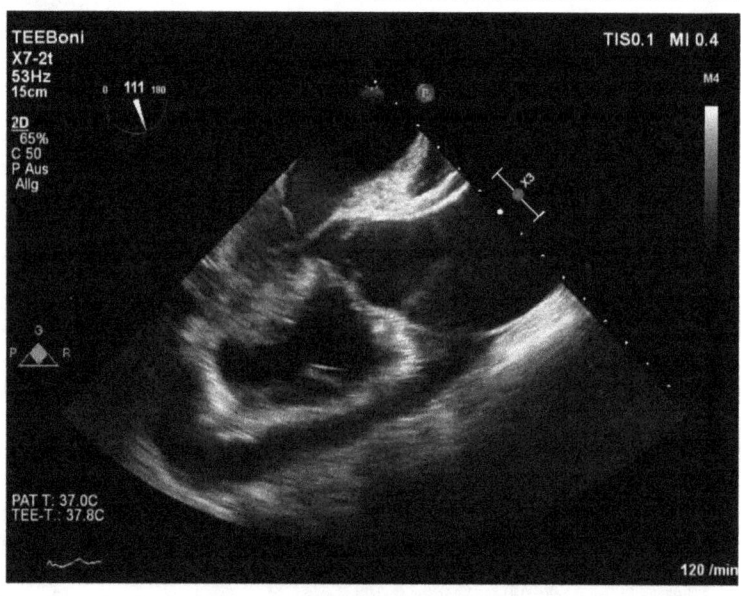

Fig. 1 Transoesophageal echocardiography demonstrating pericardial effusion and dissection

The initial postoperative period showed no complications and subsequent computer tomography of the aorta was performed. This demonstrated multiple entry sites in the descending aorta approximately 6 cm distal the left subclavian artery, with adequate perfusion of the visceral arteries and a narrowing of the true lumen following the origin of the left subclavian artery (Fig. 2). The transplanted kidney was anastomosed to the left common iliac artery with adequate perfusion. The decision was quickly made to treat the descending aorta via an endovascular stentgraft to obliterate possible retrograde perfusion to the aortic arch. Under general anaesthesia percutaneous access to the right common femoral artery was achieved. After pre-placement of sutures of Prostar XL® closure device (Abbott Vascular, Santa Clara, CA, USA), a 10F sheath was introduced and angiograms of the thoracic and abdominal aorta were performed with a pigtail catheter. A super-stiff guide wire (Back-up Meier, Boston Scientific Corporation, Marlborough, MA, USA) introduced through the pigtail catheter ensured the correct position of the guide wire in the true lumen. Consequently a Valiant Captivia thoracic stent graft (32/32/157 mm, 22F, Medtronic) system was introduced into the aortic arch and implanted in such a fashion that the covered part of the stentgraft started just distal to the origin of the left subclavian artery. The control angiogram showed adequate sealing of the descending thoracic aorta and improved flow to the true lumen of abdominal aorta (Fig. 3). The control CT examination 5 days later showed improved flow in the true lumen and abdominal. Furthermore no dissection could be demonstrated in the aortic arch.

Further hospital stay was uneventful without neurological sequelae and the patient could be discharged to the rehabilitation centre on the 18th postoperative day. The baby could be definitively extubated on the 24th postoperative day, he required phototherapy due to hyperbilirubinemia, the patent ductus could be successfully treated by Ibuprofen and the baby could be discharged home safely with a weight of 2015 g and 43 cm height after a 3 month hospital stay.

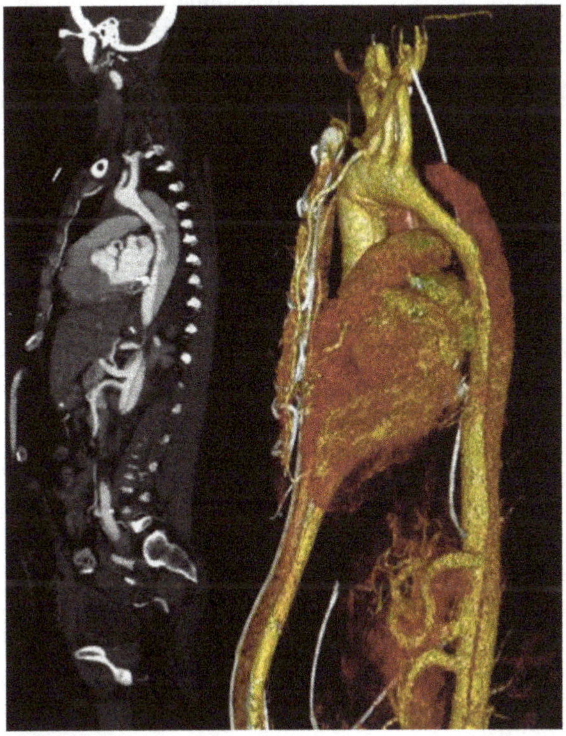

Discussion

Aortic dissection in woman under 40 years of age are associated with pregnancy in 50% of patients, often related

Fig. 2 CT scan demonstrating entry site distal to the left subclavian artery

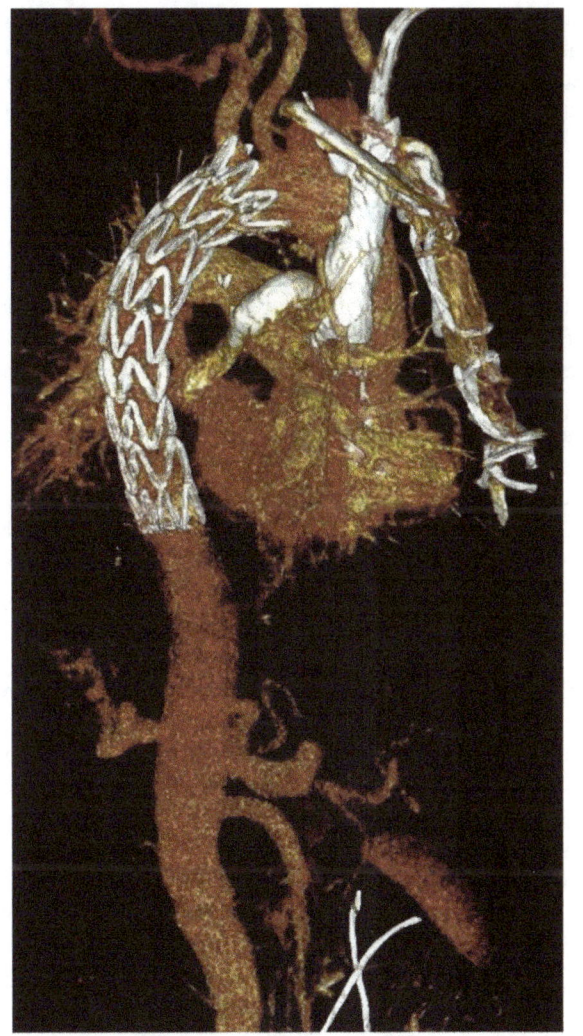

Fig. 3 Postinterventional CT scan after deployment of stentgraft

to hormonal changes with high levels of oestrogen and progesterone as well as risk factors predisposing to aortic stress such as systemic arterial hypertension, most often in the third trimester of pregnancy [2]. Tachycardia, increased cardiac output observed during pregnancy, expanded intravascular volume and position dependent compression of the distal aorta and iliac arteries by the gravid uterus stresses the proximal aorta [4]. Preeclampsia is another risk factor often associated with aortic dissection [9]. In most cases of aortic dissection the histological findings show medial degeneration with mucoid degeneration and loss of elastic fibres. Acute type A aortic dissection require emergency surgery, with restoration of blood flow, with mortality rate of untreated dissection increasing by 1-3% per hour after presentation [10].

Aortic dissection in pregnancy poses several problems in the therapeutic strategy, with understandable reluctance to perform immediate repair. In many cases described the child was delivered first and treatment of the aortic dissection was performed thereafter, usually by standard treatment of the ascending aorta and open distal anastomosis in circulatory arrest. These described cases most often present the fetus in a viable condition with a gestational age past the 34th week. Based on the experience of Zeebregts et al. following guidelines were proposed: In a pregnant patient with an acute aortic type A dissection therapy should be aimed at saving 2 lives, determined by the gestational age of the fetus. Before 28 weeks of gestation, aortic repair with the fetus kept in situ is recommended, if the fetus is viable after 32 weeks of gestation primary caesarean section followed by aortic repair is the treatment of choice [11]. These recommendations are shared by a large series by Zhu et al., prioritising maternal survival [12]. High flow high pressure cardiopulmonary bypass is recommended as safest for the fetus, moderate hemodilution (haematocrit of more than 25%) is aimed for [13]. Due to induction of fetal bradycardia by hypothermia, systemic hypothermia should be avoided, rewarming may also lead to premature intrauterine contractions. Open distal repair, which is preferable, should be avoided [14].

The patient described in this report suffered preeclampsia during the first pregnancy, which led to renal insufficiency with consecutive kidney transplant in 2014, further comorbidities included arterial hypertension, both predisposing factors to aortic dissection. Due to the early gestational period of the 24th week optimal planning was complicated, keeping the fetus in situ as recommended would have possibly led to the demise of the fetus Due to unclear dissection pathologies of the transverse aortic arch it was not possible to avoid circulatory arrest as arch inspection was necessary to rule out possible entry sites in this segment of the aorta. We recommended, as per guidelines, this form of treatment,ultimately the mother decided

on delivery of the fetus per caesarean section despite the possible detrimental consequences for the baby due to the early stages of the pregnancy.

The intraoperative suspicion of a retrograde Type A dissection after opening of the aortic arch, confirmed subsequently by CT examination, led to a dilemna for choice of optimal treatment. Antegrade stent-grafting of the descending aorta and total arch replacement would have been possible, the risk of longer circulatory arrest and their adjunct detrimental consequences had to be weighed against hemiarch replacement and subsequent stent-grafting after visualisation of the entry tears. The successful outcome using this treatment algorithm encourages us, other forms of treatment such as use of the frozen elephant trunk technique however may have led to a similar positive outcome.

The optimal interaction between cardiovascular surgeon, anaesthesiologist, paediatrician, gynaecologist and interventional radiologist was imminently important for the successful treatment of the patient. Preoperative CT scanning of the aorta would have provided valuable information for the surgical planning of treatment, however this was not possible without radiation risk and was avoided as the decision for operation was not dependent on the radiologic findings. Echocardiography diagnosed the dissection in this case, with described sensitivity and specificity up to 75 and 90% respectively. Transoesophageal echocardiography overcomes many of the limitations of transthoracic echocardiography and show sensitivity and specificity data as high as 99% and 98 respectively [15]. Intraoperative transoesophageal echocardiography was performed and entry tears were not clearly seen in the descending aorta so that the subsequent CT examination provided the necessary information for optimal treatment.

The decision of the mother to deliver the baby preoperatively was, retrospectively seen, a correct decision. The baby developed well over a 3 month hospital stay despite all possible detrimental consequences associated with such a premature birth. Clearly the excellent work of the neonatal paediatrician and nursing contributed to the successful outcome.

The diagnosis of aortic dissection is often overlooked, with misdiagnosis occurring in 85% of patients presenting with acute dissection [1]. Many case reports describe treatment of aortic dissection well postpartum due to missing of initial diagnosis. Awareness of this rare medical condition and prompt diagnosis of the referring centre was surely an optimal prerequisite for the successful outcome of this complex case.

Conclusion

Treatment of acute type A aortic dissection in pregnant patients at such an early gestational period with the first

24 weeks of pregnancy poses a grave dilemma for the optimal therapeutic strategy. Prompt diagnosis, precise coordination between all involved subspecialties and ultimately, as in this case, definitive treatment in consensus with operative and interventional departments have led to a successful outcome and encourages us in our daily struggle in this often demanding surgery.

Abbreviations
APGAR: Activity, Pulse, Grimace, Appearance and Respiration Score; INVOS: Cerebral oximetry monitoring; pH: Power of Hydrogen; SACP: Selective antegrade cerebral perfusion

Authors' contributions
JE: performed surgery, conceived of the study, drafted the manuscript. MH: participated in surgery, participated in the design of the study. BS: performed interventional treatment, helped to draft the manuscript. RT: performed interventional treatment, coordinated and revised the manuscript. SS: performed surgery and participated in the design and coordination of the study. MB: participated in surgery, coordinated the treatment, and participated in the design of the study. AW: Helped to draft the manuscript revised and coordinated the study. All authors have read and approved the final manuscript.

Competing interests
There are no financial or non-financial interests competing. The authors declare that they have no competing interests.

Author details
[1]Department of Cardiac Surgery, European Medical School Oldenburg-Groningen, University Hospital Oldenburg, Carl von Ossietzky University Oldenburg, Rahel Straus Str. 10, 26133 Oldenburg, Germany. [2]Department of Diagnostic and Interventional Radiology, European Medical School Oldenburg-Groningen, University Hospital Oldenburg, Carl von Ossietzky University Oldenburg, Oldenburg, Germany. [3]University Department of Obstetrics and Gynaecology, European Medical School Oldenburg-Groningen, University Hospital Oldenburg, Carl von Ossietzky University Oldenburg, Oldenburg, Germany. [4]Department of Anaesthesiology, Critical Care, Emergency Medicine and Pain Therapy, European Medical School Oldenburg-Groningen, University Hospital Oldenburg, Carl von Ossietzky University Oldenburg, Oldenburg, Germany.

References
1. Mészáros I, Mórocz J, Szlávi J, Schmidt J, Tornóci L, Nagy L, Szép L. Epidemiology and clinicopathology of aortic dissection. Chest. 2000;117(5): 1271–8.
2. Roberts WC. Aortic dissection: anatomy, consequences, and causes. Am Heart J. 1981;101(2):195–214.
3. Hagan PG, Nienaber CA, Isselbacher EM, Bruckman D, Karavite DJ, Russman PL, Evangelista A, Fattori R, Suzuki T, Oh JK, Moore AG, Malouf JF, Pape LA, Gaca C, Sechtem U, Lenferink S, Deutsch HJ, Diedrichs H, Marcos y Robles J, Llovet A, Gilon D, Das SK, Armstrong WF, Deeb GM, Eagle KA. The international registry of acute aortic dissection (IRAD): new insights into an old disease. JAMA. 2000;283(7):897–903.
4. Immer FF, Bansi AG, Immer-Bansi AS, McDougall J, Zehr KJ, Schaff HV, Carrel TP. Aortic dissection in pregnancy: analysis of risk factors and outcome. Ann Thorac Surg. 2003;76(1):309–14.
5. Lind J, Wallenburg HC. The Marfan syndrome and pregnancy: a retrospective study in a Dutch population. Eur J Obstet Gynecol Reprod Biol. 2001;98(1):28–35.
6. Gelpi G, Pettinari M, Lemma M, Mangini A, Vanelli P, Antona C. Should pregnancy be considered a risk factor for aortic dissection? Two cases of acute aortic dissection following cesarean section in non-Marfan nor bicuspid aortic valve patients. J Cardiovasc Surg. 2008;49(3):389–91.
7. Chow SL. Acute aortic dissection in a patient with Marfan's syndrome complicated by gestational hypertension. Med J Aust. 1993;159(11-12):760–2.
8. Manalo-Estrella P. Barker AE histopathologic findings in human aortic media associated with pregnancy. Arch Pathol. 1967;83(4):336–41.
9. Park JW, Kim SM, Yu GB, Kang YD. Aortic dissection accompanied by preeclampsia in a postpartum young woman. Obstet Gynecol Sci. 2016; 59(5):403–6.
10. Pitt MP, Bonser RS. The natural history of thoracic aortic aneurysm disease: an overview. J Card Surg. 1997;12(2 Suppl):270–8.
11. Zeebregts CJ, Schepens MA, Hameeteman TM, Morshuis WJ, de la Rivière AB. Acute aortic dissection complicating pregnancy. Ann Thorac Surg. 1997; 64(5):1345–8.
12. Khan IA, Nair CK. Clinical, diagnostic, and management perspectives of aortic dissection. Chest. 2002;122(1):311–28.
13. Becker RM. Intracardiac surgery in pregnant women. Ann Thorac Surg. 1983; 36(4):453–8.
14. Eilen B, Kaiser IH, Becker RM, Cohen MN. Aortic valve replacement in the third trimester of pregnancy: case report and review of the literature. Obstet Gynecol. 1981;57(1):119–21.
15. Zhu JM, Ma WG, Peterss S, Wang LF, Qiao ZY, Ziganshin BA, Zheng J, Liu YM, Elefteriades JA, Sun LZ. Aortic dissection in pregnancy: management strategy and outcomes. Ann Thorac Surg. 2017;103(4):1199–206. https://doi.org/10.1016/j.athoracsur.2016.08.089. Epub 2016 Nov 5

13

Spontaneous hemothorax caused by ruptured multiple mycotic aortic aneurysms

Po-Sung Li[1], Chung-Lin Tsai[2], Sung-Yuan Hu[1,3,4,5,6,8*], Tzu-Chieh Lin[1,3,5,7] and Yao-Tien Chang[1,3,5]

Abstract

Background: Mycotic aortic aneurysm (MAA) is a rare clinical entity with an incidence of 1-3%, but it is a life-threatening infection of aorta characterized by dilatation of aorta with false lumen. Multiple MAAs have been reported rarely with an incidence of 0.03% and associated with a high mortality rate of 80% if ruptured.

Case presentation: A hypertensive and diabetic 78-year-old man visited our emergency department complaining intermittent dull and tingled pain over the left flank region for 1 week. Chest X-ray showed left pleural effusion and hemothorax was confirmed by thoracocentesis. Computed tomography (CT) of chest demonstrated multiple thoracic aortic aneurysms and the pathological findings disclosed the diagnosis of multiple MAAs. He was discharged under an uneventful condition post-surgical aortic repair with adequate intravenous antibiotics for 4 weeks.

Conclusions: CT scan may make a definite diagnosis of multiple MAAs and management with surgical debridement, aortic repair and full-course antibiotics for Gram-positive coccus and/or Gram-negative bacillus is recommended.

Keywords: Computed tomography (CT), Hemothorax, Mycotic aortic aneurysm (MAA)

Background

Hemothorax is the presence of blood in the pleural space. The source of blood may be trauma to the chest wall, lung parenchyma, heart, or great vessels, infection/ inflammation, malignancy, coagulopathy or congenital arteriovenous malformations. Mycotic aortic aneurysm (MAA) is a rare clinical entity with an incidence of 1-3%, but it is a life-threatening infection of aorta characterized by dilatation of aorta with false lumen [1–5]. Multiple MAAs have been reported an incidence of 0.03% and associated with a high mortality rate of 70-80% if ruptured. Spontaneous hemothorax associated with ruptured MAAs has been reported rarely [6].

Case presentation

A 78-year-old hypertensive and diabetic man had a history of coronary artery disease with percutaneous coronary intervention in 1997. Chest X-ray (Fig. 1a) was normal 11 months ago. He denied major chest trauma recently. He suffered from intermittent low grade fever, dull and tingled pain over left flank region and progressive dyspnea for 1 week. He was brought to our emergency department. On arrival, vital signs were a respiratory rate of 22 breaths per min, a heart rate of 125 beats per min, a blood pressure of 158/79 mmHg and a body temperature of 36.6 °C. Physical examination revealed a pale conjunctiva, no heart murmur, absent breathing sound of left lower lung, and knocking pain over left costovertebral angle. Significant laboratory evaluation revealed white blood cell counts (WBCs) of 13,700/mm^3 with 76.3% of segmented neutrophils, hemoglobin of 7.8 g/dl, red blood cell counts (RBCs) of 4.26×10^6/mm^3, platelet counts of 634×10^3/mm^3, creatinine 1.5 mg/dl, albumin 2.6 g/dl, protein 7.8 g/dl, lactate

* Correspondence: song9168@pie.com.tw
[1]Department of Emergency Medicine, Taichung Veterans General Hospital, Taichung, Taiwan
[3]School of Medicine, Chung Shan Medical University, Taichung, Taiwan
Full list of author information is available at the end of the article

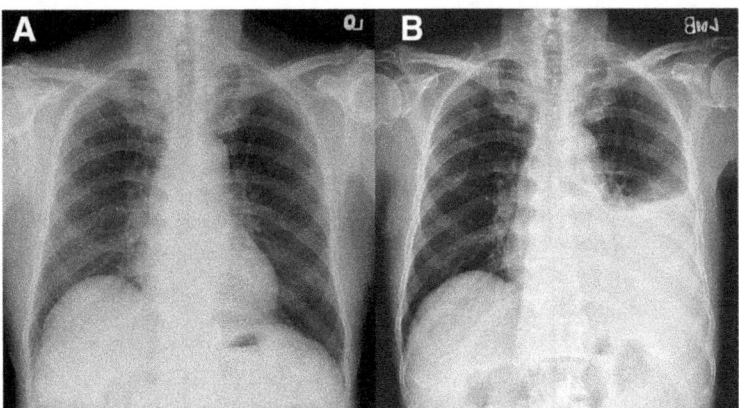

Fig. 1 Chest X-rays showed normal heart size, sharp cardiopleural angle, bare stent of coronary artery and no significant of aortic lesion (Panel **a**). Chest X-rays revealed left pleural effusion and widening of upper descending aorta (Panel **b**)

dehydrogenase (LDH) 384 U/l, glucose of 257 mg/dl, and high-sensitivity C-reactive protein (hs-CRP) of 18.6 mg/dl. Chest X-ray showed left pleural effusion and mild widening of upper descending aorta (Fig. 1b). Blood-tinged pleural effusion was confirmed via a fine-needle aspiration under sono-guide after informed consent of patient. Analysis of pleural effusion were exudative and infection of pleural effusion should be considered, including WBCs of 1625/mm³, with neutrophils of 62% and lymphocytes of 31%, RBCs of 12,500/mm³, protein of 4.5 g/dl, LDH of 266 U/l, glucose of 201 mg/dl and specific gravity of 1.030. Fever, flank pain, leukocytosis, elevated hs-CRP and hemothorax were clinical clues for high suspicion of ruptured infectious aorta. Computed tomography (CT) with intravenous contrast media depicted ruptured multiple thoracic aortic aneurysms at the level of between 8th and 11th thoracic spines with atelectasis of left lung and massive hemothorax (Fig. 2), so emergency surgical intervention with resection of fragile aorta, debridement of involved periaortic soft tissue, and reconstruction for descending aorta with Dacron graft of 20 mm was performed. Although the cultures of blood, pleural fluid, and resected aortic tissue showed no growth of bacteria or mycobacterium tuberculosis, the

pathological findings demonstrated injury of vascular wall with acute and chronic inflammatory cells infiltration, fibrinous material coated on the internal luminal surface, focal abscess formation in vascular wall (Fig. 3) and no malignancy cells or granulation tissue. The serological screen for syphilis was non-reactive. The patient recovered gradually after surgical aortic repair, intensive care and adequate intravenous antibiotics for cover Gram-positive and Gram-negative bacteria with prostaphlin 2 g per 6 h and ceftriaxone 2 g per day for 4 weeks despite of negative-culture result. He was discharged under an uneventful condition with a regular follow-up of cardiovascular out-patient department for 2 years.

Discussion

Mycotic aortic aneurysm (MAA) is a rare but life-threatening infection with an incidence of 1~3% [1–5], characterized either by bacteremic seeding from extracardiac septicemia with bacterial invasion of an atherosclerotic vascular wall, endocarditis and contiguous/direct infection, leading to weakening and dilatation of vascular wall with formation of false lumen [5–7]. Multiple MAAs had been reported an incidence of 0.03%, which had a high risk of

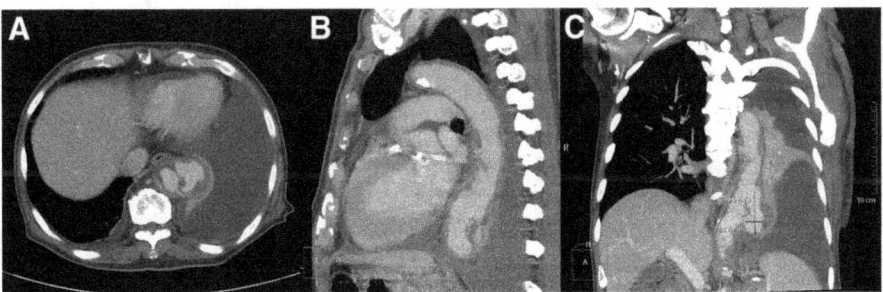

Fig. 2 Axial, sagittal and coronal views of computed tomographic scan with intravenous contrast media of chest showed irregular dumbbell-shaped aortic lesion (Panel **a**), multiple mushroom-like thoracic aortic aneurysms with the size of 8.7 mm in diameter (Panel **b**) and 46.6 mm × 22.1 mm (Panel **c**) with periaortic soft tissue density at the level of between 8th and 11th thoracic spine, massive pleural effusion and atelectasis of left lung

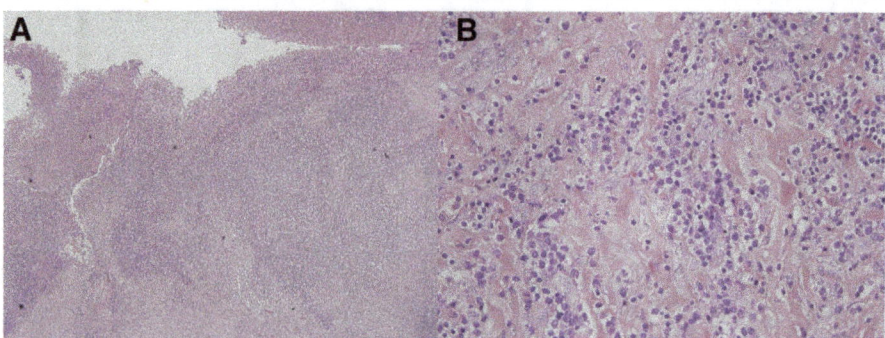

Fig. 3 Pathological findings disclosed fibrinous material coating on the internal luminal surface and formation of focal abscess was noted in the destructive vascular wall (×100) (Panel **a**). There were infiltrations of acute and chronic inflammatory cells in the damaged vascular wall (×1000) (Panel **b**)

rupture with a mortality rate of 80%. Hemothorax as a sign of ruptured multiple MAAs was extremely rare and only few cases had been reported previously [6].

The differential diagnosis of hemothorax implicated the possibility of life-threatening underlying illnesses such as trauma, coagulopathy, spontaneous pneumothorax, vascular lesions, spontaneous esophageal rupture, infectious disease (such as pneumonia, tuberculous pleurisy, fungal disease, subphrenic abscess), malignancy, connective tissue disease (lupus pleuritis, rheumatoid pleurisy, Wegener's granulomatosis), pulmonary embolism, pulmonary sequestration, and endometriosis. They are difficulty to be differentiated from chest radiographs or clinical presentations. The rupture of thoracic mycotic aortic aneurysm (MAA) should be considered in the differential diagnosis of hemothorax [1–7].

MAA can develop either by infection of arterial wall or previous aneurysm with secondary infection. They maybe have led to a true or false lumen. Blood cultures are positive in 50-75% of MAA patients [2, 5, 8]. MAA is diagnosed according to clinical presentations with triad of fever, pain and pulsatile mass; laboratory investigations of leukocytosis and elevation of inflammatory biomarkers; radiological typical findings, including mushroom-like appearance, new aneurysm formation, rapid expansion or morphological change of known aneurysms, synchronous lesions, intramural or perivascular gas, edema, soft tissue mass or stranding, ring enhancement, disruption or disappearance of aortic calcification in late stage, and extravasation in rupture; cultures of blood and/or resected aortic tissue; and the histopathological features of an acute infection, including abscess and infiltration of neutrophils [2, 5, 7].

Most common pathogens are bacteria such as *Staphylococcus* spp., *Salmonella* spp., and *Treponema pallidum*. The risk factor includes atherosclerosis, male sex, cigarette smoking, vascular abnormalities (pre-existing aneurysms), arterial trauma, old age, immunocompromised status,

intravenous drug abusers, and infectious endocarditis. Medical treatment alone can't complete cure, so cardiovascular surgeons must perform surgical debridement and reconstruction of vascular continuity for thoracic aortic multiple MAAs plus intravenous antibiotics of 4-6 weeks at least for Gram-positive coccus and Gram-negative bacillus [2, 5, 9–12].

The natural history of untreated mycotic aneurysms is of fatality from either massive hemorrhage or fulminant sepsis. Complications include 45% of rupture and 18% of fistula formation in late stage [5]. If an aortic mycotic aneurysm is diagnosed, surgical removal of an infected aneurysm must always be required because of a high mortality rate of 70-80% due to a high risk of rupture of mycotic aneurysm. Therefore undue delay of surgical intervention should be avoided. Emergency operation is recommended in those who have a ruptured aneurysm or are septic and unstable [6, 13]. The optimal timing and best surgical procedure of surgical intervention are still difficult to be determined. The timing of surgical intervention should be determined by estimated risk of aneurysm rupture and surgical risk according to the patient's underlying condition and short-interval CT re-examinations [13, 14]. The challenges of surgical intervention in patients with mycotic aneurysms are re-infection, difficulties of anastomosis lines in fragile cut-end tissue, early and late postoperative bleeding, so a wide and extensive debridement of all infected tissue and a resection back to the healthy and non-infected wall of the aorta are mandatory [15, 16]. In our case, he received emergency surgical repair immediately due to ruptured multiple MAAs after radiological and laboratory survey. He was fully recovered and received regular follow up at our hospital for 2 years.

Conclusion

Although the incidence is rare, the cause of spontaneous hemothorax should include rupture of MAA. Hold the implantation of chest tube if there is no trauma-related hemothorax. Etiologies of spontaneous hemothorax must be completed as soon as possible. Emergency surgical repair with adequate and full course of intravenous antibiotics are recommended if there is an evidence of rupture of MAA, such as hemothorax, because of high mortality. We recommend that the differential diagnosis of spontaneous hemothorax in high suspicion of infectious aorta should include MAA.

Abbreviations
CT: Computed tomography; LDH: Lactate dehydrogenase; MAAs: Mycotic aortic aneurysms; RBCs: Red blood cell counts; WBCs: White blood cell counts

Acknowledgements
Thanks for efforts of emergency resuscitation team, radiological technicians and division of infection in clinical diagnosis and management of this patient.

Funding
This research received no specific grant from any funding agency in the public, commercial, or not-for-profit sectors.

Authors' contributions
The work presented here was carried out as collaboration among all the authors. Lin TC, Tsai CL, Li PS, Chang YT, and Hu SY were clinical responsible. Hu SY, Tsai CL and Lin TC defined the research theme. Lin TC, Chang YT, and Hu SY analyzed the data, interpreted the results and wrote the paper. Lin TC and Hu SY worked together on data collection and interpretation. Hu SY, Chang YT and Li PS co-designed the study and discussed the analysis, interpretation, and presentation. All authors have read and approved the final version of the manuscript.

Competing interests
The authors declare that they have no competing interests.

Author details
[1]Department of Emergency Medicine, Taichung Veterans General Hospital, Taichung, Taiwan. [2]Division of Cardiac Surgery, Cardiovascular Center, Taichung Veterans General Hospital, Taichung, Taiwan. [3]School of Medicine, Chung Shan Medical University, Taichung, Taiwan. [4]Institute of Medicine, Chung Shan Medical University, Taichung, Taiwan. [5]Department of Nursing, College of Health, National Taichung University of Science and Technology, Taichung, Taiwan. [6]Department of Nursing, Central Taiwan Univeristy of Science and Technology, Taichung, Taiwan. [7]College of Public Health, China Medical University, Taichung, Taiwan. [8]1650 Taiwan Boulevard Sect. 4, Taichung 40705, Taiwan.

References
1. Voitle E, Hofmann W, Cejna M. Aortic emergencies-diagnosis and treatment - a pictorial review. Insights Imaging. 2015;6:17–32.
2. Stellmes A, Von Allmen R, Derungs U, et al. Thoracic endovascular aortic repair as emergency therapy despite suspected aortic infection. Interact Cardiovasc Thorac Surg. 2013;16:459–64.
3. Lee WK, Mossop PJ, Little AF, et al. Infected (mycotic) aneurysms: spectrum of imaging appearances and management. Radiographics. 2008;28:1853–68.
4. Kan CD, Lee HL, Yang YJ. Outcome after endovascular stent graft treatment for mycotic aortic aneurysm. J Vasc Surg. 2007;46:906–12.
5. Fisk M, Peck LF, Miyagi K, et al. Mycotic aneurysms: a case report, clinical review and novel imaging strategy. QJM. 2012;105:181–8.
6. Dwivedi AN, Srinivasan A, Jain S. Multiple Mycotic aneurysms of the abdominal aorta illustrated on MDCT scanner. J Clin Imaging Sci. 2015;5:49.
7. Abehsira G, Bagate F, Estagnasié P, Squara P. Multiple aortic mycotic aneurysms complicating a spondylitis without endocarditis. Intensive Care Med. 2013;39:1133.
8. Jaffer U, Gibbs R. Mycotic thoracoabdominal aneurysms. Ann Cardiothorac Surg. 2012;1:417–25.
9. Nakashima M, Usui A, Oshima H, Ueda Y. The treatment of infectious aneurysms in the thoracic aorta; our experience in treating five consecutive patients. Interact Cardiovasc Thorac Surg. 2010;10:334–7.
10. Lopes RJ, Almeida J, Dias PJ, Pinho P, Maciel MJ. Infectious thoracic aortitis: a literature review. Clin Cardiol. 2009;32:488–90.
11. Brook I. Anaerobic bacteria as a cause of mycotic aneurysm of the aorta: microbiologyand antimicrobial therapy. Curr Cardiol Rev. 2009;5:36–9.
12. Hsu PJ, Lee CH, Lee FY, Liu JW. Clinical and microbiological characteristics of mycotic aneurysms in a medical center in southern Taiwan. J Microbiol Immunol Infect. 2008;41:318–24.
13. Kim YW. Infected aneurysm: current management. Ann Vasc Dis. 2010;3:7–15.
14. Usui A. Surgical management of infected thoracic aneurysms. Nagoya J Med Sci. 2013;75:161–7.
15. Dubois M, Daenens K, Houthoofd S, Peetermans WE, Fourneau I. Treatment of mycotic aneurysms with involvement of the abdominal aorta: single-centre experience in 44 consecutive cases. Eur J Vasc Endovasc Surg. 2010;40:450–6.
16. Huang YK, Chen CL, MS L, et al. Clinical, microbiologic, and outcome analysis of mycotic aortic aneurysm: the role of endovascular repair. Surg Infect. 2014;15:290–8.

14

Right ventricular functional analysis utilizing first pass radionuclide angiography for pre-operative ventricular assist device planning

Ryan Avery[1]* (iD), Kevin Day[1], Clinton Jokerst[2], Toshinobu Kazui[3], Elizabeth Krupinski[4] and Zain Khalpey[3]

Abstract

Background: Advanced heart failure treated with a left ventricular assist device is associated with a higher risk of right heart failure. Many advanced heart failures patients are treated with an ICD, a relative contraindication to MRI, prior to assist device placement. Given this limitation, left and right ventricular function for patients with an ICD is calculated using radionuclide angiography utilizing planar multigated acquisition (MUGA) and first pass radionuclide angiography (FPRNA), respectively. Given the availability of MRI protocols that can accommodate patients with ICDs, we have correlated the findings of ventricular functional analysis using radionuclide angiography to cardiac MRI, the reference standard for ventricle function calculation, to directly correlate calculated ejection fractions between these modalities, and to also assess agreement between available echocardiographic and hemodynamic parameters of right ventricular function.

Methods: A retrospective review from January 2012 through May 2014 was performed to identify advanced heart failure patients who underwent both cardiac MRI and radionuclide angiography for ventricular functional analysis. Nine heart failure patients (8 men, 1 woman; mean age of 57.0 years) were identified. The average time between the cardiac MRI and radionuclide angiography exams was 38.9 days (range: 1 - 119 days). All patients undergoing cardiac MRI were scanned using an institutionally approved protocol for ICD with no device-related complications identified. A retrospective chart review of each patient for cardiomyopathy diagnosis, clinical follow-up, and echocardiogram and right heart catheterization performed during evaluation was also performed.

Results: The 9 patients demonstrated a mean left ventricular ejection fraction (LVEF) using cardiac MRI of 20.7% (12 – 40%). Mean LVEF using MUGA was 22.6% (12 – 49%). The mean right ventricular ejection fraction (RVEF) utilizing cardiac MRI was 28.3% (16 – 43%), and the mean RVEF calculated by FPRNA was 32.6% (9 – 56%). The mean discrepancy for LVEF between cardiac MRI and MUGA was 4.1% (0 – 9%), and correlation of calculated LVEF using cardiac MRI and MUGA demonstrated an R of 0.9. The mean discrepancy for RVEF between cardiac MRI and FPRNA was 12.0% (range: 2 – 24%) with a moderate correlation ($R = 0.5$). The increased discrepancies for RV analysis were statistically significant using an unpaired t-test ($t = 3.19$, $p = 0.0061$). Echocardiogram parameters of RV function, including TAPSE and FAC, were for available for all 9 patients and agreement with cardiac MRI demonstrated a kappa statistic for TAPSE of 0.39 (95% CI of 0.06 – 0.72) and for FAC of 0.64 (95% of 0.21 – 1.00).

(Continued on next page)

* Correspondence: ravery@radiology.arizona.edu
[1]Department of Medical Imaging, Banner - University Medical Center, 1501 N. Campbell Ave, PO Box 245067, Tucson, AZ 85724, USA
Full list of author information is available at the end of the article

(Continued from previous page)

Conclusion: Heart failure patients are increasingly requiring left ventricular assist device placement; however, definitive evaluation of biventricular function is required due to the increased mortality rate associated with right heart failure after assist device placement. Our results suggest that FPRNA only has a moderate correlation with reference standard RVEFs calculated using cardiac MRI, which was similar to calculated agreements between cardiac MRI and echocardiographic parameters of right ventricular function. Given the need for identification of patients at risk for right heart failure, further studies are warranted to determine a more accurate estimate of RVEF for heart failure patients during pre-operative ventricular assist device planning.

Keywords: Magnetic resonance imaging, First pass radionuclide angiography, Multigated acquisition radionuclide angiography, Automatic implantable cardiac device, Right ventricular ejection fraction, Left ventricular ejection fraction

Background

Advanced left heart failure therapy is focused on hospitalization and heart transplantation given the poor outcomes of medical therapy alone in these patients [1, 2]. However, the finite supply of donor hearts has limited transplantation to 4500 annual cases worldwide with 2200 of these performed in the United States [3]. The introduction of the left ventricular assist device (LVAD) has become a valuable tool providing a bridge to transplant till a donor organ becomes available, or a bridge to therapy with evidence suggesting an increased 1-year survival compared to medical management [3–6]. For patients who are not a transplant candidate, LVAD implantation has also been approved as a destination therapy offering both improved mortality rate and quality of life [7, 8].

Given the prevalence of advanced heart failure, potential LVAD recipients in the US is estimated to be 150,000 to 250,000 patients [3, 9]. Further studies have noted that despite the improvements in 1-year survival rates, LVADs continue to have significant morbidity and mortality related to development of right ventricular failure (RVF) after LVAD placement hypothesized to be related to the LVAD providing only left ventricular support [10, 11]. While the clinical decision regarding the selection of univentricular or biventricular support device is multifactorial, the risk of post-device placement RVF warrants that the size and function of the right ventricle (RV) should be an integral component in this decision-making process [12–14]. Furthermore, RV function in heart failure patients correlates with mortality risk, and is more predictive of survival than exercise testing and left ventricular ejection fraction (LVEF) [15–18]. If right ventricular function is compromised, the risk of post-procedural RVF is high, and LVAD implantation into patients needing biventricular support will result in an increased risk of right ventricular failure and poor clinical outcomes [11, 19–23].

While echocardiography is a widely available and non-invasive method of ventricular functional analysis with RV function assessed by both tricuspid annular plane systolic excursion (TAPSE) and fractional area of change (FAC), monitoring RV function and size with ultrasound parameters is not currently advocated for definitive RV evaluation [18]. Radionuclide angiography was determined to be the first, noninvasive, quantitative assessment of ventricular function [24], and more recently cardiac MRI cinematic images of the ventricles provides a level of accuracy allowing it be considered the "gold standard" for calculation of both LVEF and RVEF and ventricular volumetric parameters [25, 26].

Despite the advantages of cardiac MRI, ventricular function using radionuclide angiography continues to be favored with the multi-gated acquisition technique (MUGA) used to calculate LVEF, and the first-pass radionuclide angiography (FPRNA) technique used to calculate the RVEF. Multiple factors contribute to the continued preferred status of radionuclide angiography in societal guidelines; particularly, the limited availability of cardiac MRI, and that is contraindicated in patients with implantable cardiac devices (ICDs) [27–33].

In a continued effort for accurate assessment of both left and right ventricular function for patients prior to LVAD placement, a workflow was implemented at our institution for patients with conventional ICDs allowing for scanning with a 1.5 T MRI utilizing a published evidence-supported protocol [34–40]. Our goal was to accurately evaluate LV and RV function prior to LVAD placement by comparing the performance of radionuclide angiography to the reference standard values of cardiac MRI and other available hemodynamic and echocardiographic parameters of right ventricular functional analysis with the objective of preventing both post-LVAD implantation RVF and its associated mortality risk.

Methods
Study design

An IRB-approved, retrospective review from January 2012 through May 2014 was performed at a single US academic medical center. The review identified all adult advanced heart failure patients treated with an ICD who were being evaluated for either LVAD placement or heart transplantation. All patients were included who underwent left and right ventricular function evaluation with both cardiac MRI and radionuclide angiography within 120 days. A comparison of the calculated left and right ventricular ejection functions was performed comparing cardiac MRI with radionuclide angiography. The electronic medical record for each patient who met inclusion criteria was reviewed for the clinical course, specifically whether the patient went on to receive a LVAD. Medical record review also included performance of any echocardiogram or right heart catheterization performed during the evaluation period. While these exams do not provide a calculated ejection fraction, that right ventricular functional parameters from these exams have been shown to be predictive of post-operative right ventricular failure after LVAD placement [41].

Cardiac MRI exams included in the study required the performance of a complete short-axis series of the ventricles using cine EKG-gated sequences. Radionuclide angiography examinations included in the study required performance of both a MUGA and FPRNA exam for respective LVEF and RVEF evaluation. Right ventricular functional parameters from available echocardiograms included tricuspid annular plane systolic excursion (TAPSE) and fractional area of change (FAC), and from available right heart catheterization (RHC) parameters included central venous pressure (CVP), mean pulmonary artery pressure (MPAP), and right ventricular stroke work index (RVSWI) utilizing thermodilution.

Study population
Nine patients including 8 (89%) men and 1 (11%) woman with a mean age of the patients was 57.0 years (median: 60.0, range: 28 - 66) underwent ventricular ejection fraction evaluation with both cardiac MRI and radionuclide angiography for pre-operative heart failure evaluation for planning of LVAD placement or heart transplantation. Four patients were diagnosed with ischemic cardiomyopathy, and 5 patients were diagnosed with nonischemic cardiomyopathy. The average time interval between the cardiac MRI and radionuclide angiography (MUGA and FPRNA) was 38.9 days (range: 1 - 119 days). The average dose of intravenously administered technetium-99 m labeled RBCs for radionuclide angiography was 23.0 mCi (range 20.1 – 25.0 mCi).

All patient had a transthoracic echocardiogram performed during their evaluation with the average time between echocardiogram and cardiac MRI of 41 days (range: 1 – 125 days). Additionally, 7 of the 9 patients underwent RHC with an average time between RHC and cardiac MRI of 47 days (range 1-125 days).

All patients evaluated had previously undergone ICD placement prior to cardiac MRI examination, which was performed using an institutionally approved ICD safe protocol. There were no device-related complications from cardiac MRI in our study population.

Cardiac magnetic resonance examination acquisition and analysis
All patients were screened by a multi-specialty team prior to performance of the MRI. Screening required a cardiology evaluation consisting of electrophysiology laboratory interrogation of the ICD. The approved selection criteria required all cardiac leads in place for more than 6 weeks; stable pace, sense, and impedance parameters, normal battery function, and a stable non-paced heart rhythm with a heart rate greater than 50 beats per minute. If any of parameters were unable to be achieved, the patient was unable to undergo an MRI.

Prior to the MRI examination, the ICD was programmed to a sensing-only mode without cardiac pacing within the EP laboratory by electrophysiology-specialized cardiologists. Ventricular tachycardia and ventricular fibrillation detection, a feature in implantable defibrillators, was also turned off if applicable. The patient was monitored during the entire exam, and after the MRI was performed the patient was immediately returned to the electrophysiology laboratory where the ICD was reprogrammed to its original settings. Performance of the Cardiac MRI was done under the supervision of a dedicated advanced cardiac imaging radiologist and an MRI physicist who were both present for the entirety of each examination.

Each cardiac MRI was performed using a 1.5 T Siemens Magnetom Aera (Siemens Healthcare, Erlangen, Germany) with a multiphase array body coil. Specific absorption rate was limited to 1.5 W/kg for a maximum of 30 min. Gradient recalled echo (GRE) images were obtained for all bright blood and cine gated images to minimize susceptibility artifact related to the ICD battery pack. All images were obtained during breath hold. GRE cine gated images of the LV long-axis were performed in the 2, 3, and 4 chamber orientations for ventricular assessment. For complete ventricular analysis, GRE cine gated short axis series including complete coverage both ventricles were performed. The short axis series consisted of a stack of 8 mm thick images with a 10% distance factor between images. No gadolinium-based contrast agents were administered during the examination.

Cardiac MRI interpretation and offline post-processing analysis (CVI42, Circle Cardiovascular Imaging, Calgary, Canada) of ventricular ejection fractions was performed by consensus between two fellowship trained cardiovascular radiologists. Ventricular ejection fraction calculations were performed by manual contouring of the endocardial border of both ventricles during both end-diastole and end-systole utilizing all relevant sequences of the short axis series. Offline post-processing analysis also calculated end diastolic, end systolic, and stroke volumes of both ventricles. The results of the original studies were collected retrospectively, and were not reinterpreted.

Multi gated acquisition scan acquisition and analysis

Ventricular ejection fraction determined by radionuclide angiography was performed using an intravenous injection of Technetium-99 m-tagged red blood cells (RBC). Radiopharmaceutical tagging was performed using an in vitro labelling technique to ensure a high percentage of RBC tagging, and to prevent the injection of free Technetium-99 m. The RBCs for tagging were acquired from a 1 - 3 mL intravenous blood sample from the patient, which was subsequently tagged with radiopharmaceutical by a commercial tagging kit (UltraTag™, Mallinckrodt Pharmaceuticals, Maryland Heights, MO) prior to reinjection. After tagged RBC reinjection, the FPRNA examination was performed by obtaining dynamic nuclear angiography images in the RAO 30° projection at a rate of 50 msec/frame for a total acquisition of 440 frames. Additional, gated planar images in the RAO 30° projection were subsequently obtained for 300 s. After the FPRNA examination was performed, the MUGA portion of the radionuclide angiography examination was performed for LVEF evaluation. The MUGA images were acquired with gated images performed in the LAO 45° projection for 10 min.

RVEF was calculated by performance of computer contouring of the right ventricle in the RAO 30° position throughout the cardiac cycle and computer detection of the end diastole (ED) and end systole (ES) frames. Right ventricular contouring was performed by identification of the tagged RBC within the RV cavity and contouring of the endocardial border of the RV while excluding the right atrium and main pulmonary artery (Fig. 1). LVEF

was calculated by the MUGA portion of the examination that was performed in a similar fashion by contouring the endocardial border of the LV throughout the cardiac cycle in either the LAD 45° or 70° projection given the anatomic position of the heart, and computer detection of ED and ES. All contouring was performed an experience nuclear technologist, and two fellowship trained nuclear medicine radiologists confirmed exam quality and interpreted the FPRNA and MUGA images. The results were obtained retrospectively and were not reinterpreted.

Echocardiographic acquisition and analysis

All patients underwent a comprehensive 2D transthoracic echocardiographic examination performed during rest from the left parasternal, apical and subcostal windows using the GE ultrasound (Chicago, IL). RV assessment included TAPSE, which was measured by M-mode to assess RV longitudinal function by tracing movement of the tricuspid valve annulus from end diastole to end systole. RV area was measured by planimetry of the RV cavity in the apical view along the RV free wall to the apex and back to the tricuspid annulus for both systole and diastole to obtain the end-systolic area (ESA) and end-diastolic areas (EDA) respectively. Fractional area change (FAC) was calculated as [(EDA-ESA)/EDA] × 100.

Invasive hemodynamic measurements

RHC was performed through the right internal jugular or femoral approach in 7 subjects at rest using the Swan-Ganz pulmonary artery catheter in the supine position. Direct measurements of RAP, pulmonary artery systolic pressure, PA diastolic pressure (PADP), mean PA pressure (MPAP), cardiac output (CO) by thermodilution, cardiac index (CI) and pulmonary artery wedge pressure (PAWP) were obtained and real-time tracings

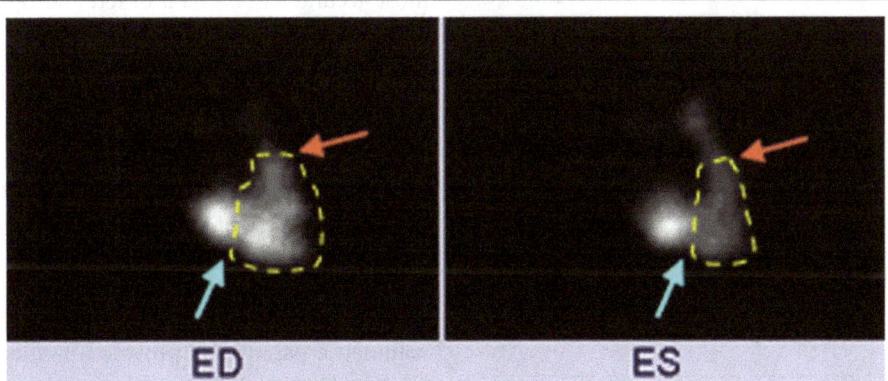

Fig. 1 Images of end diastole (ED) and end systole (ES) from a first pass radionuclide angiography. Images were obtained in the 30° RAO position, and computer contouring of the right ventricle was manually performed (yellow dashed line). Attention to including the right ventricular outlow tract to the pulmonary valve (red arrow) and base of the right ventricle to the right atrium (blue arrow) was performed

were displayed on a monitor. Right ventricular stroke work index (RVSWI) was calculated as (CI/HR) x MPAP × 0.0144.

Results

Statistical analysis ventricular ejection fractions of the nine patients who met inclusion criteria included calculation of discrepancies and correlation coefficient between the ejection fractions provided by cardiac MRI and radionuclide angiography, which provided LVEF by MUGA and RVEF by FPRNA. Discrepancy values were evaluated for statistical significance using an unpaired t-test.

The mean RVEF using cardiac MRI was 28.3% (median 27.0%, range: 16 – 43%). The mean RVEF calculated using FPRNA was 32.6% (median 32.0%, range: 9 – 56%). The mean LVEF calculated using cardiac MRI was 20.7% (median 21.0%, range: 12 – 40%), and mean LVEF calculated using MUGA was 22.6% (median 19.0%, range: 12 – 49%).

The mean RVEF discrepancy between cardiac MRI and FPRNA was 12.0% (median 13.0%, range: 2 – 24%). The mean LVEF discrepancy between cardiac MRI and MUGA was 4.1% (median 3.0%, range: 0 – 9%). The difference in discrepancies between the two modalities for RV and LV analysis was statistically significant using an unpaired t-test (t = 3.19, p = 0.006) (Table 1). The correlation coefficient between FPRNA generated RVEF and cardiac MRI RVEF was 0.5 (Fig. 2). The correlation coefficient between LVEF calculated using MUGA and cardiac MRI was 0.9 (Fig. 3).

Agreement of ventricular function using reference standard cardiac MRI to echocardiogram was performed for all 9 patients by performed by calculation of a Kappa statistic comparing mild, moderate, and severe RV

dysfunction for both TAPSE and FAC to mild, moderate, and severe RV dysfunction determined by calculated RVEFs determined by cardiac MRI [42, 43] (Table 2). The kappa statistic for RV function agreement between echocardiogram TAPSE agreement and cardiac MRI was 0.39 with a 95% CI of 0.06 - 0.72. The kappa statistic between echocardiogram FAC and Cardiac MRI showed a higher agreement of 0.64 with a 95% CI of 0.21 - 1.00. RHC parameter comparison demonstrated abnormal CVP, MPAP, and RVSWI in 6 of the 7 patients who had underwent RHC during heart failure evaluation (Table 3).

Of the nine patients in this study, three patients subsequently received an LVAD (HeartMate II Ventricular Assist Device, Thoratec Corporation, Pleasanton, California) for left ventricular support. One of the patients who underwent LVAD implantation was successfully bridged to transplant while the other two are still awaiting transplant. One patient identified for LVAD placement did not receive their LVAD secondary to complications from ischemic bowel disease that resulted in the patient expiring prior to LVAD placement. One patient identified for LVAD placement was deemed unsuitable for transplant due to lack of social support and inability to comply with smoking cessation program. Three patients improved clinically on optimal medical therapy and optimized medical management was pursued. One patient was discovered to have arrhythmogenic right ventricular dysplasia (ARVD) based on the MRI findings and improved on optimal medical therapy (Table 4).

Discussion

Patients with advanced heart failure being evaluated for LVAD placement require reliable and reproducible evaluation of right ventricular size and function given the high risk of mortality associated with RVF after LVAD placement. Despite evidence that cardiac MRI provides the most accurate assessment of left and right ventricular size and function, it has not been readily available for heart failure patients given that many of these patients have previously undergone placement of ICD. Despite the recent approval of the first conditional ICD by the FDA, current societal guidelines regard all current, conventional ICDs as a relative contraindication to MRI [44, 45] leading to the continued use of radionuclide angiography.

In our study, we compare the benefits of right ventricular evaluation cardiac MRI for "gold standard" calculation of RVEF with the additional functional and volumetric parameters provided by this modality against ejection fraction calculated by radionuclide angiography. While LVEF calculation using MUGA demonstrated an expected strong correlation (R of 0.9) with cardiac MRI, our research demonstrated only a moderate correlation

Table 1 Discrepancies between left and right ventricular ejection fraction calculated by both MUGA and FPRNA radionuclide angiography and cardiac MRI demonstrated

Pt	FPRNA RVEF (%)	MRI RVEF (%)	Discrepancy (%)	MUGA LVEF (%)	MRI LVEF (%)	Discrepancy (%)
1	9	23	14	12	12	0
2	56	43	13	15	21	6
3	16	27	11	19	21	2
4	42	25	17	16	13	3
5	32	34	2	22	13	9
6	22	16	6	49	40	9
7	24	32	8	19	21	2
8	44	31	13	24	23	1
9	48	24	24	27	22	5
Mean	32.6	28.3	12	22.6	20.7	4.1

FPRNA tended to over-estimate RVEF. Correlation between RVEFs from CARDIAC MR and FPRNA was 0.5. Correlation between LVEFs from CARDIAC MR and MUGA was 0.9. The degree of discrepancy in RVEF between FPRNA and CARDIAC MR was statistically significant (p = 0.006) relative to the degree of discrepancy in LVEF between MUGA and CARDIAC MR

Right ventricular functional analysis utilizing first pass radionuclide angiography for pre-operative...

91

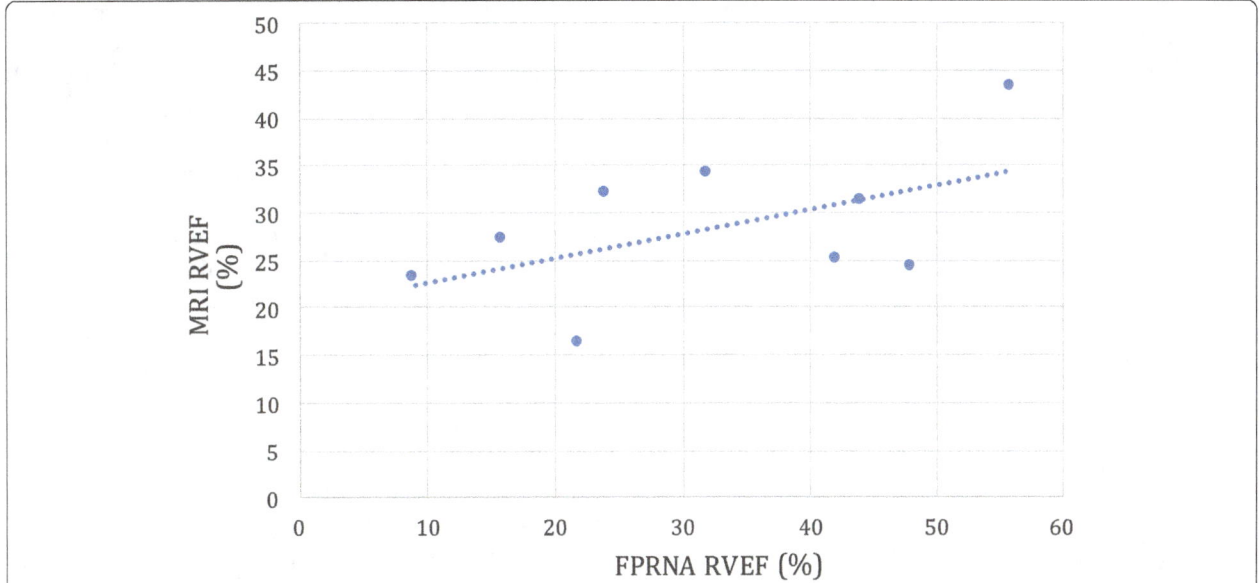

Fig. 2 Correlation of MRI derived right ventricular ejection fraction (MRI RVEF) to radionuclide derived right ventricular ejection fraction utilizing a first-pass radionuclide angiography (MUGA RVEF). A moderate correlation (*R* = 0.5) was determined when comparing RVEF calculated by both modalities

(R of 0.5) between RVEF using FPRNA compared to cardiac MRI. Additionally, the discrepancy between RVEF calculated by cardiac MRI and radionuclide angiography was larger than LVEF values from cardiac MRI and MUGA.

Previous studies have shown that non-invasive echocardiographic assessments of such as FAC and TAPSE show a strong correlation to RVEF calculated with radionuclide angiography [42], and while our small study population was unable to produce strong correlation between

radionuclide angiography calculated RVEF and echocardiographic parameters, our findings demonstrated a similar agreement between RV functional assessment performed with cardiac MRI when compared to both FAC and TAPSE assessments of RV function with FAC demonstrating a 'moderate agreement' and TAPSE demonstrating a 'fair' agreement. The agreement of echocardiographic parameters of RV function, especially FAC, suggest that while echocardiography may not provide a calculated RVEF it may serve as an

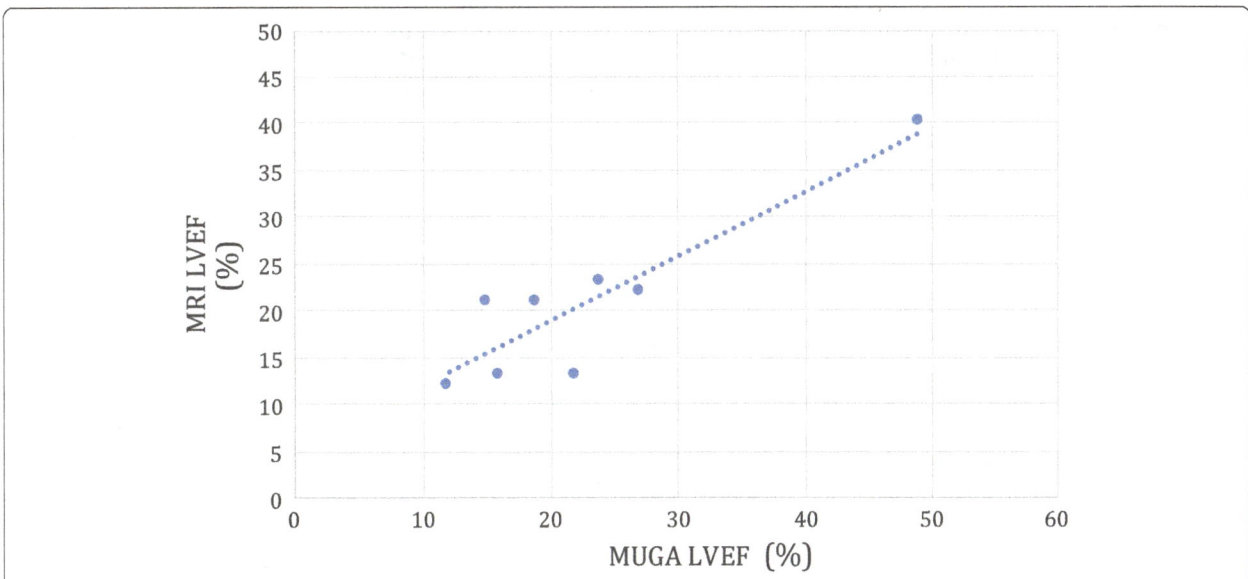

Fig. 3 Correlation of MRI derived left ventricular ejection fraction (MRI LVEF) to radionuclide derived left ventricular ejection fraction utilizing a multi-gated acquisition (MUGA LVEF). Correlation between the 2 modalities demonstrates a strong correlation (*R* = 0.9)

Table 2 The agreement between RV functional analysis determined by cardiac MRI was calculated for both echocardiographic tricuspid annular systolic excursion (TAPSE) and fractional area of change (FAC)

Patient	MRI RVEF (%)	Echo TAPSE (mm)	Echo FAC (%)	Days between Echo and MRI Exams
1	23	26	17	120
2	43	20	27	51
3	27	16	21	20
4	25	12	24	1
5	34	15	13	37
6	16	< 8	15	0
7	32	12	16	0
8	31	12	24	12
9	24	< 8	13	125
Kappa (95% CI)	–	0.39 (0.06 - 0.72)	0.64 (0.21 - 1.00)	

While FAC demonstrated a moderate correlation with FAC (Kappa of 0.69) to cardiac MRI, TAPSE (Kappa of 0.39) only demonstrated a fair agreement
TAPSE abnormal values: mild: 1.3 - 1.5 cm; moderate: 1.0 - 1.2 cm; severe: <1.0 cm
FAC abnormal values: mild: 25 - 31%; moderate: 18 - 24%; severe ≤17%

acceptable substitute for FPRNA, which can routinely be performed as a part of echocardiographic assessment of heart failure. Furthermore, while only 7 patients underwent RHC during heart failure evaluation, RHC parameters of RV function (i.e., CVP, MPAP, and RVSWI) were able to detect RV failure 6 of the 7 cases suggesting a supporting role for RHC.

Since the calculation of ventricular ejection fraction using cardiac MRI has been accepted as the most accurate assessment of ventricular function, our results suggest that the use of an RVEF calculated by FPRNA may not be the optimum method for patient risk stratification prior to LVAD implantation given the high risk of mortality in patients who progress to RVF. Conversely,

our results validate that LVEF calculation determined by radionuclide angiography is acceptable for calculation of left ventricular EF given the strong correlation (R of 0.9) when compared to cardiac MRI. However, the inability of MUGA to provide additional functional parameters; e.g., left ventricular end-diastolic and end-systolic volumes, stroke volume, etc., should foster continued research for evaluation of left ventricular functional and volumetric assessment in patients with ICDs.

Given the evidence supporting heart failure severity with increasing RV chamber size and the increased mortality with the development of RVF after LVAD implantation, we suggest that further investigation of cardiac MRI for RVEF assessment is warranted given the high discrepancy and a moderate correlation of RVEFs acquired by gold-standard cardiac MRI and the more widely utilized FPRNA. Also, given the utility of RHC for detecting of RV failure, further studies to categorize the severity of RHF into a mild, moderate, and severe classification system of these parameters may provide further utility for pre-operative assessment of RV function.

While cardiac MRI is still limited by both the availability and the complexities of ICD safe MRI protocols, our data suggests that further investigation for surrogate measurements is warranted. Given echocardiographic and hemodynamic examinations both provide multiparametric right ventricular function analysis, our study suggest further study of these parameter may provide a equivocal or improved RV functional assessment compared to first-pass radionuclide angiography techniques when compared to 'gold standard' MRI derived values. Also, further study of RV volumetric assessments utilizing echocardiogram and/or cardiac MRI may also be useful given that studies demonstrated that multiple echocardiographic parameters, including smaller RV chamber size or abnormal RV short-

Table 3 Right heart catheterization was performed in 7 of the 9 subjects during heart failure evaluation for pre-operative planning for LVAD or heart transplantation

Patient	MRI RVEF (%)	CVP (mmHg)	MPAP (mmHg)	RVSWI – thermodilution (gm-m/m2/beat)	Days between RHC and MRI Exams
1	23	20	44.67	13.92	117
2	43	12	27.33	17.21	49
3	27	–	–	–	–
4	25	9	26.67	14.12	2
5	34	10	41.67	24.29	22
6	16	*8*	*12.67*	*7.97*	0
7	32	–	–	–	–
8	31	25	45.33	12.17	11
9	24	12	37.00	9.64	125

While patients demonstrated abnormal RV function ranging from mild to severe, RHC parameters used to predict postoperative RVF (i.e., central venous pressure (CVP), mean pulmonary pressure (MPAP), and right ventricular stroke work index (RVSWI)) demonstrated abnormal values in 6 of the 7 patients evaluated with RHC. Italicized values are within normal limits
Normal values: CVP = 3 - 8 mmHg, MPAP = < 25 mmHg, RVSWI = 5 - 10 g-m/m2/beat

Table 4 Patient diagnoses and clinical follow-up

Pt	Sex	Age	Diagnosis	Follow-up
1	M	60	NICM	Ischemic bowel; patient expired prior to therapy
2	M	51	ICM	LVAD placed for bridge to therapy
3	M	64	ICM	No device placed; lack of social and unable to quit smoking
4	M	66	NICM	Improved on optimal medical therapy
5	F	59	NICM	LVAD place for bridge to therapy
6	M	64	NICM	Diagnosed with ARVD with cardiac MR
7	M	63	ICM	Improved on optimal medical therapy
8	M	28	NICM	Improved on optimal medical therapy
9	M	58	ICM	LVAD for bridge to therapy; definitive therapy with OHT

Nine patients with diagnosed with advanced heart failure, related to ischemic (ICM) or nonischemic cardiomyopathy (NICM) were retrospectively studied. All patients underwent both cardiac MRI and radionuclide angiography to calculate left and right ventricular function. Clinical follow-up is listed

axis to long-axis ratio, have been a significant predictor of post-operative RVF after LVAD placement [46].

Although this study showed statistically significant discrepancy between RVEFs calculated using cardiac MRI compared to FPRNA, our findings are limited since it was a retrospective study with a small sample population due to the inclusion criteria applied to the study, which required a careful and strict screening to ensure safe performance of MRI with ICD. Given the small patient population we attempted to strengthen our finding by comparing additional available parameters of RV functional assessment including echocardiography and RHC. Furthermore, continued research into cardiac MRI derived right ventricle metrics, such as echocardiographic stroke volume index or end diastolic volume index, may provide further insight into proper risk stratification of patients being evaluated for the either a left-sided or biventricular assist device thus minimizing the morbidity and mortality associated with post-LVAD implantation RVF.

Conclusions

Advanced heart failure patients are increasingly being treated with left ventricular assist device placement; however, definitive evaluation of both left and right ventricular function is required due to the increased mortality rate associated with right heart failure after LVAD placement. Our results suggest that FPRNA only has a moderate correlation with RVEF calculated using cardiac MRI. Furthermore, echocardiographic parameters of RV function including TAPSE and FAC demonstrated a fair and moderate agreement, respectively, compared to cardiac MRI suggesting a possible substitute for FPRNA. With the increasing need for identification of patients at risk for right heart failure, further studies are warranted to find a more accurate estimate of RVEF. Since this study and prior studies comparing radionuclide or echocardiographic RV function analysis to cardiac MRI-derived RVEFs produced at best a

moderate agreement/correlation, investigation in how these methodologies attempt to reduce the complicated anatomy of RV into a planar measurement would be helpful. Furthermore, refinement of these planar measurements and improved quality control regarding attention to anatomic boundaries may increase agreement with MRI allowing for a more readily available noninvasive assessment of RV function.

The expected increase in availability of MRI-conditional ICDs suggests that evaluation of advanced heart failure patients with cardiac MRI also should be further investigated as a definitive assessment for both left and right ventricular function prior to left ventricular assist device placement, and that cardiac MRI data may serve as the most accurate standard for RV volume and functional analysis for determination of the optimal pre-operative planning technique for patients undergoing LVAD implantation for bridge to transplant or destination therapy, or for other advanced devices such as a BiVAD or TAH.

Abbreviations
ARVD: Arrhythmogenic right ventricular dysplasia; BiVAD: Bi-ventricular assist device; CVP: Central venous pressure; EDA: End- diastolic area; ESA: End-systolic areas; FAC: Fractional area of change; FPRNA: First pass radionuclide angiography techniques; ICD: Automatic implantable cardiac devices; ICM: Ischemic cardiomyopathy; LVAD: Left ventricular assist device; LVEF: Left ventricular ejection fraction; MPAP: Mean pulmonary artery pressure; MRI: Magnetic resonance imaging; MUGA: Multigated acquisition; NICM: Non-ischemic cardiomyopathy; RHC: Right heart catheterization; RVEF: Right ventricular ejection fraction; RVF: Right ventricular failure; RVSWI: Right ventricle stroke work index; TAH: Total artificial heart; TAPSE: Tricuspid annular plane systolic excursion

Funding
Not Applicable.

Authors' contributions
TK and ZK were members of the surgical team. RA, IO, and CJ were RA, KD, EK and CJ were involved in drafting and critical revisions. All authors read and approved the final manuscript.

Competing interests

The authors declare that they have no competing interests. The work was primarily performed at the University of Arizona, which has a master research agreement with Siemens Healthcare, Erlangen, Germany.

Author details

[1]Department of Medical Imaging, Banner - University Medical Center, 1501 N. Campbell Ave, PO Box 245067, Tucson, AZ 85724, USA. [2]Department of Radiology, Mayo Clinic Hospital – Phoenix, Phoenix, AZ, USA. [3]Department of Surgery, Division of Cardiothoracic Surgery, Banner – University Medical Center, Tucson, AZ, USA. [4]Department of Radiology and Imaging Science, Emory University Hospital, Atlanta, US, Georgia.

References

1. Yancy CW, Jessup M, Bozkurt B, Butler J, Casey DE, Drazner MH, et al. 2013 ACCF/AHA guideline for the Management of Heart Failure: executive summary: a report of the American College of Cardiology Foundation/American Heart Association task force on practice guidelines. Circulation. 2013;128:1810–52.
2. Hunt SA, Baker DW, Chin MH, Cinquegrani MP, Feldman AM, Francis GS, et al. ACC/AHA guidelines for the evaluation and Management of Chronic Heart Failure in the adult: executive summary a report of the American College of Cardiology/American Heart Association task force on practice guidelines (committee to revise the 1995 guidelines for the evaluation and Management of Heart Failure): developed in collaboration with the International Society for Heart and Lung Transplantation; endorsed by the Heart Failure Society of America. Circulation. 2001;38(7):2101–13.
3. Miller LW, Guglin M. Patient selection for ventricular assist devices: a moving target. J Am Coll Cardiol. 2013;61(12):1209–21.
4. Slaughter MS, Rogers JG, Milano CA, et al. Advanced heart failure treated with continuous-flow left ventricular assist device. N Engl J Med. 2009;361:2241–51.
5. Starling RC, Naka Y, Boyle AJ, et al. Results of the post-U.S. Food and Drug Administration-approval study with a continuous flow left ventricular assist device as a bridge to heart transplantation: a prospective study using the INTERMACS (interagency registry for mechanically assisted circulatory support). J Am Coll Cardiol. 2011;57:1890–8.
6. John R, Naka Y, Smedira NG, et al. Continuous flow left ventricular assist device outcomes in commercial use compared with the prior clinical trial. Ann Thorac Surg. 2011;92:1406–13. discussion 1413
7. Stewart GC, Givertz MM. Mechanical circulatory support for advanced heart failure: patients and Technology in Evolution. Circulation. 2012;125(10):1304–15.
8. Capdeville M, Smedira NG. Advances and future directions for mechanical circulatory support. Anesthesiol Clin. 2013;31(2):321–53.
9. Miller LW. Left ventricular assist devices are underutilized. Circulation. 2011; 123:1552–8. discussion 1558
10. Kormos RL, Gasior TA, Kawai A. Transplant Candidate's clinical status rather than right ventricular function defines need for Univentricular versus biventricular support. J Thorac Cardiovasc Surg. 1996;111:773–82.
11. Kormos RL, Teuteberg JJ, Pagani FD. Right ventricular failure in patients with the Heartmate II continuous-flow left ventricular assist device: incidence, risk factors, and effect on outcomes. J Thorac Cardiovasc Surg. 2010;139:1316–24.
12. Dandel M, Potapov E, Krabatsch T, Stepanenko A, Löw A, Vierecke J, Knosalla C, Hetzer R. Load dependency of right ventricular performance is a major factor to be considered in decision making before ventricular assist device implantation. Circulation. 2013;128(11 Suppl 1):S14–23.
13. Fitzpatrick JR 3rd, Frederick JR, Hiesinger W, Hsu VM, McCormick RC, Kozin ED, Laporte CM, O'Hara ML, Howell E, Dougherty D, Cohen JE, Southerland KW, Howard JL, Paulson EC, Acker MA, Morris RJ, Woo YJ. Early planned institution of biventricular mechanical circulatory support results in improved outcomes compared with delayed conversion of a left ventricular assist device to a biventricular assist device. J Thorac Cardiovasc Surg. 2009;137(4):971–7.
14. Matthews JC, Koelling TM, Pagani FD, Aaronson KD. The right ventricular failure risk score a pre-operative tool for assessing the risk of right ventricular failure in left ventricular assist device candidates. J Am Coll Cardiol. 2008;51(22):2163–72.
15. Zornoff LA, Skali H, Pfeffer MA. Right ventricular dysfunction and risk of heart failure and mortality after myocardial infarction. SAVE Investigators J Am Coll Cardiol. 2002;39:450–5.
16. Ghio S, Gavazzi A, Campana C, et al. Independent and additive prognostic value of right ventricular systolic function and pulmonary artery pressure in patients with chronic heart failure. J Am Coll Cardiol. 2001;37:183–8.
17. Di Salvo TG, Mathier M, Semigran MJ, et al. Preserved right ventricular ejection fraction predicts exercise capacity and survival in advanced heart failure. J Am Coll Cardiol. 1995;25:1143–53.
18. Ramani GV, Gurm G, Dilsizian V, Park MH. Noninvasive assessment of right ventricular function: will there be resurgence in radionuclide imaging techniques? Curr Cardiol Rep. 2010;12(2):162–9.
19. Patlolla B, Beygui R, Haddad F. Right-ventricular failure following left ventricle assist device implantation. Curr Opin Cardiol. 2013;28(2):223–33.
20. Kalogeropoulos AP, Kelkar A, Weinberger JF, Morris AA, Georgiopoulou VV, Markham DW, Butler J, Vega JD, Smith AL. Validation of clinical scores for right ventricular failure prediction after implantation of continuous-flow left ventricular assist devices. J Heart Lung Transplant. 2015;34(12):1595–603.
21. Sitbon O, Humbert M, Nunes H, et al. Long-term intravenous Epoprostenol infusion in primary pulmonary hypertension: prognostic factors and survival. J Am Coll Cardiol. 2002;40:780–8.
22. D'Alonzo GE, Barst RJ, Ayres SM, et al. Survival in patients with primary pulmonary hypertension: results from a National Prospective Registry. Ann Intern Med. 1991;115:343–9.
23. Voelkel NF, Quaife RA, Leinwand LA, et al. Right ventricular function and failure: report of a National Heart, Lung, and Blood Institute working group on cellular and molecular mechanisms of right heart failure. Circulation. 2006;114:1883–91.
24. Strauss HW, Zaret BL, Hurley PJ, et al. A Scintigraphic method for measuring left ventricular ejection fraction in man without cardiac catheterization. Am J Cardiol. 1971;28:575–80.
25. Geva T. MRI is the preferred method for evaluating right ventricular size and function in patients with congenital heart disease. Circulation Card Imaging. 2014;7(1):190–7.
26. Puchalski MD, Williams RV, Askovich B, Minich LL, Mart C, Tani LY. Assessment of right ventricular size and function: Echo versus magnetic resonance imaging. Congenit Heart Dis. 2007;2(1):27–31.
27. Brent BN, Mahler D, Matthay RA, et al. Noninvasive diagnosis of pulmonary arterial hypertension in chronic obstructive pulmonary disease: right ventricular ejection fraction at rest. Am J Cardiol. 1984;53:1349–53.
28. Pasque MK, Trulock EP, Kaiser LR, et al. Single lung transplant for pulmonary hypertension: three month hemodynamic follow-up. Circulation. 1991;84:2275–9.
29. Tobinick E, Schelbert HR, Henning H, et al. Right ventricular ejection fraction in patients with acute inferior and anterior myocardial infarction assessed by radionuclide angiography. Circulation. 1978;57:1078–84.
30. Starling MRI, Dell'Italia LJ, Chaudhuri TK, et al. First transit and equilibrium radionuclide angiography in patients with inferior Transmural myocardial infarction: criteria for the diagnosis of associated Hemodynamically significant right ventricular infarction. J Am Coll Cardiol. 1984;4:923–30.
31. Hansen CL, Goldstein RA, Akinboboye OO, et al. Myocardial perfusion and function: single photon emission computed tomography. ASNC Imaging Guidelines J Nucl Cardiol. 2007;14:e39–60.
32. Ramani GV, Gurm G, Dilsizian V, Park MH. Noninvasive assessment of right ventricular function: will there be resurgence in radionuclide imaging techniques? Curr Cardiol Rep. 2010;12(2):162–9. doi:10.1007/s11886-010-0092-y. Review. PubMed PMID: 20425172
33. Van Wolferen SA, Marcus JT, Boonstra A, et al. Prognostic value of right ventricular mass, volume, and function in idiopathic pulmonary arterial hypertension. Eur Heart J. 2007;28:1250–7.
34. Roguin A, Zviman MM, Meininger GR, et al. Modern pacemaker and implantable Cardioverter/defibrillator systems can be magnetic resonance imaging safe: in vitro and in vivo assessment of safety and function at 1.5 T. Circulation. 2004;110(5):475–82.
35. Naehle CP, Kreuz J, Strach K, et al. Safety, feasibility, and diagnostic value of cardiac magnetic resonance imaging in patients with cardiac pacemakers and implantable Cardioverters/defibrillators at 1.5 T. Am Heart J. 2011;161(6):1096–105.
36. Nazarian S, Roguin A, Zviman MM, et al. Clinical utility and safety of a protocol for noncardiac and cardiac magnetic resonance imaging of

patients with permanent pacemakers and implantable-Cardioverter defibrillators at 1.5 Tesla. Circulation. 2006;114(12):1277–84.

37. Sommer T, Naehle CP, Yang A, et al. Strategy for safe performance of Extrathoracic magnetic resonance imaging at 1.5 Tesla in the presence of cardiac pacemakers in non-pacemaker-dependent patients: a prospective study with 115 examinations. Circulation. 2006;114(12):1285–92.

38. Luechinger R, Duru F, Scheidegger MB, et al. Force and torque effects of a 1.5-Tesla MRI scanner on cardiac pacemakers and ICDs. Pacing Clin Electrophysiol. 2001;24(2):199–205.

39. Kaasalainen T, Pakarinen S, Kivistö S, et al. MRI with cardiac pacing devices - safety in clinical practice. Eur J Radiol. 2014;83(8):1387–95.

40. Kalin R, Stanton MS. Current clinical issues for MRI scanning of pacemaker and defibrillator patients. Pacing Clin Electrophysiol. 2005;28(4):326–8.

41. Armstrong HF, Schulze PC, Kato TS, Bacchetta M, Thirapatarapong W, Bartels MN. Right ventricular stroke work index as a negative predictor of mortality and initial hospital stay after lung transplantation. J Heart Lung Transplant. 2013;32(6):603–8. doi:10.1016/j.healun.2013.03.00.

42. Roberts JD, Forfia PR. Diagnosis and assessment of pulmonary vascular disease by Doppler echocardiography. Pulm Circ. 2011;1(2):160–81. doi:10.4103/2045-8932.83446.

43. Lang RM, Bierig M, et al. American Society of Echocardiography's nomenclature and standards committee; task force on chamber quantification; American College of Cardiology Echocardiography Committee; American Heart Association; European Association of Echocardiography, European Society of Cardiology. Recommendations for chamber quantification. Eur J Echocardiogr. 2006;7(2):79–108. Epub 2006 Feb 2

44. Kypta A, Blessberger H, Hoenig S, Saleh K, Lambert T, Kammler J, Fellner F, Lichtenauer M, Steinwender C. Clinical safety of an MRI conditional implantable Cardioverter defibrillator system: a prospective Monocenter ICD-magnetic resonance imaging feasibility study (MIMI). J Magn Reson Imaging. 2016;43(3):574–84.

45. Expert Panel on MRI Safety, Kanal E, Barkovich AJ, Bell C, Borgstede JP, Bradley WG Jr, Froelich JW, Gimbel JR, Gosbee JW, Kuhni-Kaminski E, Larson PA, Lester JW Jr, Nyenhuis J, Schaefer DJ, Sebek EA, Weinreb J, Wilkoff BL, Woods OT, Lucey L, Hernandez D. ACR Guidance Document on MRI safe Practices: 2013. J Magn Reson Imaging. 2013;37(3):501–30.

46. Neyer J, Arsanjani R, Moriguchi J, Siegel R, Kobashigawa J. Echocardiographic parameters associated with right ventricular failure after left ventricular assist device: a review. J Heart Lung Transplant. 2016;35(3):283–93. doi:10.1016/j.healun.2015.12.018.

15

Reoperation for a giant arch anastomotic pseudoaneurysm eleven years after total arch replacement with island reconstruction

Ryohei Matsuura [1,2]*⦿, Yasushi Tsutsumi [1], Osamu Monta [1], Hisazumi Uenaka [1], Kenji Tanaka [1], Takaaki Samura [1] and Hirokazu Ohashi [1]

Abstract

Background: The long-term effects of some surgical treatment procedures of arch replacement for aortic dissection or aortic aneurysm are unknown.

Case presentation: The present study reports the case of a 68-year-old man admitted to our hospital for aortic arch anastomotic pseudoaneurysm with concomitant aortic root enlargement and coronary artery stenosis. Eleven years ago, at the age of 56 years, he underwent total arch replacement with island reconstruction for chronic aortic dissection. We performed a second total arch replacement, aortic root replacement, and coronary artery bypass, using a cardiopulmonary bypass with cannulation through the right subclavian artery, femoral artery, and femoral vein prior to re-sternotomy. We also used selective cerebral perfusion. Postoperatively, the patient temporarily required reintubation; however, he was discharged in good condition on the fiftieth postoperative day.

Conclusions: This case suggests that island reconstruction has the potential to cause arch anastomotic pseudoaneurysms, particularly after a long postoperative period.

Keywords: Island reconstruction, Pseudoaneurysm, Arch replacement

Background

Along with recent progress in aortic surgery, the number of patients undergoing thoracic aortic aneurysm surgery has increased, with evident improvements in long-term performance [1, 2]. However, some cases require reoperation long after the initial surgery [3–5]. We experienced a rare case of pseudoaneurysm in the arch anastomotic region in the eleventh year after a total arch replacement with island reconstruction.

Case presentation

A 68-year-old man was admitted to our hospital due to aortic arch anastomotic pseudoaneurysm with concomitant aortic root enlargement and coronary artery stenosis. At 56 years of age, the patient had undergone a total arch

replacement at another hospital, with three-branched island reconstruction performed using the T-graft technique for a chronic aortic dissection, expanding from the ascending aorta to distal aortic arch (Figs. 1 and 2). In the aortic arch island reconstruction, the adventitia and intima of the arteries were combined and reinforced externally by a felt, and end-to-end anastomosis was performed with a 30-mm synthetic vascular graft with one branch. Thereafter, the patient was followed up by a local physician; however, a computed tomography (CT) scan was not performed, as no relevant symptoms were observed. A CT scan at another hospital, however, showed a giant pseudoaneurysm at the site of the island reconstruction 11 years later. Though endovascular repair was considered, the patient was ultimately determined to be inoperable by the other hospital, as enlargement of the aortic root was also observed. He was subsequently referred to our hospital and he opted to undergo surgery at our institution.

At the time of presentation, the patient was 168 cm in height and weighed 71 kg. His vital signs were as

* Correspondence: r-matsuura@surg1.med.osaka-u.ac.jp
[1]Department of Cardiovascular Surgery, Fukui Cardiovascular Center, 2-228 Shinbo, Fukui 910-0833, Japan
[2]Department of Cardiovascular Surgery, Osaka University Graduate School of Medicine, 2-2 E1, Yamadaoka, Suita-shi, Osaka 565-0871, Japan

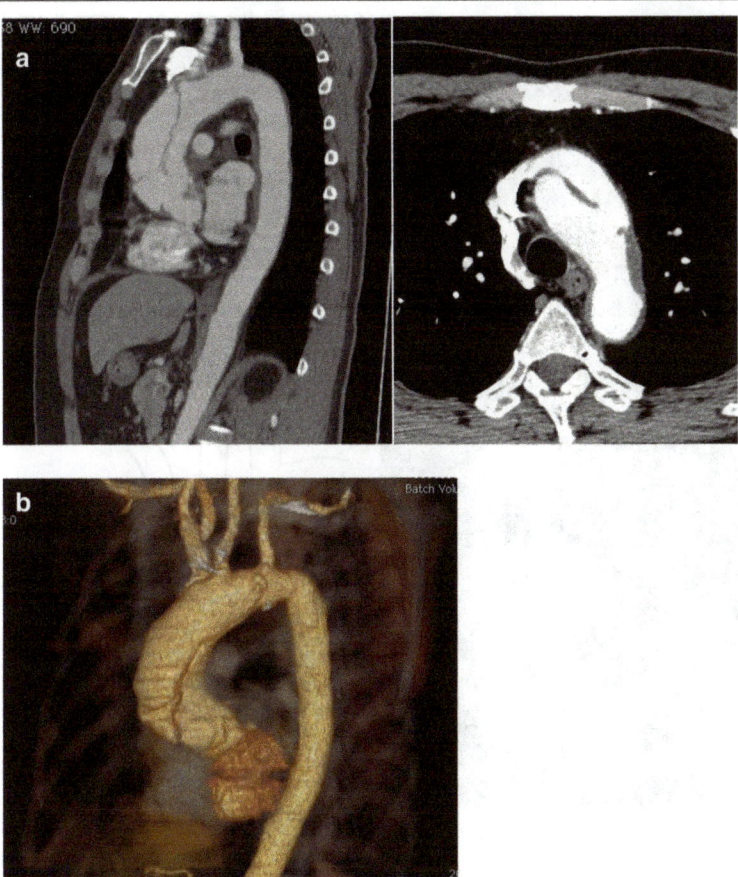

Fig. 1 CT scan showing a Stanford type A aortic dissection. **a** Multiplanar reconstruction view of CT angiogram of the thoracic aorta. The maximum diameter of the ascending aorta was 51 mm. The entry was at the ascending aorta and the reentry was between the left common carotid artery and left subclavian artery. **b** Preoperative multi detector computed tomography

follows: body temperature, 36.1 °C; blood pressure, 120/60 mmHg (no difference between left and right arms); pulse rate, 70 bpm (regular); and SpO$_2$, 100% (room air). Upon physical examination, his consciousness was clear, but expressed hoarseness in his voice. The patient had a median sternotomy scar. A diastolic murmur was detected in the third intercostal space at the left sternal border on thoracic auscultation. Breath sounds were normal, and the abdomen was soft and flat. An electrocardiogram showed normal sinus rhythm. A chest X-ray revealed enlargement of the left 1st arch and elevation of the left diaphragm. His cardio-thoracic ratio was 55.4%.

There were no abnormal laboratory findings nor did echocardiography reveal abnormal cardiac function upon admission.

Contrast-enhanced CT (Fig. 3) showed that a giant arch pseudoaneurysm (81 mm wide) had formed in the island-shaped arch branch. No false lumen was observed in the aneurysm, and its enlargement was omnidirectional. The diameter of the aortic root was also enlarged

to approximately 56 mm in size. In addition, coronary angiography indicated that there was 99% stenosis of the left anterior descending coronary artery at #7, collateral circulation from the right coronary artery, and 75% stenosis of the left circumflex artery at #13.

Based upon these observations, the patient underwent a repeat total arch replacement, aortic root replacement (i.e., Bentall procedure), and coronary artery bypass grafting [the left internal thoracic artery (LITA) and saphenous vein graft (SVG) were used]. Under general anesthesia, extracorporeal perfusion was initiated. We re-performed a median sternotomy and successfully opened the thorax without causing any damage to the aneurysm, while gradually decreasing the rectal temperature to 28 °C while sending blood to the right femoral artery and right axillary artery, while removing blood from the right femoral vein. We were able to switch the cannula from the femoral vein to the superior and inferior vena cava, as needed. After removing the previously used vascular graft, the coronary ostia on the right and left were confirmed and excised in the shape

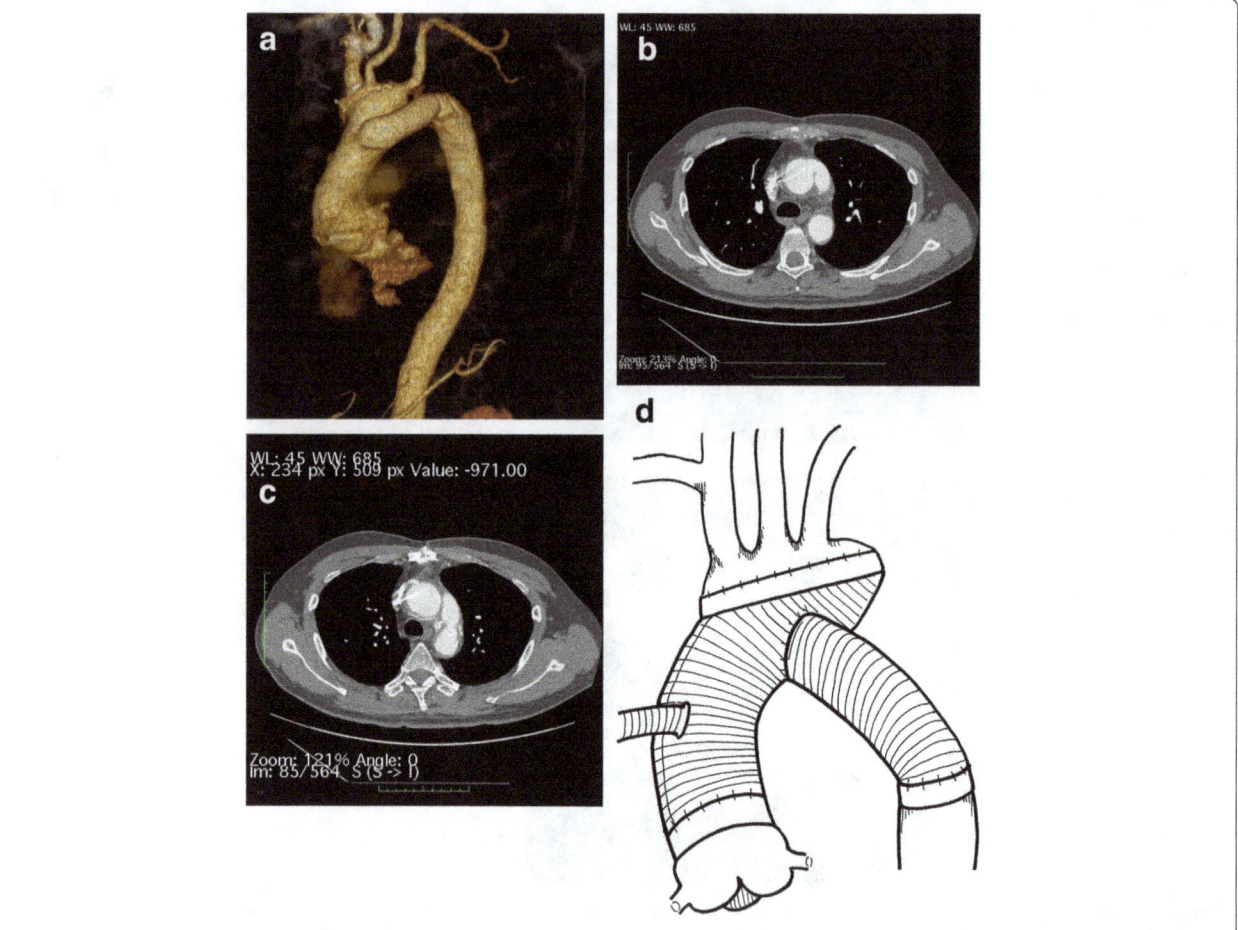

Fig. 2 Postoperative multidetector computed tomography (MDCT) showing total aortic arch replacement with island reconstruction using the T-graft technique. It also shows that no false lumens remained after the first surgery. **a** Synthetic image, (**b-c**) axial view, and (**d**) scheme of the procedure. The diameter of the graft: proximal, 30 mm; distal, 18 mm

of a button. A 23 mm Carpentier-Edwards Perimount (CEP)® bovine pericardial bioprosthesis (Edwards Life Science, Irvine, CA) and a 28 mm Vascutek® Gelweave Valsalva Graft (Terumo Vascutek, Renfrewshire, Scotland, UK) were combined with a running suture, and the skirt portion and the aortic valve annulus were attached with a 3–0 PROLENE running suture (Ethicon, Somerville, NJ, USA), with a felt strip between them. The right and left coronary arteries were continuously sutured with 5–0 PROLENE (Ethicon, Somerville, NJ, USA) for reconstruction of the Carrel patch. When the rectal temperature reached 28 °C, circulation of the lower body was arrested and antegrade selective cerebral perfusion was initiated by the insertion of balloon-occludable catheters to each cervical branch of the aorta. Upon incision of the aneurysm, it was revealed that the inner wall was covered by atheroma, although no false lumen was observed inside the aneurysm or arch branches. After removing as much of the aneurysm as possible, three separate perfusions of cervical branches were performed. On the distal side, another

vascular graft was retained and connected to a 26 mm, four-branched synthetic vascular graft (J-graft SHIELD NEO®, Japan Lifeline, Japan) with 3–0 PROLENE (Ethicon, Somerville, NJ, USA) using the open distal technique. After a restart of blood flow from the synthetic vascular graft branch, the left subclavian artery was reconstructed. In addition, the SVG and LITA were sutured to #14 and #8, respectively, and the Valsalva graft and the 26 mm J-graft were attached with running sutures of 4–0 PROLENE (Ethicon, Somerville, NJ, USA). The central side of the SVG was then anastomosed to the J-graft to allow the release of the aorta clamp. Finally, the left common carotid artery and brachiocephalic artery were reconstructed.

The operation was completed under stable hemodynamics. The operation time was 660 min, extracorporeal circulation time was 363 min, aortic clamp time was 172 min, circulatory arrest time was 38 min, the lowest rectal temperature was 27.6 °C, and intraoperative bleeding was 3240 mL.

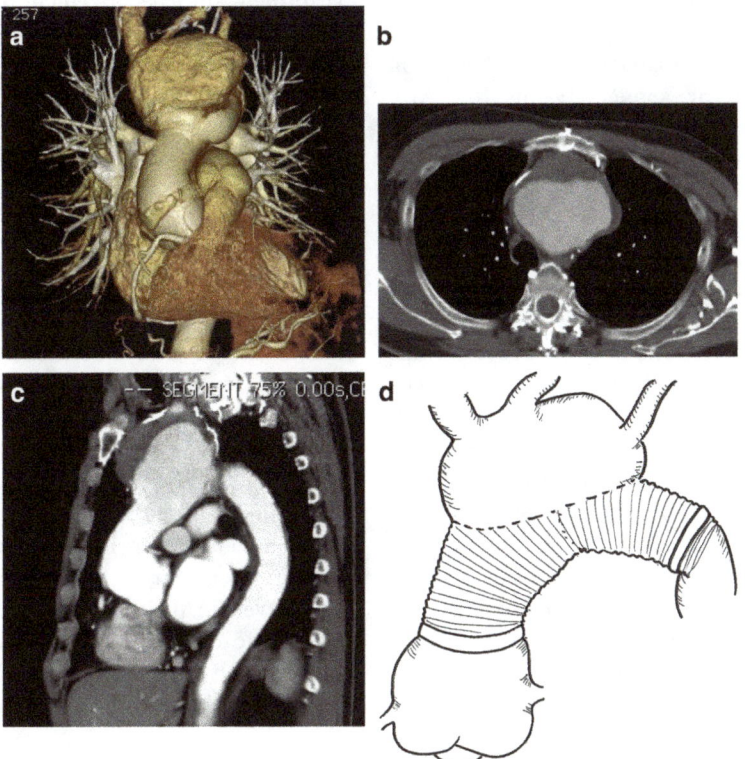

Fig. 3 Multidetector computed tomography (MDCT) 11 years after the previous surgery. The MDCT demonstrates a giant arch anastomotic pseudoaneurysm, aortic root enlargement and coronary artery stenosis, and shows no re-dissection in the pseudoaneurysm. **a** Synthetic image, (**b-c**) axial view, and (**d**) scheme of the aneurysm

Although the patient was re-intubated on the fourth postoperative day after extubation for ventilator failure, he was extubated again and discharged from the ICU on the eighth postoperative day. An indwelling pacemaker was inserted on the 40 s postoperative day due to sick sinus syndrome and the patient was ultimately discharged from the hospital on the fiftieth postoperative day (Fig. 4). He has been visiting the hospital as an outpatient and is in favorable condition.

Discussion

A wide range of arch replacement reconstruction techniques have been reported, including the open distal technique, arch-first technique (AFT), and hypothermic circulatory arrest (HCA)/simple clamping. Moreover, there are several techniques for cerebral perfusion, such as antegrade selective cerebral perfusion (SCP), and retrograde cerebral perfusion (RCP). Therefore, the choice of reconstruction techniques or supplemental

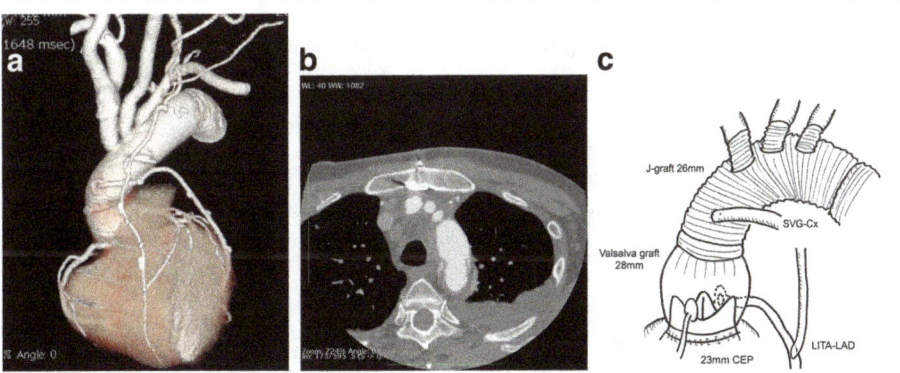

Fig. 4 Postoperative multidetector computed tomography (MDCT) scan showing redo total arch replacement, aortic root replacement and coronary artery bypass (LITA-LAD, Ao-SVG-PL). LITA: left internal thoracic artery, LAD: left descending artery, Ao: Aorta, SVG: saphenous vein graft, PL: posterior lateral. **a** Synthetic image, (**b**) axial view, and (**c**) scheme of the aneurysm

devices for perfusion depends on the patient condition, surgeon preference, and institution policy. To reduce the duration of non-physiologic circulation when performing RCP, AFT is employed by some surgeons [6]. AFT shortens cerebral ischemia time and ensures a favorable surgical field. It is also reported to reduce the occurrence of cerebral complications [7]. Other measures have been taken to shorten the cerebral ischemia time, among which arch branched island reconstruction is believed to be a simpler procedure, entailing the requirements of relatively less effort with fewer movements and opportunities for error during operation [8]. In this case, this reconstruction is performed as part of the T-graft technique. In addition to ensuring secure cerebral perfusion, the use of two synthetic vascular grafts with different diameters can provide flexibility in selecting the desired graft diameter when an apparent discrepancy is observed in the proximal and distal sides [9].

Notably, we observed in this case that residual vessel diseases induced the formation of a giant pseudoaneurysm in the eleventh postoperative year. While the formation of a pseudoaneurysm after thoracic aorta synthetic vascular graft replacement is rare, it is a possibly fatal complication once it develops. Reported causes of pseudoaneurysm formation include synthetic vascular graft infection, deterioration/enlargement of synthetic vascular graft, deterioration of suture thread, hypertension, aortic dissection, mechanical stress at the anastomotic site, and tissue necrosis due to the excessive use of gelatin resorcin formalin (GRF) glue [3, 4, 10]. Consequently, the pseudoaneurysm in this case had no obvious cause. Regarding aortic aneurysms, there are some reports that residual weak vessel diseases often necessitate reoperation, even in cases of true aneurysms; thus, a dissected aorta is used in most instances of cervical anastomosis (island reconstruction), including in this case [5]. In the vascular structure reconstructed during the first surgery, blood pumped from the heart was applying pressure directly to the weak anastomotic site, and hence it may have been more likely to form an aneurysm. In cases such as ours, with dissection advanced to the distal aortic arch, employing a reconstruction technique that can remove the weakened aortic wall as much as possible during the first surgery is important.

Treatment using stent grafts for pseudoaneurysms has been reported, but treatment of postoperative aortic arch pseudoaneurysms is difficult due to the complicated shape [11]. However, branch TEVAR is challenging in terms of device preparation. In the debranching and TEVAR technique, re-thoracotomy is necessary, and difficulties in placement and anastomosis of the debranched graft, plus in ensuring exposure of the carotid artery, are to be expected in the case of a giant pseudoaneurysm. In this case, repair with re-thoracotomy was performed since enlargement of the aortic root and complications of other coronary diseases were observed in addition to the presence of non-anatomical reconstruction using the T-graft technique.

During reoperation for thoracic aortic aneurysm, the patient will be at risk if the pseudoaneurysm is ruptured during a median sternotomy; hence, the re-operation is more carefully performed than a general thoracotomy. The effectiveness of extracorporeal circulation using the femoral artery and vein with HCA in performing reoperation for thoracic aortic aneurysm has been reported; thus, it should always be a possibility for consideration, although operative invasiveness must be taken into account [10, 12, 13].

Although five- to 10-year operative outcomes of thoracic aortic surgeries have improved over time, they are still poorly understood due to the scarcity of reports of long-term outcomes over 10 years. In the increasingly aging population, promising long-term prognoses are anticipated, even in patients with Marfan syndrome or those with aortic disease that developed at a relatively young age. As such, reconstruction techniques must be examined in consideration of longer prognoses in the future.

Conclusions

We experienced a case requiring reoperation for aortic arch pseudoaneurysm 11 years after a total arch replacement with island reconstruction for chronic aortic dissection. We believe that sufficient examination of reconstruction techniques is necessary, particularly in cases of relatively young patients who are expected to have a favorable long-term prognosis.

Abbreviations

AFT: Arch-first technique; GRF: Gelatin resorcin formalin; HCA: Hypothermic circulatory arrest; LITA: Left internal thoracic artery; RCP: Retrograde cerebral perfusion; SCP: Selective cerebral perfusion; SVG: Saphenous vein graft; TEVAR: Thoracic endovascular aortic repair

Acknowledgements

The authors would like to thank Paul Shelton and Editage for English language review.

Funding

The authors have no funding, financial relationships.

Declarations

This case report is based on a study first reported in the Japanese Journal of Cardiovascular Surgery 2015;44(4):232-236.

Authors' contributions

All authors have read and approved the final manuscript.

Reoperation for a giant arch anastomotic pseudoaneurysm eleven years after total arch replacement...

101

Competing interests

The authors declare that they have no competing interests.

References

1. Di Eusanio M, Berretta P, Cefarelli M, Castrovinci S, Folesani G, Alfonsi J, et al. Long-term outcomes after aortic arch surgery: results of a study involving 623 patients. Eur J Cardiothorac Surg. 2015;48(3):483–90.
2. Li B, Ma WG, Liu YM, Sun LZ. Is extended arch replacement justified for acute type a aortic dissection? Interact Cardiovasc Thorac Surg. 2015;20(1):120–6.
3. Kimura S, Ueno Y. Redo total arch replacement for a patient with pseudoaneurysm of the thoracic aortic graft. Jpn. J Cardiovasc Surg. 2012; 41:29–32.
4. Izumiyama O, Yamashita A, Sugimoto S, Baba M. A case of anastomotic pseudoaneurysm at an anastomosis between two woven Dacron prostheses following aortic arch replacement. Jpn J Cardiovasc Surg. 2000; 29:191–4.
5. Sasaki A, Sakata J, Satou H, Kazui T. A case of descending graft replacement of the anastomotic aneurysm using simple hypothermic retrograde cerebral circulation 9 years after surgery of the distal aortic arch. Jpn J Cardiovasc Surg. 2002;31:311–3.
6. Rokkas CK, Kouchoukos NT. Single-stage extensive replacement of the thoracic aorta: the arch-first technique. J Thorac Cardiovasc Surg. 1999;117:99–105.
7. Sasaki M, Usui A, Yoshikawa M, Akita T, Ueda Y. Arch-first technique performed under hypothermic circulatory arrest with retrograde cerebral perfusion improves neurological outcomes for total arch replacement. Eur J Cardiothorac Surg. 2005;27(5):821–5.
8. Ishida N, Shimabukuro K, Matsuno Y, Takemura H. Ascending aorta and total arch replacement in a Stanford type a aortic dissection with island reconstruction for an isolated left vertebral artery. Jpn. J Cardiovasc Surg. 2010;39(6):318–20.
9. Ohtake H, Kimura K, Yashiki Y, Yamaguchi S, Tomita S, Watanabe G. T-graft technique under antegrade cerebral perfusion for aortic arch aneurysm. Ann Thorac Surg. 2010;90(5):1721–3.
10. Katsumata T, Moorjani N, Vaccari G, Westaby S. Mediastinal false aneurysm after thoracic aortic surgery. Ann Thorac Surg. 2000;70(2):547–52.
11. Ikeda O, Ideta I, Kunitomo R, Utsunomiya D, Urata J, Hirayama T, et al. Management of endovascular repair for anastomotic pseudoaneurysm after surgical reconstruction. Jpn. J Vasc Surg. 2009;18(5):573–9.
12. Malvindi PG, van Putte BP, Sonker U, Heijmen RH, Schepens MA, Morshuis WJ. Reoperation after acute type a aortic dissection repair: a series of 104 patients. Ann Thorac Surg. 2013;95(3):922–7.
13. Malvindi PG, van Putte BP, Heijmen RH, Schepens MA, Morshuis WJ, et al. Reoperations for aortic false aneurysms after cardiac surgery. Ann Thorac Surg. 2010;90(5):1437–43.

Impact of prosthesis-patient mismatch after mitral valve replacement in rheumatic population: Does mitral position prosthesis-patient mismatch really exist?

Seung Hyun Lee, Byung Chul Chang, Young-Nam Youn, Hyun Chel Joo, Kyung-Jong Yoo and Sak Lee[*]

Abstract

Background: Prosthesis-patient mismatch (PPM) is characterised by the effects of inadequate prosthesis size relative to body surface area (BSA).The purpose of this study was to determine the impact of PPM on late clinical outcomes after mitral valve replacement (MVR) in rheumatic population.

Methods: From 2000 to 2013, a total of 445 patients (mean age 54.2 ± 11.7 years) underwent isolated MVR ($\pm$tricuspid annuloplasty) for rheumatic disease were investigated. Effective orifice area (EOA) was determined by the continuity equation and PPM was defined as indexed EOA (EOA/BSA) ≤ 1.2 cm^2/m^2. Clinical and echocardiographic follow-up (mean follow up 8.7 ± 4.0 years) results were compared.

Results: 37% of patients ($n = 165$) had PPM. There were no significant differences in baseline and operative characteristics between patients with and without PPM except age and IEOA. A significant decrease in mean trans-valvular pressure gradient (MPG) over time following MVR, however the change of MPG showed no differences between groups (No PPM vs. PPM: 8.9 ± 4.7 mmHg $\rightarrow 3.6 \pm 1.2$ mmHg vs. 8.7 ± 4.5 mmHg $\rightarrow 3.8 \pm 1.4$ mmHg, p-value $= 0.28$). In all patients, there was a reduction of left atrium dimension (58.6 ± 12.0 mm $\rightarrow 53.2 \pm 12.0$ mm vs. 57.9 ± 8.9 mm $\rightarrow 52.2 \pm 8.9$ mm, p-value $= 0.68$) and left ventricular end diastolic diameter (49.9 ± 5.7 mm $\rightarrow 48.9 \pm 5.7$ mm vs. 49.7 ± 6.0 mm $\rightarrow 48.3 \pm 5.0$ mm, $p = 0.24$) without statistical significance. Freedom from TR progression rates at 3 and 5 years (99% vs.98%, 99% vs. 98%, p-value $= 0.1$), and overall survival rates at 3 and 5 years (97% vs. 96%, 94% vs. 94%, p-value $= 0.7$) were similar.

Conclusion: This study shows that mitral PPM is not associated with atrial /ventricular remodeling and might not influence late clinical outcome including late TR progression, survival in rheumatic population.

Keywords: Heart valve prosthesis, Hemodynamics, Mitral valve, Mortality, Surgery, Valves

Background

Previous studies reported that prosthesis–patient mismatch (PPM) in aortic valve position is strongly associated with worse hemodynamics, less regression of left ventricular hypertrophy, more cardiac events, and higher mortality rates after aortic valve replacement [1–3]. However, PPM following mitral valve replacement (MVR)

has been still less investigated. Previous studies reported that mitral PPM is various, from 30 to 85% when in vivo evaluation of effective orifice area (EOA) is performed [4–6]. Some studies on the clinical impact of PPM following MVR on survival have reported conflicting results, although two recent trials showed that PPM in the mitral position independently affects long-term survival.

Dumesnil et al. have addressed that indexed EOA derived from in vivo postoperative measures is the only parameter that can consistently be correlated with postoperative gradients as well as clinical outcomes in defining PPM [7]. Mitral PPM can be equated to residual mitral stenosis

* Correspondence: Sak911@yuhs.ac
Division of Thoracic and Cardiovascular Surgery, Severance Cardiovascular Hospital, Yonsei Cardiovascular Research Institute, Yonsei University, College of Medicine, 250 Seongsanno, Seodaemun-gu, Seoul 03722, Republic of Korea

resulting in increased trans-mitral gradients, increased left atrial pressure, and pulmonary hypertension (PH). These factors may lead to right ventricular dilatation/ dysfunction and to atrial fibrillation, which may, in turn, lead to tricuspid annulus dilatation and functional tricuspid regurgitation (fTR).

However, despite of small sized mitral prosthesis implantation such as 25 mm, we can easily find that no occurrence of TR after MVR during follow duration. In Asian rheumatic population, mitral annuls size is relatively small compared with western mitral disease, so we can easily meet the patients with small sized mitral prosthesis replacement and collect many cases. The objective of this study was to investigate the impact of mitral PPM on late clinical outcomes including TR progression and survival following MVR in rheumatic population.

Methods

Patient population

We retrospectively reviewed a consecutive series of 445 patients who underwent elective isolated MVR with or without TAP (tricuspid annuloplasty) for rheumatic mitral valve disease at Severance Cardiovascular Hospital, University of Yonsei, from Jan 2000 to Dec 2013. Patients with concomitant aortic valve, coronary artery bypass and aorta surgery were excluded. In cases of TAP, if residual TR grade after TAP were 2,3 and 4, they were also excluded for minimizing the confusion of TR progression analysis. Data were retroprospectively collected and recorded in an electronic database, and clinical follow-up was completed with routine outpatient clinics. Patients who did not present at the visit were contacted by telephone, and all symptoms, mortality, and any complications that occurred during follow-up were recorded. This study was approved by the Institutional Review Board of Yonsei University College of Medicine. Individual patient consent was waived because this study did not interfere with patient treatment, and the database was designed so that individual patients could not be identified. All baseline and clinical characteristics were obtained from the medical record of patients.

All patients underwent a full median sternotomy and operation performed on cardio-pulmonary bypass. The prostheses were used in as followings:

- Mechanical prosthesis: St. Jude Medical Standard Mechanical (St. Jude Medical Inc., St. Paul, MN) ($n = 140$), MIRA (Edwards Lifesciences; Irvine, Calif) ($n = 54$), ATS (Medtronic, Minneapolis, MN) ($n = 85$), Sorin (Sorin Biomedica, Saluggia, Italy) ($n = 11$), ON-X (On-X Life Technology, Austin, TX) ($n = 61$), CarboMedics Mechanical (Sulzer CarboMedics, Austin, TX) ($n = 12$).

- Bioprosthesis: Perimount Magna (Edwards Lifesciences LLC, Irvine, CA) ($n = 49$), Epic (St. Jude Medical Inc., St. Paul, MN) ($n = 17$), Hancock (Medtronic, Minneapolis, MN) ($n = 7$), Biocor (St. Jude Medical Inc., St. Paul, MN) ($n = 11$). In all cases, posterior chordal preservation was attempted as a routine maneuver.

Doppler-echocardiographic assessment

Clinical and echocardiographic assessment was performed prior to MVR and 12–60 months after operation. The echocardiographic images of the included patients were reanalyzed by 2 experienced echocardiographers who were unaware of the patient's clinical data. LV internal diameter, septal thickness, and LV posterior wall thickness were measured at end-diastole. LV mass was calculated using the formula developed by Devereux et al. [8], and LV mass was indexed for the body surface area. The left atrial volume was calculated from the parasternal long-axis view and apical four-chamber view using the prolate ellipse method [9]. The severity of TR was assessed using color flow imaging and regurgitant jet area [10]. Doppler color flow mapping was used to assess the competency of the prosthetic valves.

EOA calculation and definition of PPM

The in-vivo prosthetic valve effective orifice area (EOA) was calculated with the use of the continuity equation, using the stroke volume measured in the LV outflow tract divided by the integral of themitral valve transprosthetic velocity-time integral during diastole. The indexed EOA (IEOA) was calculated by dividing the measured EOA by the patient's body surface area (BSA) at the time of follow-up. Indexed EOA was used to define PPM as significant if ≤ 1.2 cm^2/m^2, moderate if > 0.9 cm^2/m^2 and ≤ 1.2 cm^2/m^2, and severe if ≤ 0.9 cm^2/m^2 [4].

Statistical analysis

Data were prospectively collected and recorded in an electronic database; statistical analysis was performed using the Statistical Package for the Social Sciences, version 11.0 (SPSS, Chicago, IL). Continuous data are expressed as the mean and standard deviation; categorical data are expressed as the percentage, comparisons were made using the 2-sample t and the χ2 or the Fischer exact tests, respectively. We gain the optimal cutoff value of IEOA for late TR progression and mortality, receiver operating curve (ROC) method was used. Comparison between group with or without PPM, Kaplan Meyer survival analysis was used and p value $<$ 0.05 was considered statistically significant.

Results

Mitral valve patient–prosthesis mismatch

Of the 445 study patients, PPM was in 165 (37.1%), severe in only 8 by the definition of PPM. The proportion of patients with PPM was lower in those with mechanical valves ($n = 362$) than those with bioprosthesis ($n = 83$) ($n = 116$, 32% vs. $n = 49$, 59%, $p < 0.01$). An IEOA of patients with mechanical valves had a higher than those with bioprosthesis (1.41 ± 0.31 vs. 1.15 ± 0.21, $p < 0.01$). The clinical characteristics of the patients are shown in Table 1. Female portion of patients with PPM were similar (52, 31.5% vs. 69, 24.6%, $p = 0.09$) and PMV (Percutaneous mitral valvuloplasty) history were also not significantly different between groups (37, 8.3% vs. 66, 14.8%, $p = 0.8$). However, the age (55.96 ± 12.36 vs. 53.28 ± 10.82, $p < 0.01$) and BSA (body surface area, m^2) in PPM group (1.61 ± 0.14 vs. 1.55 ± 0.15, $p < 0.01$) was significantly higher than no PPM group regardless gender. Tissue valve portion was meaningfully higher in PPM group compared with No PPM group (29.7% vs. 12.1%).

Perioperative data and early clinical outcomes

Perioperative and early outcomes including postoperative echocardiography data are shown in Table 2. Thirty-day mortality was similar between groups (0% vs. 0.2%, $p = 1.0$), and postoperative CVA (cerebrovascular accidents) was also not different (0% vs. 0.2%, $p = 1.0$). There were also similar rates of other morbidities (postoperative bleeding: 1.8% vs. 1.1%, $p = 0.08$, acute renal failure: 0.2% vs. 0.7%) between groups.

The mean prosthesis size (mm) in No PPM group was significantly bigger than PPM group (27.89 ± 1.55 vs. 27.58 ± 1.57, $p = 0.03$). Values of EOA (2.38 ± 0.41 vs. 1.69 ± 0.15, $p < 0.01$) and IEOA (1.55 ± 0.25 vs. 1.06 ± 0.08, $p < 0.01$) in No PPM group were also siginificantly bigger than PPM group (Table 2). The ealry change of

Table 1 Basic preoperative charateristics

Preoperative parameters

	PPM ($n = 165$)	No PPM ($n = 280$)	p value
Age (years)	55.96 ± 12.36	53.28 ± 10.82	0.02
Gender (Female, n, %)	52 (31.5%)	69 (24.6%)	0.09
BSA (cm/m²)	1.61 ± 0.14	1.55 ± 0.15	< 0.01
Valve type (Tissue No, %)	49 (29.7%)	34 (12.1%)	< 0.01
Previous PMV Hx. (n, %)	37 (8.3%)	66 (14.8%)	0.82
LVEF (%)	62.70 ± 9.28	60.71 ± 9.52	0.31
LVEDD (mm)	48.27 ± 5.06	48.98 ± 5.72	0.23
LVESD (mm)	32.98 ± 5.17	33.8 ± 6.25	0.19
LAD (AP, mm)	52.29 ± 8.98	53.42	0.38
MPG (mmHg)	8.7 ± 4.52	8.91 ± 4.71	0.38

BSA body surface area, *PMV* percutaneous mitral valvuloplasty, *LVEF* left ventricular ejection fraction, *LVEDD* left ventricular end diastolic dimension, *LVESD* left ventricular end systolic dimension, *MPG* mean pressure gradient

Table 2 Early clinical outcomes and the the change of hemodynamics parameters

Perioperative and postoperative parameters

	PPM ($n = 165$)	No PPM ($n = 280$)	p value
30 days mortlaity	0 (0%)	1 (0.2%)	1.0
CVA (n, %)	0 (0%)	1 (0.2%)	1.0
ARF (n,%)	1 (0.2%)	3 (0.7%)	1.0
Postoperative Bleeding (n,%)	8 (1.8%)	5 (1.1%)	0.08
Prosthesis size (mm)	27.58 ± 1.57	27.89 ± 1.55	0.03
EOA (cm²)	1.69 ± 0.15	2.38 ± 0.41	< 0.01
IEOA	1.06 ± 0.08	1.55 ± 0.25	< 0.01
The change of RVSP (mmHg)	10.85 ± 14.75	9.91 ± 14.75	0.53
The change of MPG (mmHg)	4.7 ± 4.5	5.3 ± 5.0	0.34

CVA cerebral vascular event, *ARF* acute renal failure, *EOA* effective orifice area, *IEOA* indexed effective orifice area, *RVSP* right ventricular systolic pressure, *MPG* mean pressure gradient

MPG (mmHg) (4.7 ± 4.5 vs. 5.3 ± 5.0, $p = 0.34$) and right ventricular systolic pressure (RVSP, mmHg) (10.85 ± 14.75 vs. 9.91 ± 14.75, $p = 0.53$) after MVR was similar between groups.

Late clinical outcomes including postoperative echocardiography data, TR progression and survival

Mean echocardiography follow up duration was 8.4 ± 3.7 (0.3–15.2) years. Left ventricular ejection fraction (LVEF, %), left ventricular end systolic dimension (LVESD, mm), left ventricular end systolic dimension (LVEDD, mm), left atrim size (anterior-posterior distance, mm), and mean pressure gradient (MPG, mmHg) were routinely checked during follow up for analyzing ventricular remodeling. LVEF improvement in No PPM group was significantly better than PPM group (Δ: 0.83 ± 13.77 vs. 0.98 ± 9.70, $p = 0.89$). Left atrium (Δ LAD: 11.0 ± 18.8 vs. 13.5 ± 19.1, $p = 0.19$) and ventricular remodeling (Δ LVESD: 5.6 ± 12.4 vs. 4.1 ± 11.7, $p = 0.2$ and Δ LVEDD: 8.3 ± 17.8 vs. 5.7 ± 16.0, $p = 0.13$) were similar between groups. The reduction of right ventricular systolic pressure (RVSP, mmHg) (8.75 ± 8.2 vs. 10.7 ± 17.9 $p = 0.30$) and the MPG change (4.9 ± 4.5 vs. 5.3 ± 5.0, $p = 0.34$) were also not siginicantly different between groups (Table 3).

Freedom from TR progression (3,4) rate at 3, 5, and 10 years was 99%, 98%, and 93%, respectively. Freedom from TR progression (3,4) rate in patients with PPM at 3, 5, and 10 years was similar to that of patients without PPM (98%, 98%, 98% vs. 99%, 99%, 91%, respectively, $P = 0.09$) (Fig. 1a). After including TR grade 2, freedom from TR progression (2,3,4) in patients with PPM at 3, 5, and 10 years was similar to that of patients without PPM (98%, 96%, 94% vs. 98%, 96%, 85%, respectively, $P = 0.10$) (Fig. 1b).

Table 3 Serial change of hemodynamic characteristic and remodelling data

		Preoperative	Immediate postoperative	Last followup
LVEF (%)	No PPM	60.71	60.30	62.09
	PPM	61.70	61.60	62.68
LVESD (mm)	No PPM	34.64	34.21	33.48
	PPM	33.76	33.08	33.09
LVEDD (mm)	No PPM	49.92	48.67	48.69
	PPM	49.30	47.94	48.06
LAD (AP, mm)	No PPM	58.12	51.32	52.62
	PPM	57.88	51.03	52.17
MPG (mmHg)	No PPM	8.99	3.59	3.76
	PPM	8.83	4.01	4.02
RVSP (mmHg)	No PPM	42.33	31.82	32.96
	PPM	43.75	32.56	33.02

LVEF left ventricular ejection fraction, *LVEDD* left ventricular end diastolic dimension, *LVESD* left ventricular end systolic dimension, *LAD* left atrium dimension, *MPG* mean pressure gradient, *RVSP* right ventricular systolic pressure

Overall 3, 5, and 10-year survivals were 97%, 94%, and 88%, respectively. Patients with PPM had similar 3, 5, and 10-year survivals compared with no PPM patients (96%, 94% and 88% vs. 97%, 94% and 88%, respectively, $P = 0.80$) (Fig. 2).

Sub-analysis of severe PPM patients was as followings: Total eight patients had severe PPM (definition: IEOA ≤ 0.9 cm2/m2) and average age was 62.63 years (37 ~ 71). BSA was 1.7 (1.56 ~ 1.81) and preoperative TR were all under mild (Gr1). EF was 58.5% (36 ~ 71%), LVEDD was 52.5 mm (47 ~ 59 mm) and LA size (AP diameter, mm) was 59.3 mm (51 ~ 65 mm). Average IEOA was 0.85 (0.82~0.88). Five were Hancock ($n = 2/27$ mm, $n = 3/$ 29 mm, Medtronic, Minneapolis, MN), 2 were Epic ($n =$

2/29 mm, St. Jude Medical Inc., St. Paul, MN) and 1 was Perimount Magna ($n = 1/25$ mm, Edwards Lifesciences LLC, Irvine, CA). There was no in-hospital mortality and postoperative newly onset TR was none in all cases. There was just one case of late mortality after postoperative 6 years due to stomach cancer, but this was not correlated with cardiac death or TR progression.

For the gaining optimal IEOA cut value of TR progression, we used ROC method and 1.38 was determined as a cut value (new PPM value) for TR progression (Fig. 3). We divided two groups based on 1.38 (IEOA, new PPM) and compared late TR progression and cumulative survival. But against our expectation, the larger IEOA group (1.39 ≤, No PPM) showed inferior tendency of freedom

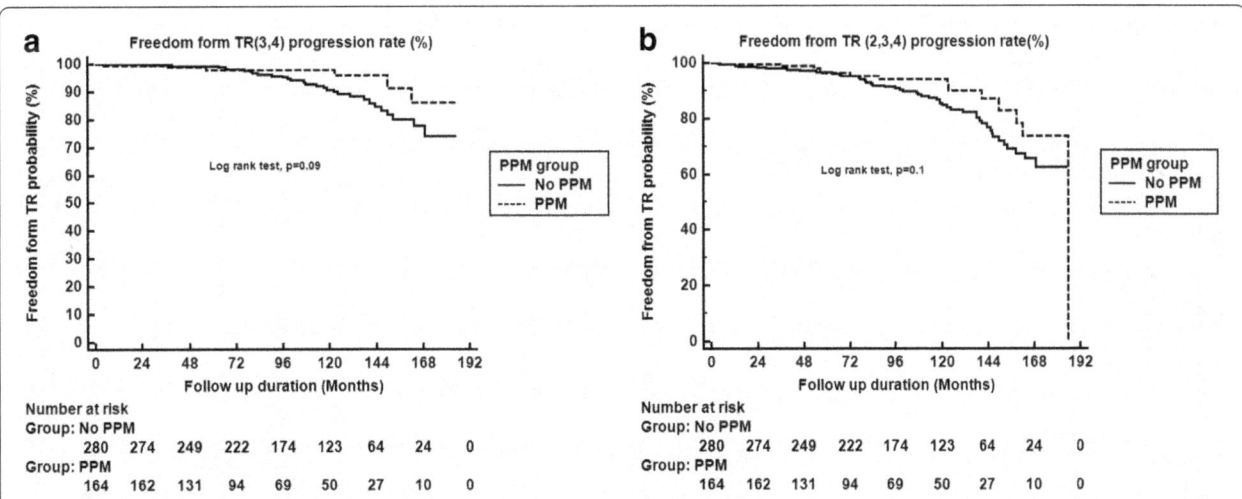

Fig. 1 Freedom from TR progression rate at 3, 5, and 10 years between groups (PPM vs. No PPM). **a** Freedom from TR progression (3,4) rate at 3, 5, and 10 years was 99%, 98%, and 93%, respectively. Freedom from TR progression (3,4) rate in patients with PPM at 3, 5, and 10 years was similar to that of patients without PPM (98%, 98%, 98% vs. 99%, 99%, 91%, respectively, $P = 0.09$). **b** Freedom from TR progression (2,3,4) in patients with PPM at 3, 5, and 10 years was similar to that of patients without PPM (98%, 96%, 94% vs. 98%, 96%, 85%, respectively, $P = 0.10$)

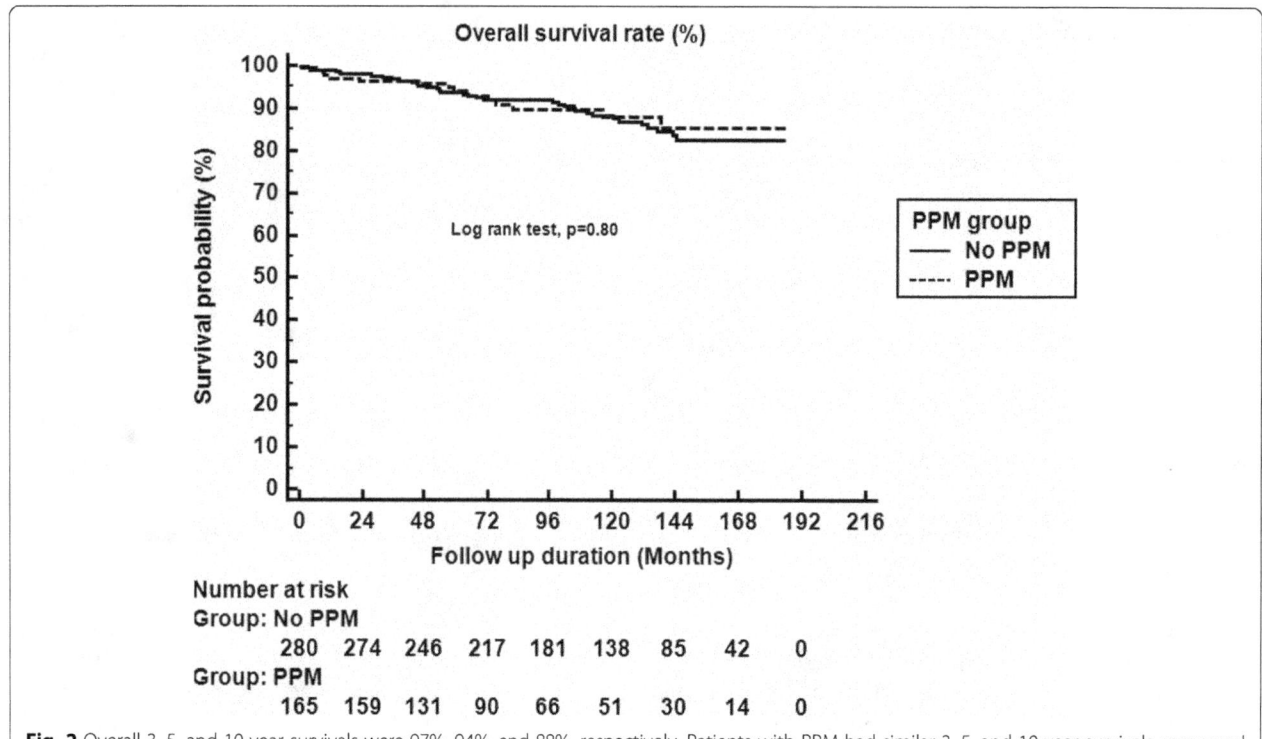

Fig. 2 Overall 3, 5, and 10-year survivals were 97%, 94%, and 88%, respectively. Patients with PPM had similar 3, 5, and 10-year survivals compared with no PPM patients (96%, 94% and 88% vs. 97%, 94% and 88%, respectively, $P = 0.80$)

from TR progression at 3,5 and 10 years (99, 99% and 88% vs. 99%, 98% and 97%, respectively, $P = 0.08$) (Fig. 4a). For survival, Patients with PPM had similar 3, 5, and 10-year survivals compared with no PPM patients (96%, 92% and 86% vs. 97%, 96% and 89%, respectively, $P = 0.16$) (Fig. 4b).

Considering valve type such as mechanical and tissue, late bleeding event related with warfarin intake showed higher in mechanical prosthesis group ($n = 11$, 3.1%)

compared with tissue prosthesis ($n = 2$, 2.4%) as expected. Late CVA incidence was 6.3% in mechanical and 10.8% in tissue prosthesis group. Reoperation related with degeneration was 1.1% in mechanical and 3.6% in tissue prosthesis group.

Discussion

The main findings of the present study are as followings: (1) the incidence of PPM after MVR in patients with

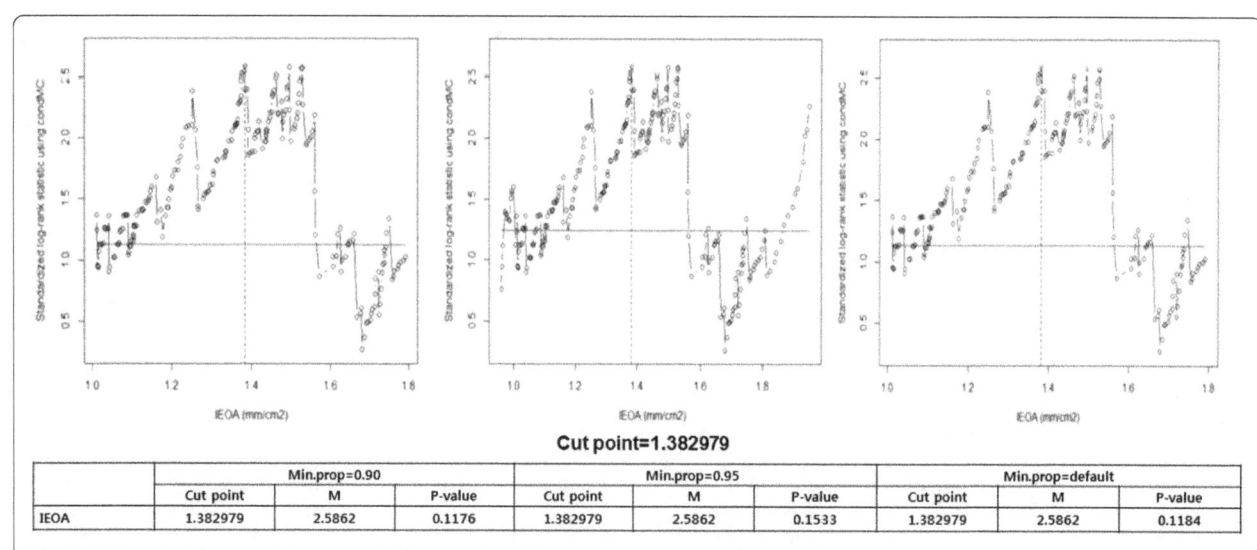

	Min.prop=0.90			Min.prop=0.95			Min.prop=default		
	Cut point	M	P-value	Cut point	M	P-value	Cut point	M	P-value
IEOA	1.382979	2.5862	0.1176	1.382979	2.5862	0.1533	1.382979	2.5862	0.1184

Fig. 3 ROC method for the gaining optimal IEOA cut value of TR progression 1.38 was determined as a cut value (new PPM value) for TR progression

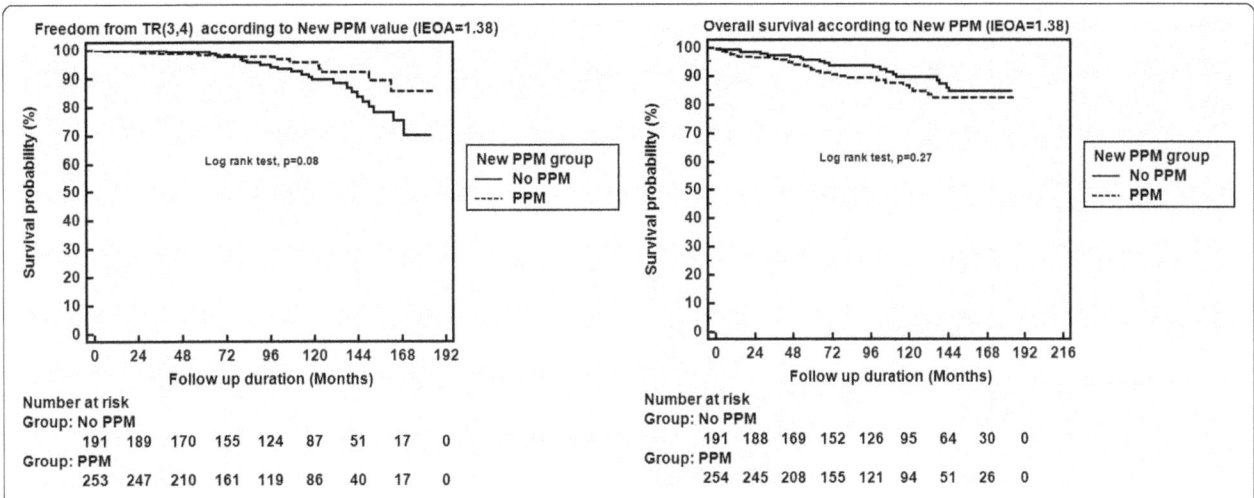

Fig. 4 Freedom from TR progression and overall survival at 3,5 and 10 years. **a** Freedom from TR progression at 3,5 and 10 years (99, 99% and 88% vs. 99%, 98% and 97%, respectively, P = 0.02). **b** Freedom from all cause mortality at 3, 5, and 10-year (96%, 92% and 86% vs. 97%, 96% and 89%, respectively, P = 0.16)

rheumatic mitral stenosis was relatively high against our expectation; (2) mitral position PPM was not correlated with late clinical result including late TR progression and survival; (3) the larger IEOA, the more TR progression tendency ($p = 0.08$), ironically.

Since first described in 1978 [11], PPM after MVR has been suggested to be correlate with poor clinical outcomes including persistent pulmonary hypertension and late functional tricuspid regurgitation [2, 12]. Until now, well described mechanism of the adverse effect of PPM was originated from high residual transvalvular pressure gradients, which is same with residual mitral stenosis with similar consequences (ie, the persistence of abnormally high mitral gradients and increased left atrial and pulmonary arterial pressures). The major consequence of pulmonary hypertension is right ventricular failure, which generally results from chronic pressure overload and associated volume overload with the development of tricuspid regurgitation. Hence, the persistence of left atrial and pulmonary hypertension associated with PPM is likely the main factor responsible for the increased mortality observed in the patients with severe PPM [4].

However, some reports suggested that PPM did not affect survival after MVR [13, 14], although several recent trials showed that mitral PPM independently affects long-term survival [4, 5]. Mitral valve replacement itself should ideally improve pulmonary hypertension and tricuspid regurgitation without increasing operative times and risk. The negative effects of aortic valve PPM on left ventricular remodeling, functional status, early mortality, and late survival have been extensively corroborated. [1, 15–17] What remains uncertain is whether clinically deleterious effects of PPM could be encountered after MVR.

Actually, there has been a recent rising interest in mitral PPM, which has been well documented in the pediatric population from small BSA and limited size of prosthesis according to growth potential. A variety of factors have been used in an attempt to define the concept of clinical PPM in children: These have included size/weight ratios, Z scores, maximum transprosthesis velocity (Vmax), and 2.5 times increase in body weight from the time of implant. In all instances, these factors have been correlated with outcomes (early mortality, survival, and PTH) [18, 19]. Adult mitral PPM was the subject of an original case report in 1981 [20], it has subsequently been theorized, through in vitro pulse duplicator analysis, that an indexed geometrical area (IGOA) less than 1.3 to 1.5 cm2/m2 could potentially leave the patient with high postoperative trans-mitral gradients. In a clinical study, a good correlation between elevated transprosthetic mitral gradient and in vivo IEOA was demonstrated by the use of the continuity eq. (CE) during echocardiographic assessment of porcine mitral prostheses [7]. In this report, an IEOA of 1.3 to 1.5 cm2/m2 or less at rest was associated with a mean mitral gradient of 4 mmHg; with every 10% increase in stroke volume (maximum 50%), there was a proportional increase of the mean mitral gradient.

However, in our study, there was very weak relation between trans-mitral gradients and IEOA induced from correlation coefficient analysis ($r = -0.08$, $p = 0.07$) (Fig. 5). It means that postoperative decrease of MPG was induced well regardless of IEOA and there was no problematic residual pressure gradients which can make physiologic mitral stenosis (Fig 6a). Also we found that BSA did not show strong correlation with IOEA ($r = 0.27$) and PPM incidence was not significantly different

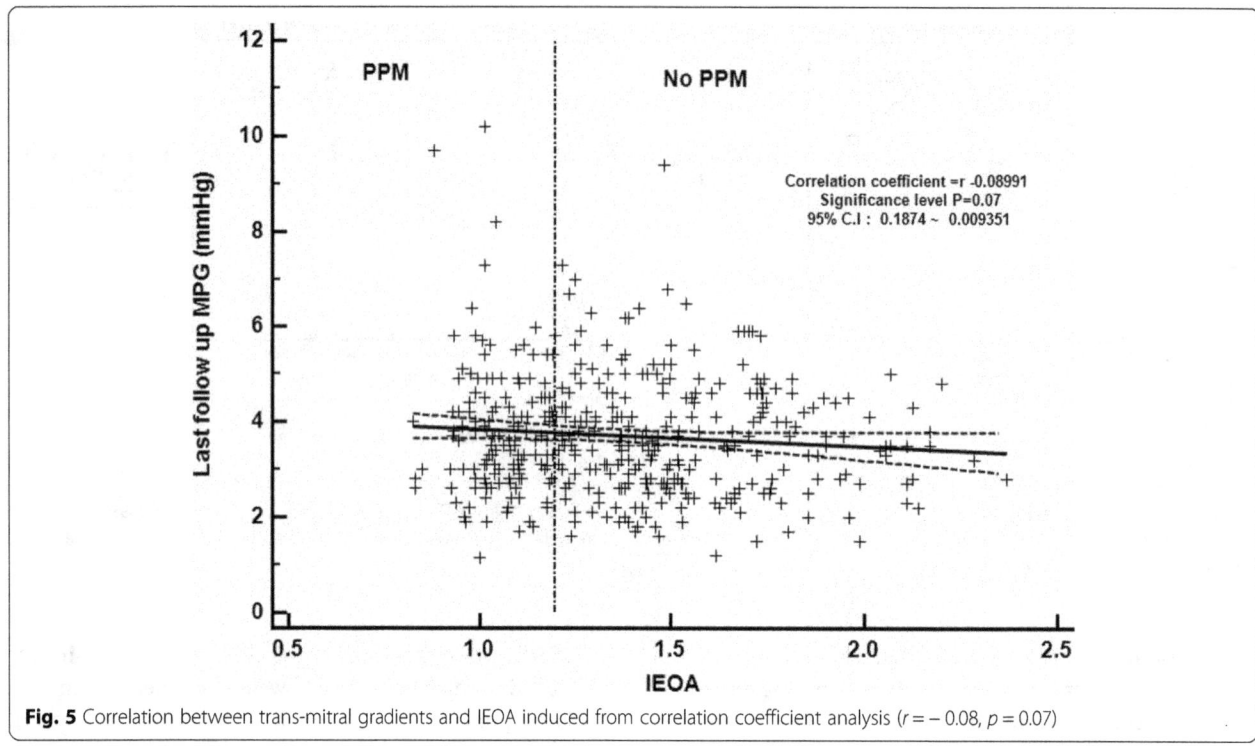

Fig. 5 Correlation between trans-mitral gradients and IEOA induced from correlation coefficient analysis ($r = -0.08$, $p = 0.07$)

under 29 mm sized population using same correlation coefficient analysis ($r = 0.17$) (Fig. 6b). In asian population, small size mitral implantation might be considered generally to be occured more frequently rather than western population, however implantation prosthesis size was not so strongly associated with BSA. Mitral prosthesis size in No PPM group was slightly bigger than PPM group (27.89 ± 1.55 vs. 27.58 ± 1.57, $p = 0.03$), but after exclusion of 31 mm size implanted patients, there was no significant different between groups (27.44 ± 1.42 vs. 27.69 ± 1.35, $p = 0.08$). From the

analysis of TR progression rate, we found contradictory result that PPM group showed superior freedom from TR progression rate in both classic IEOA classficaiton (1.25) and newly gained IEOA (1.38) classification. This doesn't necessarily mean that the bigger mitral prosthesis, the better clinical outcomes. Bigger mitral implantation might mean two things: 1) Big BSA or 2) Heart enlargement, however, from our result, big BSA doesn't necessarily mean bigger mitral implantation (Fig. 6a, $r = 0.27$). Then mitral annulus enlargement from heart failure might be strong candidate for bigger

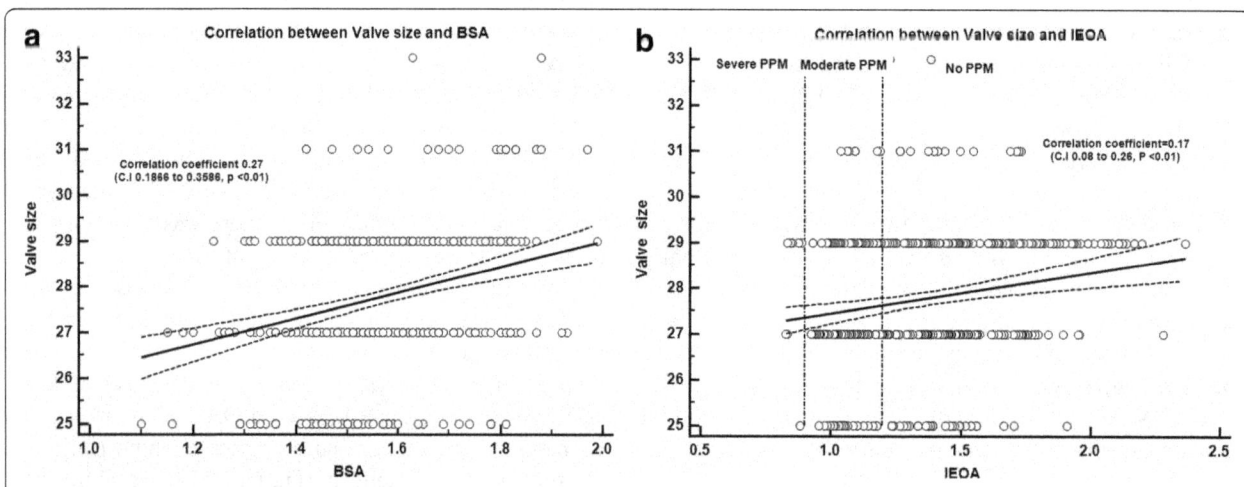

Fig. 6 Correlation between valve implantation size and BSA, IEOA. **a** Correlation between valve implantation size and BSA ($r = 0.27$, $p < 0.01$). **b** Correlation between valve implantation size and IEOA ($r = 0.17$, $p < 0.01$)

prosthesis implantation. Actually mitral annulus enlargement sometimes closely connected with heart dysfunction and TR can be more frequently progressed in this group. Recently published study about mitral PPM suggested mitral PPM significantly affects longterm outcomes after mitral valve replacement in terms of longterm survival and freedom from cardiac death [21], however this study was just analyzed by reference values and very limited old types of valves.

Study limitations

Our study has limitations that must be recognized. First, this study was a retrospective study, although all consecutive patients who underwent MVR for rheumatic population during the study period were enrolled. Second, this study was limited in rheumatic population in order to increase the possibility of mitral PPM under hypothesis that rheumatic mitral stenosis actually showed small mitral annulus compared with other mitral pathologies. Threfore, further evaluation for the extension of population should be needed.

Conclusions

PPM is not an independent predictor of late onset TR progression and long term survival rate after MVR. Hemodynamic positive change and remodeling were similar regardless of PPM. Also contrary to expectations, BSA was not so strongly correlated with EOA and the bigger IEOA showed close correlation with TR progression tendency. So we suggest that mitral PPM might have not clinical significance in real world and the most important thing in MVR is safe implantation by appropriate sizing.

Abbreviations

ARF: Acute renal failure; BSA: Body surface area; CE: Continuity equation; CVA: Cerebral vascular event; EOA: Effective orifice area; fTR: Functional tricuspid regurgitation; IGOA: Indexed geometrical area; LVEDD: Left ventricular end diastolic dimension; LVEF: Left ventricular ejection fraction; LVESD: Left ventricular end systolic dimension; MPG: Mean pressure gradient; MPG: Mean trans-valvular pressure gradient; MVR: Mitral valve replacement; PH: Pulmonary hypertension; PMV: Percutaneous mitral valvuloplasty; PPM: Prosthesis-patient mismatch; ROC: Receiver operating curve; RVSP: Right ventricular systolic pressure; TAP: Tricuspid annuloplasty

Acknowledgements

Not applicable.

Funding

No funding was received.

Authors' contributions

SHL, SL firstly involved in study design; YNY, HCJ collected the data from medical charts; KJY and BCC reviewed the manuscript, and all authors contributed each with important intellectual content during the manuscript writing and approved the final version.

Competing interests

The authors declare that they have no competing interests.

References

1. Pibarot P, Dumesnil JG. The relevance of prosthesis-patient mismatch after aortic valve replacement. Nat Clin Pract Cardiovasc Med. 2008;5(12):764–5.
2. Angeloni E, Melina G, Pibarot P, Benedetto U, Refice S, Ciavarella GM, Roscitano A, Sinatra R, Pepper JR. Impact of prosthesis-patient mismatch on the regression of secondary mitral regurgitation after isolated aortic valve replacement with a bioprosthetic valve in patients with severe aortic stenosis. Circ Cardiovasc Imaging. 2012;5(1):36–42.
3. Melina G, Angeloni E, Benedetto U, Refice S, Miceli A, Miele C, Ciavarella GM, Sinatra R. Relationship between prosthesis-patient mismatch and pro-brain natriuretic peptides after aortic valve replacement. J Heart Valve Dis. 2010;19(2):171–6.
4. Magne J, Mathieu P, Dumesnil JG, Tanne D, Dagenais F, Doyle D, Pibarot P. Impact of prosthesis-patient mismatch on survival after mitral valve replacement. Circulation. 2007;115(11):1417–25.
5. Lam B-K, Chan V, Hendry P, Ruel M, Masters R, Bedard P, Goldstein B, Rubens F, Mesana T. The impact of patient–prosthesis mismatch on late outcomes after mitral valve replacement. J Thorac Cardiovasc Surg. 2007;133(6):1464–1473.e1463.
6. Jamieson WRE, Germann E, Ye J, Chan F, Cheung A, MacNab JS, Fradet GJ, Stanford EA, Bryson LA, Lichtenstein SV. Effect of prosthesis-patient mismatch on long-term survival with mitral valve replacement: assessment to 15 years. Ann Thorac Surg. 2009;87(4):1135–42.
7. Dumesnil JG, Pibarot P. Prosthesis-patient mismatch: an update. Curr Cardiol Rep. 2011;13(3):250–7.
8. Devereux RB, Alonso DR, Lutas EM, Gottlieb GJ, Campo E, Sachs I, Reichek N. Echocardiographic assessment of left ventricular hypertrophy: comparison to necropsy findings. Am J Cardiol. 1986;57(6):450–8.
9. Sanfilippo AJ, Abascal VM, Sheehan M, Oertel LB, Harrigan P, Hughes RA, Weyman AE. Atrial enlargement as a consequence of atrial fibrillation. A prospective echocardiographic study. Circulation. 1990;82(3):792–7.
10. Zoghbi WA, Enriquez-Sarano M, Foster E, Grayburn PA, Kraft CD, Levine RA, Nihoyannopoulos P, Otto CM, Quinones MA, Rakowski H, et al. Recommendations for evaluation of the severity of native valvular regurgitation with two-dimensional and Doppler echocardiography. J Am Soc Echocardiogr. 2003;16(7):777–802.
11. Rahimtoola SH. The problem of valve prosthesis-patient mismatch. Circulation. 1978;58(1):20–4.
12. Li M, Dumesnil JG, Mathieu P, Pibarot P. Impact of valve prosthesis-patient mismatch on pulmonary arterial pressure after mitral valve replacement. J Am Coll Cardiol. 2005;45(7):1034–40.
13. Sakamoto H, Watanabe Y. Does patient-prosthesis mismatch affect long-term results after mitral valve replacement? Ann Thorac Cardiovasc Surg. 2010;16(3):163–7.
14. Shi WY, Yap CH, Hayward PA, Dinh DT, Reid CM, Shardey GC, Smith JA. Impact of prosthesis–patient mismatch after mitral valve replacement: a multicentre analysis of early outcomes and mid-term survival. Heart. 2011;97(13):1074–81.
15. Blais C, Dumesnil JG, Baillot R, Simard S, Doyle D, Pibarot P. Impact of valve prosthesis-patient mismatch on short-term mortality after aortic valve replacement. Circulation. 2003;108(8):983–8.
16. Rao V, Jamieson WR, Ivanov J, Armstrong S, David TE. Prosthesis-patient mismatch affects survival after aortic valve replacement. Circulation. 2000;102(19 Suppl 3):III5–9.
17. Ruel M, Rubens FD, Masters RG, Pipe AL, Bedard P, Hendry PJ, Lam BK, Burwash IG, Goldstein WG, Brais MP, et al. Late incidence and predictors of persistent or recurrent heart failure in patients with aortic prosthetic valves. J Thorac Cardiovasc Surg. 2004;127(1):149–59.

18. Caldarone CA, Raghuveer G, Hills CB, Atkins DL, Burns TL, Behrendt DM, Moller JH. Long-term survival after mitral valve replacement in children aged < 5 years: a multi-institutional study. Circulation. 2001;104(12 Suppl 1):I143–7.

19. Friedman S, Edmunds LH Jr, Cuaso CC. Long-term mitral valve replacement in young children. Influence of somatic growth on prosthetic valve adequacy. Circulation. 1978;57(5):981–6.

20. Rahimtoola SH, Murphy E. Valve prosthesis–patient mismatch. A long-term sequela. Br Heart J. 1981;45(3):331–5.

21. Hwang HY, Kim YH, Kim KH, Kim KB, Ahn H. Patient-prosthesis mismatch after mitral valve replacement: a propensity score analysis. Ann Thorac Surg. 2016;101(5):1796–802.

17

Adding left atrial appendage closure to open heart surgery provides protection from ischemic brain injury six years after surgery independently of atrial fibrillation history

Jesper Park-Hansen[1,2], Susanne J.V. Holme[3], Akhmadjon Irmukhamedov[4], Christian L. Carranza[3], Anders M. Greve[1,2], Gina Al-Farra[5], Robert G. C. Riis[6], Brian Nilsson[7], Johan S.R. Clausen[1,2], Anne S. Nørskov[1,2], Christina R. Kruuse[8], Egill Rostrup[9] and Helena Dominguez[1,2*] (iD)

Abstract

Background: Open heart surgery is associated with high occurrence of atrial fibrillation (AF), subsequently increasing the risk of post-operative ischemic stroke. Concomitant with open heart surgery, a cardiac ablation procedure is commonly performed in patients with known AF, often followed by left atrial appendage closure with surgery (LAACS). However, the protective effect of LAACS on the risk of cerebral ischemia following cardiac surgery remains controversial. We have studied whether LAACS in addition to open heart surgery protects against post-operative ischemic brain injury regardless of a previous AF diagnosis.

Methods: One hundred eighty-seven patients scheduled for open heart surgery were enrolled in a prospective, open-label clinical trial and randomized to concomitant LAACS vs. standard care. Randomization was stratified by usage of oral anticoagulation (OAC) planned to last at least 3 months after surgery. The primary endpoint was a composite of post-operative symptomatic ischemic stroke, transient ischemic attack or imaging findings of silent cerebral ischemic (SCI) lesions.

Results: During a mean follow-up of 3.7 years, 14 (16%) primary events occurred among patients receiving standard surgery vs. 5 (5%) in the group randomized to additional LAACS (hazard ratio 0.3; 95% CI: 0.1–0.8, $p = 0.02$). In per protocol analysis ($n = 141$), 14 (18%) primary events occurred in the control group vs. 4 (6%) in the LAACS group (hazard ratio 0.3; 95% CI: 0.1–1.0, $p = 0.05$).

Conclusions: In a real-world setting, LAACS in addition to elective open-heart surgery was associated with lower risk of post-operative ischemic brain injury. The protective effect was not conditional on AF/OAC status at baseline.

Keywords: Atrial fibrillation, Heart surgery, Left atrial appendage closure, Stroke

* Correspondence: mdom0002@regionh.dk
[1]Department of Cardiology, Bispebjerg and Frederiksberg University Hospital, Nordre Fasanvej 57, DK-2000 Frederiksberg, Denmark
[2]Department of Biomedicine, University of Copenhagen, Copenhagen, Denmark
Full list of author information is available at the end of the article

Background

Atrial fibrillation (AF) is a common complication after open heart surgery and is associated with both early perioperative and late post-operative stroke [1–5]. Previous studies report incident AF in 10 to 65% of patients after open heart surgery [1, 6], with highest incidences after a combination of coronary artery bypass grafting (CABG) and valve surgery [7]. In patients with non-operative AF, the risk of ischemic stroke is markedly reduced by adequate OAC [8]. However, the management of post-operative AF is still a challenge and is by some regarded as a transient phenomenon not requiring intervention [9, 10]. The risk of bleeding poses a significant limitation to the use of OAC, which consequently increases focus on left atrial appendage (LAA) closure [11, 12], as the LAA is a predilection site for thrombus formation during AF [13, 14]. Importantly, the patient population undergoing open heart surgery is often frail and carry comorbidities such as hypertension and chronic obstructive pulmonary disease, which add risk of future AF and stroke complications [15]. Moreover, a large fraction of these elderly individuals also have subclinical AF that portends an adverse prognosis comparable to recognized AF [16]. It is therefore conceivable that LAACS in conjunction with open heart surgery could mitigate the risk of stroke both in patients with and without overt AF at time of surgery. Notwithstanding, the evidence for routine use of LAACS during elective open-heart surgery is controversial. Accordingly, the primary aim of this study was to investigate the long-term effect of LAACS on cerebral ischemia following scheduled open-heart surgery. We hypothesized that surgical LAACS protects against cerebral ischemia in the following years regardless of AF status at time of surgery.

Methods

Study design

From August 2010 to September 2015, we conducted a prospective, randomized, open label study on patients scheduled for open heart surgery to receive either concomitant LAACS or standard care. The LAACS study is registered at clinicaltrials.gov (NCT02378116). The study was initiated at the Department of Thoracic Surgery, University Hospital of Gentofte, Denmark. During 2010, the Department of Thoracic Surgery was transferred and merged with the equivalent department at Rigshospitalet, Copenhagen, where the study continued. Patients were randomized the day before surgery after signing informed consent. To ensure a balanced distribution of patients receiving OAC between the two study-arms, randomization was stratified according to ongoing use of anti-coagulation. This included patients undergoing surgical biological valve replacement until January 2012, as post-operative anti-coagulation was no longer recommended [17].

Patients were randomized 1:1 by a computer-generated randomization in blocks of 16 patients. Since we expected substantial cross-over, procedures were monitored at the end of each operation for cross-over. If one of the study groups reached a discrepancy of 4 between randomization allocation and the actual operation, the randomization block was suspended and substituted by a 3:1 randomization in the next block (n 16) to compensate for the difference.

The study protocol recommended double closure with both purse string and running suture, although this closure method was not mandatory. Patients were invited to pre-surgery magnetic resonance imaging (MRI) scan (MRI-0) whenever possible. Immediately after discharge, all patients were invited for a post-operative baseline brain MRI scan (MRI-1) scheduled between 2 and 4 weeks after discharge and a follow-up MRI (MRI-2) performed at least 6 months after surgery.

Study population

Consecutive patients undergoing planned first-time open-heart surgery (CABG, valve surgery or a combination of both) during the study period were asked to participate in the trial, provided that their residence was within 40 km radius from the hospital. Major exclusion criteria included endocarditis and implanted pacemaker (see Additional file 1: Table S1 for full inclusion and exclusion criteria). All patients in the LAACS arm were invited to undergo post-operative transesophageal echocardiography (TEE) by a senior cardiologist to visualize the LAA and the quality of the closure. Patients could decline TEE and remain in the study for follow-up.

MRI analyses

The brain MRI included imaging of cerebrum, cerebellum and brainstem. All MRIs were reviewed by a fellow in radiology with years of experience, and the possibility of consulting unclear cases with a neuro radiologist. Radiologists were blinded to randomization. MRI-criteria for silent cerebral infarcts (SCI) were equivalent to those in the Framingham offspring study, i.e., cavitating lesions ≥ 3 mm with CSF-like signal intensities on T1, T2 and FLAIR [17]. Both acute and old SCIs were included. Differentiation from dilated Virchow-Robins spaces (dVRS) was attempted using the location criterion (i.e., excluding lesions along perforating or medullary arteries or in the lower third of the basal ganglia) and shape criterion (i.e. oval lesions criteria along the penetrating arteries with intensity close to CSF were considered dVRS) [18].

Endpoint definitions

The pre-specified endpoint protocol was post-operative cerebral ischemic events defined as a composite of first ischemic stroke or transient ischemic attack (ICD-10: DG450–9), increased amount of SCI between MRI-1 and MRI-2 and post-operative findings of SCI by brain imaging (computed tomography [CT] or MRI) performed in clinical settings unrelated to study enrollment.

Secondary outcomes were strict symptomatic ischemic strokes. That is, ischemic stroke or transient ischemic attack, excluding cerebral ischemic events classified solely on imaging findings and all-cause mortality. We followed all patients for at least 1 year after surgery. The clinical outcomes Ischemic stroke and transient ischemic attack were ascertained by following the patient's electronic records yearly. Patients vital status were obtained using data from the Central Office of Civil Registration, which comprises all citizens in Denmark. Additionally, telephone interviews were performed after minimum 1 year to ascertain whether the patients had experienced signs of clinically unrecognized cerebral ischemia. If so, it would be registered as a transient ischemic attack.

Power calculation

We based our power calculations on the incidence of AF among patients undergoing open heart surgery and the expected variation in a combined end-point of clinical stroke, transitory ischemic attack (TIA), and occurrence of silence infarctions, which included findings of newly silent lacunar infarctions with imaging in clinical settings and changes on number of lacunar infarctions from baseline MRI (at discharge) to MR2. Incident stroke occurs in 1–5% of heart surgery patients [19–21], often within the first months following surgery [22]. At the initiation of the study, there were almost no studies with long-term MRI follow-up after open heart surgery [23]. Around 50% of patients undergoing surgery of carotid arteries have lacunar infarctions on MRI [24], and the presence of AF roughly doubles the risk of strokes [25]. We assumed an equivalent prevalence of 50–70% of infarctions counting both subclinical and clinical perioperative strokes/TIA. This is equivalent to findings on CABG surgery [26] and valve surgery [23], respectively, where MRI changes occur in 40–70% of patients. Therefore, we assumed that closure of the LAA would reduce findings on MRI scans and clinical strokes/TIA from a total of 60 to 35% with a 5% margin. With a significance level of 5%, we calculated that we could demonstrate this benefit with a 5% margin and 90% power by including 90 patients. After the initiation of the study, it became apparent that MRI scans were not feasible for many patients. Hence, we recalculated the number of patients needed based on newer data on occurrence of stroke after heart surgery [27–30], considering a three-

to five-fold increased risk of stroke in patients with non-contracting, patent LAA who had undergone MAZE-procedure during surgery [31] combined with an occurrence of images of infarction after CABG over 20% [32], the latter including MRI changes [23, 26]. Without other available evidence on truly long-term follow-up studies after heart surgery associated to AF, we calculated that we could investigate the protective effect of LAACS based on any signs of cerebral infarction (stroke, TIA or imaging evidence of silent cerebral ischemia) through randomization of 400 patients, if LAACS could reduce events from 65 to 45% with a significance level of 5 and 91% power. With 88% power, a second calculation showed a necessity of including 100 patients in each group. Therefore, we maintained our plan to randomize 200 patients.

Statistical analysis

All analyses were performed using SAS statistical software package version 9.4 (SAS Institute Inc., Cary, NC). Continuous variables are presented as mean±standard deviation and categorical variables as number and percentages. After inspection for normality, differences between the LAACS and control group were evaluated by Student's t-test (continuous variables) and by Chi-square and Fisher's exact test (categorical variables) where appropriate. Cause specific Cox time to event analysis was used to estimate the rate ratios for incident stroke and all-cause mortality according to randomization. A cumulative probability plot of incident stroke according to randomization was generated by Fine and Gray competing risk regression using death as a competing event [33]. All outcome analyses were performed as intention to treat and per protocol. Patients were considered to have complied with the treatment protocol when LAAC was performed according to randomization. A sensitivity analysis was performed to evaluate model dependence on imaging findings by comparing overall results with a model that only included events due to symptomatic ischemic stroke or transient ischemic attack. A two-tailed p-value < 0.05 was regarded as statistically significant.

Ethics

The project was approved by Regional Ethics Committee of Capital Region Denmark (protocol number H-3-2010-017) and follows the Helsinki declaration.

Results

Of 914 patients invited to participate, 205 (22.4%) were enrolled. Of those, 187 (91.2%) were randomized and 141 (75.4%) ultimately followed the treatment protocol (see Additional file 2: Figure S1). During the second year of the study, discrepancy between randomization and performed procedure reached a difference of four (due to overweight of patients randomized to LAACS who did not undergo closure), and the following randomization blocks of 16 patients were switched to 3:1 randomization. The rest of the study randomization continued 1:1.

Two patients randomized to additional LAACS crossed over due to technical difficulties during the operation, and the LAACS procedure was avoided. In five patients with known paroxysms of AF, the surgeons changed the planned operation adding intra-operative ablation and closing the left appendage, despite randomization to the control group. Baseline characteristics of randomized participants are showed in Table 1. No adverse events such as bleeding due to LAACS procedure were recorded. 75 (40%) patients underwent both of the planned brain MRIs. Thirty patients had brain infarctions in pre-surgery MRI. Of 74 patients who underwent subsequent MRI shortly after discharge, 11 had SCI at post-discharge MRI. Among 75 available sets of post-discharge and long-term MRI, only two had new SCI, one in each group.

There were no detectable differences in randomization to LAACS, age or gender between patients that had the planned brain MRI scans vs. those that did not (all $p > 0.35$, Additional file 3: Table S2). 10 patients from the LAACS group accepted the invitation to undergo TEE (mean 524 days after surgery date). In none of the cases could the lumen of the LAA or any flow from the appendage orifice be identified.

Clinical outcomes

Follow up was up to 6 years, mean 3.7 ± 1.6 years (totaling 684 patient years of follow-up). End of study was 1 year after reaching our pre-specified sample size of 200 patients. Five patients were lost to follow-up for the primary endpoint and 24 (13%) died. At end of study telephone-interviews, no patient was suspected to have suffered a clinically unrecognized ischemic cerebral event. In the intention-to-treat analysis, there were 5 (5%) primary events in the LAACS-group and 14 (16%) in the control group (hazard ratio 0.3; 95% CI: 0.1–0.8, $p = 0.02$, Table 2, Fig. 1 and Additional file 4: Table S3 Contingency table of individual events). Tests of interaction revealed no dependency of the preventative effect of LAACS on baseline AF status, CHA_2DS_2-VASc score or use of OAC ($p = 0.55$, $p = 0.56$ and $p = 0.49$ for interaction, respectively). Secondary outcome analysis revealed no detectable difference in all-cause mortality ($p = 0.79$) between the LAACS group ($n = 12$, 12%) vs. the controls ($n = 12$, 14%, Table 2). Similarly, in a sensitivity analysis that excluded the eight patients that underwent primary events only based on radiological findings, there was a trend but no longer a significant

Table 1 Baseline characteristics according to randomized left atrial appendage closure

Variable	Not closed (n = 86)	Closed (n = 101)
Age – years	69.3 ± 8.8	67.6 ± 9.6
Men - n (%)	75 (87.2)	84 (83.2)
Clinical characteristics		
Congestive heart failure - n (%)	15 (17.9)	16 (15.8)
Atrial fibrillation - n (%)	12 (12.8)	18 (16.8)
Diabetes - n (%)	19 (22.1)	31 (30.7)
Hypertension - n (%)	60 (69.8)	75 (74.3)
CHADS-VASc – unit	2.9 ± 1.4	2.9 ± 1.5
Prior stroke - n (%)	15 (17.4)	11 (10.9)
Chronic kidney disease[a] - n (%)	14 (16.3)	15 (14.9)
Medicine		
ASA - n (%)	69 (80.2)	75 (74.3)
Clopidogrel - n (%)	14 (16.3)	19 (18.8)
OAC		
VKA - n (%)	26 (30.2)	36 (35.6)
NOAC - n (%)	2 (2.2)	2 (2.0)
Beta-blocker - n (%)	47 (54.7)	61 (60.4)
Verapamil - n (%)	4 (4.5)	2 (2.0)
Calcium-blocker - n (%)	19 (21.3)	34 (33.7)
Digoxin - n (%)	5 (5.6)	3 (3.0)
Renin-angiotensin system blocker - n (%)	40 (46.5)	54 (53.5)
Amiodarone - n (%)	23 (26.7)	18 (17.8)
Statin - n (%)	74 (86.0)	81 (80.2)
Procedural characteristics		
Surgery type		
AVR only - n (%)	17 (19.1)	17 (16.8)
AVR with CABG - n (%)	20 (22.5)	22 (21.8)
AVR with aortic surgery - n (%)	1 (1.1)	1 (1.0)
AVR with MVR - n (%)	0 (0)	2 (2.0)
Aortic surgery only - n (%)	1 (1.1)	0 (0)
CABG only - n (%)	40 (46.5)	50 (49.5)
CABG with MVR - n (%)	2 (2.3)	2 (2.0)
MVR only - n (%)	4 (4.5)	7 (6.9)
Tricuspid surgery only - n (%)	1 (1.2)	0 (0)
Perioperative atrial fibrillation - n (%)	52 (60.5)	50 (50.0)

Abbreviations CHADS-VASc Congestive heart failure, hypertension, age [≥75 years], diabetes, stroke – peripheral vascular disease, age [≥65 years], sex-category, *OAC* Oral anticoagulation, *VKA* Vitamin K-antagonist, *NOAC* Novel oral anticoagulation, IQR: interquartile range
[a]eGFR< 30 ml/min

reduction in ischemic strokes among patients randomized to LAACS ($p = 0.08$, Table 2 and Fig. 2).

In the per protocol sensitivity analysis (Table 3), there were 4 (6%) primary events in the LAACS group vs. 14 (18%) in the control arm (hazard ratio 0.3; 95%

Table 2 Proportion of patients meeting endpoints according to randomized left atrial appendage closure, stratified by use of anti-coagulants

Endpoint	Not closed (n = 86)	Closed (n = 101)	Hazard ratio	P-value
Primary events[a]	14 (16.3%)	5 (5.0%)	0.3 [95% CI: 0.1–0.8]	0.0168
Clinical stroke[b]	8 (10.0%)	3 (3.0)	0.3 [95% CI: 0.1–1.1]	0.0763
Death	12 (14.0%)	12 (11.9%)	0.8 [95% CI: 0.43–1.9]	0.6562

[a]Defined as first of postoperative symptomatic ischemic stroke, transient ischemic attack or imaging evidence of new silent infarct
[b]Excluding 8 patients that were classified as primary events due to imaging findings

CI: 0.1–1.0, $p = 0.05$). Of note, in the control group, 9 (64%) of the 14 primary events occurred beyond the first year of follow-up (Fig. 1). Secondary outcome analyses again revealed no detectable difference in overall survival or strict symptomatic ischemic strokes between the two study-arms (Table 3).

The datasets used during the current study are available from the corresponding author on reasonable request.

Discussion

This is the first randomized study where LAACS in addition to first-time open-heart surgery (CABG, valve or combination of both) seems to protect against postoperative cerebral ischemic events several years after surgery. Despite a substantial number of cross-overs, results were consistent in the intention-to-treat and per-

protocol analyses. Furthermore, the impact during long-term follow-up should become visible in patients with AF, which may be offset with effective anticoagulation.

Thus, LAACS seems as a safe, low cost and easily feasible procedure that may mitigate risk of postoperative cerebral ischemia among patients undergoing planned heart surgery.

Although encouraging, these results must be interpreted cautiously. The study is not powered to demonstrate a protection against stroke. Furthermore, the rationale for including SCI in the composite primary endpoint is rather indirect [34, 35]. Yet, we found a trend towards higher stroke and TIA events in the control group ($p = 0.07$), which seems to support the relevance of SCI as true brain damage.

Comparing our findings to available literature, it is generally accepted that there is very little evidence on the effects of surgical closure of the LAA [36]. A previous study from 2000 by Johnson et al. showed no safety issues regarding LAACS among the 437 patients included, where of which 43 appendages were stapled and 391 were sutured. [37] In a recent systematic review of LAA closure, the authors concluded that there are no randomized clinical trials and that published evidence is insufficient to assess the benefits of LAACS but there is seemingly no adverse risk associated with the procedure [36].

Of note, most of the primary events in the present control group were late ischemic strokes well clear of the time of surgery and the complex array of risk

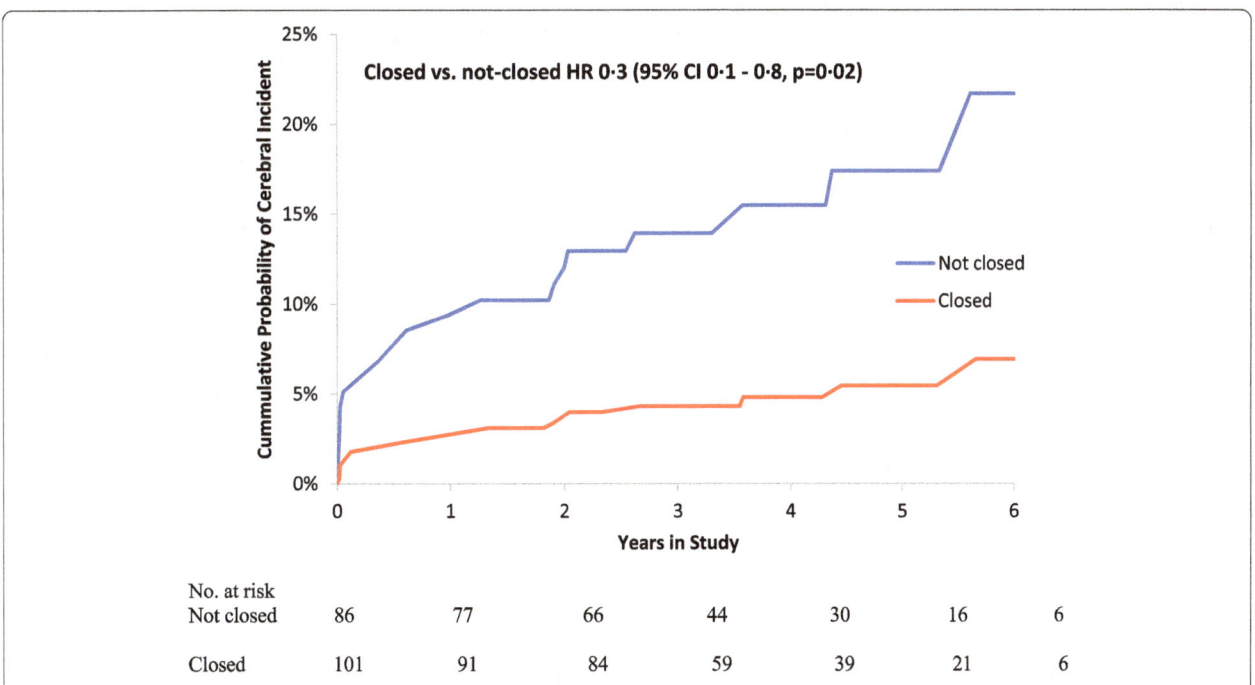

Fig. 1 Cumulative probability of primary events (combined ischemic stroke, transitory ischemic stroke or silent ischemic images) according to randomized LAACS (left atrial appendage closure with surgery)

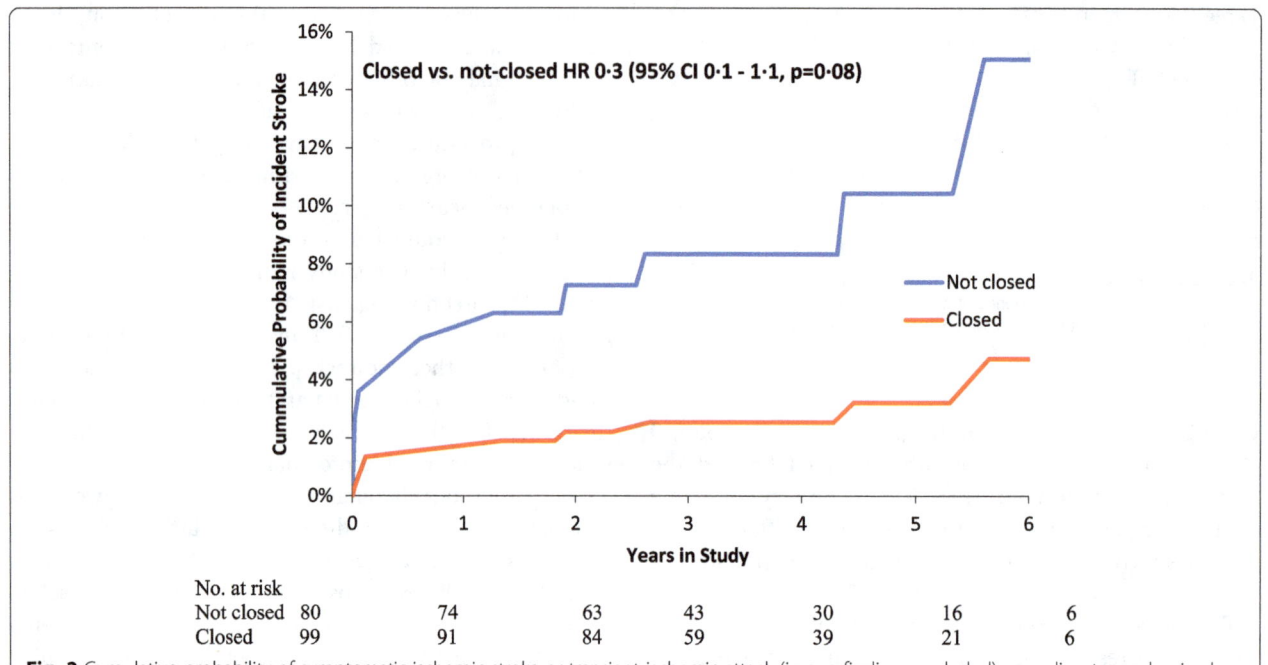

Fig. 2 Cumulative probability of symptomatic ischemic stroke or transient ischemic attack (image findings excluded) according to randomized LAACS (left atrial appendage closure with surgery)

factors related to perioperative stroke. This is in support of the theory that post-operative ischemic events by large are unrelated to the surgical procedure per se, but instead originate from LAA thrombus formation induced by AF. The facts that LAA is a prevalent site of thrombus formation during AF and that the incidence of AF after open heart surgery is as high as 50–60% further supports this hypothesis [38]. In turn, this may also explain why the effect of LAACS was not altered by baseline AF status, as there is a general consensus that post-operative AF is associated with late post-operative stroke [1, 22, 39]. Thus, LAACS may act by blocking a causal mechanism for late ischemic strokes induced by either pre- or post-operative AF.

A major concern of surgical versus percutaneous LAA closure is the risk of incomplete closure [40], although there is very little evidence that supports

this notion [11]. In our study, we found no signs of incomplete LAACS among the 10 participants that underwent TEE. With any of the surgical techniques, there is a risk of incomplete LAACS, though it varies greatly depending upon the surgical technique utilized and the definition of surgical failure [41]. Nevertheless, a recent experimental study in vitro comparing epicardial closure supports double closure with both purse string and running suture as recommended in our protocol [42].

Study limitations
The study was halted before reaching the planned randomization of 200 patients due to competing studies recruiting patients for heart surgery. Nevertheless, according to our findings, it would be sufficient to include 35 patients in each group with 90% power to find a difference on the combination of stroke, TIA and SCI 2 years after surgery with a significance level of 5%. Furthermore, due to the frailty of the patients included, the discomfort of cerebral MRI and the physically- and mentally challenging period postoperatively, it was only possible to perform full sets of MRI scans in 75 patients. However, the patients who were not able to participate in all MRI scans agreed to stay active in the study for future clinical follow up. The fact that all patients did not undergo the planned MRI scans may have introduced a selection-bias, as frail patients may be more prone to decline the brain MRI scans. However, results from sensitivity analyses restricted to symptomatic ischemic strokes

Table 3 Proportion of patients meeting endpoints according to per-protocol left atrial appendage closure stratified by use of anti-coagulants

Endpoint	Not closed (n = 77)	Closed (n = 64)	Hazard ratio	P-value
Primary events[a]	14 (18.2%)	4 (6.3%)	0.3 [95% CI: 0.1–0.9]	0.0237
Clinical stroke[b]	8 (11.3%)	2 (3.2%)	0.3 [95% CI: 0.1–1.3]	0.0907
Death	10 (13.0%)	6 (9.4%)	0.7 [95% CI: 0.3–2.3]	0.7067

[a]Defined as first of postoperative symptomatic ischemic stroke, transient ischemic attack or imaging evidence of new silent infarct
[b]Excluding 8 patients that were classified as primary events due to imaging findings

support the results that included imaging findings. Another limitation is the fact that only 10 patients accepted postoperative TEE. An unnoticed incomplete LAA closure, may thus have provoked events.

Conclusion

In a real-world setting, LAACS during elective open-heart surgery was associated with a lower risk of ischemic cerebral events following open heart surgery.

Additional files

Additional file 1: Table S1. Complete inclusion/exclusion criteria. Table listing inclusion and exclusion criteria.

Additional file 2: Figure S1. Flow-chart. Figure showing the flow-chart from screening until randomization

Additional file 3: Table S2. Baseline characteristics among patients that underwent planned brain MRI scans vs. those that did not. Table showing characteristics of patients who underwent MRI compared to those who did not.

Additional file 4: Table S3. Breakdown of primary events according to randomized treatment. Table showing brake-down of events in patients with closed LAA compared with the control group where LAA remained open.

Abbreviations

AF: Atrial fibrillation; CABG: Coronary artery bypass grafting; CI: Confidence interval; CT: Computed tomography; dVRS: Dilated Virchow-Robins spaces; eGFR: Estimated glomerular filtration rate; HR: Hazard ratio; ICD: International classification of diseases; IQR: Inter-quartile range; LAA: Left atrial appendage; LAACS: Left atrium appendage closure with surgery; MRI: Magnetic resonance imaging; NOAC: Novel oral anticoagulation; OAC: Oral anticoagulants; SCI: Silent cerebral infarcts; TEE: Transesophageal echocardiography; TIA: Transitory ischemic attack (TIA); VKA: Vitamin K-antagonist

Acknowledgements

The study group would like to thank senior radiographer Jakob Moeller for his extraordinary work and advise with the MRI part of the study. Thanks to neuro-radiologist Dr. Bodil Damgaard for consultancy regarding MRI analysis. We would also like to thank Dr. Mie Jonsson for assisting with patient recruitment and senior neurologist Dr. Thomas Truelsen for consultancy regarding follow-up.

Funding

Det Medicinske Selskab i København (research grant), Research Council in Herlev Hospital (research grant) and Research Council in Bispebjerg and Frederiksberg Hospital (research grant). Pfizer sponsored one of the meetings of the LAACS group.

Authors' contributions

All authors meet ICMJE guidelines for contribution: made substantial contributions to conception and design, or acquisition of data, or analysis and interpretation of data. HD conceived the research. HD and AI designed the study, with subsequent collaboration from SVJH, CLC, CK and ER. AMG and HD performed statistical analysis. JPH, HD, SVJH, CLC, BN, JSRC, ASN and RGCR gathered data. Each author has participated sufficiently in the work to take public responsibility for appropriate portions of the content; and agreed to be accountable for all aspects of the work in ensuring that questions related to the accuracy or integrity of any part of the work are appropriately investigated and resolved. All authors read and approved the final manuscript.

Competing interests

The authors declare that they have no competing interests.

Author details

[1]Department of Cardiology, Bispebjerg and Frederiksberg University Hospital, Nordre Fasanvej 57, DK-2000 Frederiksberg, Denmark. [2]Department of Biomedicine, University of Copenhagen, Copenhagen, Denmark. [3]Department of Thoracic Surgery, Rigshospitalet, Copenhagen, Denmark. [4]Department of Thoracic Surgery, Odense University Hospital, Odense, Denmark. [5]Department of Radiology, Herlev Gentofte University Hospital, Herlev, Denmark. [6]Department of Radiology, Bispebjerg and Frederiksberg Hospital, Frederiksberg, Denmark. [7]Department of Cardiology, Hvidovre University Hospital, Copenhagen, Denmark. [8]Department Neurology, Neurovascular Research Unit, Herlev Gentofte Hospital, Herlev, Denmark. [9]Mental Health Center Glostrup, Copenhagen, Denmark.

References

1. McDonagh DL, Berger M, Mathew JP, Graffagnino C, Milano CA, Newman MF. Neurological complications of cardiac surgery. Lancet Neurol. 2014; 13(5):490–502.
2. Murdock DK, Rengel LR, Schlund A, Olson KJ, Kaliebe JW, Johnkoski JA, Riveron FA. Stroke and atrial fibrillation following cardiac surgery. WMJ. 2003;102(4):26–30.
3. Lubitz SA, Yin X, Rienstra M, Schnabel RB, Walkey AJ, Magnani JW, Rahman F, McManus DD, Tadros TM, Levy D, et al. Long-term outcomes of secondary atrial fibrillation in the community: the Framingham heart study. Circulation. 2015;131(19):1648–55.
4. Saxena A, Dinh D, Dimitriou J, Reid C, Smith J, Shardey G, Newcomb A. Preoperative atrial fibrillation is an independent risk factor for mid-term mortality after concomitant aortic valve replacement and coronary artery bypass graft surgery. Interact Cardiovasc Thorac Surg. 2013;16(4):488–94.
5. Ahlsson A, Fengsrud E, Bodin L, Englund A. Postoperative atrial fibrillation in patients undergoing aortocoronary bypass surgery carries an eightfold risk of future atrial fibrillation and a doubled cardiovascular mortality. Eur J Cardiothorac Surg. 2010;37(6):1353–9.
6. Maisel WH. Left atrial appendage occlusion – closure or just the beginning? N Engl J Med. 2009;360(25):2601-3.
7. Maesen B, Nijs J, Maessen J, Allessie M, Schotten U. Post-operative atrial fibrillation: a maze of mechanisms. Europace. 2012;14(2):159–74.
8. Aguilar MI, Hart R. Oral anticoagulants for preventing stroke in patients with non-valvular atrial fibrillation and no previous history of stroke or transient ischemic attacks. Cochrane Database Syst Rev. 2005;3:CD001927.
9. Frendl G, Sodickson AC, Chung MK, Waldo AL, Gersh BJ, Tisdale JE, Calkins H, Aranki S, Kaneko T, Cassivi S, et al. 2014 AATS guidelines for the prevention and management of perioperative atrial fibrillation and flutter for thoracic surgical procedures. J Thorac Cardiovasc Surg. 2014;148(3):e153–93.
10. Kowey PR, Stebbins D, Igidbashian L, Goldman SM, Sutter FP, Rials SJ, Marinchak RA. Clinical outcome of patients who develop PAF after CABG surgery. Pacing Clin Electrophysiol. 2001;24(2):191–3.
11. Garcia-Fernandez MA, Perez-David E, Quiles J, Peralta J, Garcia-Rojas I, Bermejo J, Moreno M, Silva J. Role of left atrial appendage obliteration in stroke reduction in patients with mitral valve prosthesis: a transesophageal echocardiographic study. J Am Coll Cardiol. 2003;42(7):1253–8.
12. Reddy VY, Doshi SK, Sievert H, Buchbinder M, Neuzil P, Huber K, Halperin JL, Holmes D, Investigators PA. Percutaneous left atrial appendage closure for stroke prophylaxis in patients with atrial fibrillation: 2.3-year follow-up of the PROTECT AF (watchman left atrial appendage system for embolic protection in patients with atrial fibrillation) trial. Circulation. 2013;127(6):720–9.
13. Freedman B, Potpara TS, Lip GY. Stroke prevention in atrial fibrillation. Lancet. 2016;388(10046):806–17.
14. Lin AC, Knight BP. Left atrial appendage closure. Prog Cardiovasc Dis. 2015; 58(2):195–201.
15. Mathew JP, Fontes ML, Tudor IC, Ramsay J, Duke P, Mazer CD, Barash PG, Hsu PH, Mangano DT. A multicenter risk index for atrial fibrillation after cardiac surgery. JAMA. 2004;291(14):1720–9.
16. Sanna T, Diener HC, Passman RS, Di Lazzaro V, Bernstein RA, Morillo CA, Rymer MM, Thijs V, Rogers T, Beckers F, et al. Cryptogenic stroke and underlying atrial fibrillation. N Engl J Med. 2014;370(26):2478–86.

17. Das RR, Seshadri S, Beiser AS, Kelly-Hayes M, Au R, Himali JJ, Kase CS, Benjamin EJ, Polak JF, O'Donnell CJ, et al. Prevalence and correlates of silent cerebral infarcts in the Framingham offspring study. Stroke. 2008; 39(11):2929–35.

18. Giele JL, Witkamp TD, Mali WP, van der Graaf Y, Group SS. Silent brain infarcts in patients with manifest vascular disease. Stroke. 2004;35(3):742–6.

19. Lahtinen J, Biancari F, Salmela E, Mosorin M, Satta J, Rainio P, Rimpilainen J, Lepojarvi M, Juvonen T. Postoperative atrial fibrillation is a major cause of stroke after on-pump coronary artery bypass surgery. Ann Thorac Surg. 2004;77(4):1241–4.

20. Blackshear JL, Odell JA. Appendage obliteration to reduce stroke in cardiac surgical patients with atrial fibrillation. Ann Thorac Surg. 1996;61(2):755–9.

21. Salazar JD, Wityk RJ, Grega MA, Borowicz LM, Doty JR, Petrofski JA, Baumgartner WA. Stroke after cardiac surgery: short- and long-term outcomes. Ann Thorac Surg. 2001;72(4):1195–201. discussion 1201-1192

22. Kollar A, Lick SD, Vasquez KN, Conti VR. Relationship of atrial fibrillation and stroke after coronary artery bypass graft surgery: when is anticoagulation indicated? Ann Thorac Surg. 2006;82(2):515–23.

23. Knipp SC, Matatko N, Schlamann M, Wilhelm H, Thielmann M, Forsting M, Diener HC, Jakob H. Small ischemic brain lesions after cardiac valve replacement detected by diffusion-weighted magnetic resonance imaging: relation to neurocognitive function. Eur J Cardiothorac Surg. 2005;28(1):88–96.

24. Wilson DA, Mocco J, D'Ambrosio AL, Komotar RJ, Zurica J, Kellner CP, Hahn DK, Connolly ES, Liu X, Imielinska C, et al. Post-carotid endarterectomy neurocognitive decline is associated with cerebral blood flow asymmetry on post-operative magnetic resonance perfusion brain scans. Neurol Res. 2008;30(3):302–6.

25. Harthun NL, Stukenborg GJ. Atrial fibrillation is associated with increased risk of perioperative stroke and death from carotid endarterectomy. J Vasc Surg. 2010;51(2):330–6.

26. Floyd TF, Shah PN, Price CC, Harris F, Ratcliffe SJ, Acker MA, Bavaria JE, Rahmouni H, Kuersten B, Wiegers S, et al. Clinically silent cerebral ischemic events after cardiac surgery: their incidence, regional vascular occurrence, and procedural dependence. Ann Thorac Surg. 2006;81(6):2160–6.

27. Garg S, Sarno G, Gutierrez-Chico JL, Garcia-Garcia HM, Gomez-Lara J, Serruys PW, investigators A-I. Five-year outcomes of percutaneous coronary intervention compared to bypass surgery in patients with multivessel disease involving the proximal left anterior descending artery: an ARTS-II sub-study. EuroIntervention. 2011;6(9):1060–7.

28. Hedberg M, Boivie P, Engstrom KG. Early and delayed stroke after coronary surgery - an analysis of risk factors and the impact on short- and long-term survival. Eur J Cardiothorac Surg. 2011;40(2):379–87.

29. Bucerius J, Gummert JF, Borger MA, Walther T, Doll N, Onnasch JF, Metz S, Falk V, Mohr FW. Stroke after cardiac surgery: a risk factor analysis of 16,184 consecutive adult patients. Ann Thorac Surg. 2003;75(2):472–8.

30. Korn-Lubetzki I, Oren A, Asher E, Dano M, Bitran D, Fink D, Steiner-Birmanns B. Strokes after cardiac surgery: mostly right hemispheric ischemic with mild residual damage. J Neurol. 2007;254(12):1708–13.

31. Buber J, Luria D, Sternik L, Raanani E, Feinberg MS, Goldenberg I, Nof E, Gurevitz O, Eldar M, Glikson M, et al. Left atrial contractile function following a successful modified maze procedure at surgery and the risk for subsequent thromboembolic stroke. J Am Coll Cardiol. 2011;58(15):1614–21.

32. Gottesman RF, Sherman PM, Grega MA, Yousem DM, Borowicz LM Jr, Selnes OA, Baumgartner WA, McKhann GM. Watershed strokes after cardiac surgery: diagnosis, etiology, and outcome. Stroke. 2006;37(9):2306–11.

33. Jason P, Fine RJG. A Proportional Hazards Model for the subdistribution of a competing risk. J Am Stat Assoc. 1999;94(446):496–509.

34. Gaita F, Corsinovi L, Anselmino M, Raimondo C, Pianelli M, Toso E, Bergamasco L, Boffano C, Valentini MC, Cesarani F, et al. Prevalence of silent cerebral ischemia in paroxysmal and persistent atrial fibrillation and correlation with cognitive function. J Am Coll Cardiol. 2013;62(21):1990–7.

35. Stefansdottir H, Arnar DO, Aspelund T, Sigurdsson S, Jonsdottir MK, Hjaltason H, Launer LJ, Gudnason V. Atrial fibrillation is associated with reduced brain volume and cognitive function independent of cerebral infarcts. Stroke. 2013;44(4):1020–5.

36. Noelck N, Papak J, Freeman M, Paynter R, Low A, Motu'apuaka M, Kondo K, Kansagara D. Effectiveness of left atrial appendage exclusion procedures to reduce the risk of stroke: a systematic review of the evidence. Circ Cardiovasc Qual outcomes. 2016;9(4):395–405.

37. Johnson WD, Ganjoo AK, Stone CD, Srivyas RC, Howard M. The left atrial appendage: our most lethal human attachment! Surgical implications. Eur J Cardiothorac Surg. 2000;17(6):718–22.

38. Patel D, Gillinov MA, Natale A. Atrial fibrillation after cardiac surgery: where are we now? Indian Pacing Electrophysiol J. 2008;8(4):281–91.

39. Creswell LL, Schuessler RB, Rosenbloom M, Cox JL. Hazards of postoperative atrial arrhythmias. Ann Thorac Surg. 1993;56(3):539–49.

40. Aryana A, d'Avila A. Incomplete closure of the left atrial appendage: implication and management. Curr Cardiol Rep. 2016;18(9):82.

41. Katz ES, Tsiamtsiouris T, Applebaum RM, Schwartzbard A, Tunick PA, Kronzon I. Surgical left atrial appendage ligation is frequently incomplete: a transesophageal echocardiograhic study. J Am Coll Cardiol. 2000;36(2):468–71.

42. Mirow N, Vogt S, Irqsusi M, Moosdorf R, Kirschbaum A. Epicardial left atrial appendage closure-comparison of surgical techniques in an ex vivo model. J Thorac Dis. 2017;9(3):757–61.

18

Epicardial infrared ablation to create a linear conduction block on a beating right atrium

Hiroshi Kubota[*] , Hidehito Endo, Hikaru Ishii, Hiroshi Tsuchiya, Yusuke Inaba, Yu Takahashi and Katsunari Terakawa

Abstract

Background: It is still difficult to create a secure linear conduction block on a beating heart from the epicardial side. To overcome this drawback we developed an infrared coagulator equipped with a cuboid light-guiding quartz rod. This study was designed to electrophysiologically confirm the efficacy of a new ablation probe using infrared energy in a clinical case.

Methods: The infrared light from a lamp is focused into the newly developed cuboid quartz rod, which has a rectangular distal exit-plane that allows 30 mm × 10 mm linear photocoagulation. Two pairs of electrodes were attached to the right atrium of a patient who was undergoing surgery. Each pair of electrodes was placed 10 mm from an ablation line. The change in conduction time between the two pairs of electrodes was measured during ablation. The predicted conduction time delay ratio was 1.54.

Results: The actual conduction time after ablation was 1.38–1.43 times longer than the pre-ablation conduction time.

Conclusions: The infrared ablation using a newly developed cuboid probe made it possible to create a linear conduction block on the beating right atrial free wall clinically.

Keywords: Atrial fibrillation, Ablation, Coagulator, Energy source, Electrophysiology, Arrhythmia treatment, Infrared, Minimally invasive surgery, Maze procedure, Photocoagulation

Background

The newly developed infrared coagulator, named the "Kyo-Co (Photon incorporation, Saitama, Japan)", contains a reflector that focuses light from a tungsten-halogen lamp into a light-conducting 30 mm × 10 mm cuboid quartz rod, and the light emerges as 35 W/cm^2 of near-infrared light energy (wavelength: 400 nm to approximately 1600 nm; peak wavelength: 850 nm). The distal exit-plane of the light-conducting rod has a rectangular plane surface (30 × 10 mm) (Fig. 1).

Methods

In a preliminary experiment, the probe applied to a specimen of chicken muscle tissue, and the muscle tissue was ablated for a total of 28 s (4 s × 5 times at 2 s intervals) ($n = 5$). Tissue temperature with time was measured with a thermometer Ti480® (Fluke Corporation, WA, U.S.A.). The maximum temperature of muscle tissue was measured. After ablation of the chicken muscle the depth of the lesion was measured macroscopically.

The maximum temperature of the chicken muscle was 97.9 + 2.1 °C, and the depth of the lesion was 8.7 + 0.8 mm (Fig. 2).

Clinical experience

In 2014, the ethics committee of Kyorin University approved a clinical and epidemiologic study entitled, Surgical treatment of arrhythmias, infectious endocarditis, infected aortic aneurysms, and cardiac tumors with an infrared coagulator. Written consent was obtained from the patient.

We hypothesized that when a rectangular transmural lesion is created in the same shape as the exit plane of

* Correspondence: kub@ks.kyorin-u.ac.jp
Department of Cardiovascular Surgery, Kyorin University, 6-20-2, Shinkawa, Mitaka, Tokyo 181-8611, Japan

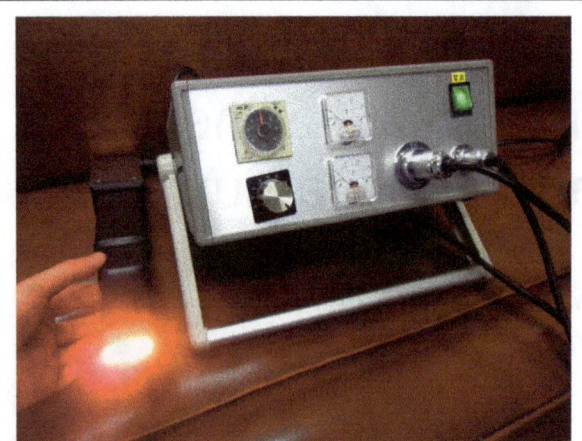

Fig. 1 Infrared coagulator "Kyo-co". The cuboid quartz rod exit plane has a rectangular (30 mm × 10 mm) surface designed to enable creation of a linear lesion. Light from a tungsten-halogen lamp emerges as 35 W/cm^2 of near-infrared light energy (wavelength: 400 to approximately 1600 nm; peak wavelength: 850 nm)

the cuboid quartz rod, the translesion conduction time would be prolonged. We predicted that the conduction time prolongation ratio (post-ablation conduction time/pre-ablation conduction time) would be directly proportional to the conduction distance prolongation ratio (post-ablation conduction distance/pre-ablation conduction distance). The predicted conduction prolongation ratio was 46.1/30.0 mm = 1.54 (Fig. 3). After obtaining written informed consent from the patient, in August 2016 mitral and tricuspid valve plasty and a maze procedure were performed on a 64-year-old man with infectious endocarditis, severe mitral regurgitation, moderate tricuspid regurgitation, and paroxysmal atrial fibrillation. After a median sternotomy, the pericardium was opened, and the epicardial atrial ablation and electrophysiological study were performed before

commencing the cardiopulmonary bypass. Two pairs of alligator clip electrodes were attached to the right atrium 10 mm from the expected ablation line. The pair of electrodes attached on the dorsal side of the ablation line was used to pace the right atrium, and the pair of electrodes attached on the ventral side of the ablation line was used as sensing electrodes to record the atrial potential. The cuboid 30 mm long 10 mm wide quartz rod of the infrared coagulator was applied epicardially to create a linear lesion on the free wall of the beating right atrial free wall as part of the incision line of the maze procedure (Fig. 3). The total duration of each ablation was 28 s applied in a 5 series of 4.0 s each at 2.0 s intervals. The pacing rate was set to 90 bpm. An electrocardiogram (ECG) and atrial potentials were recorded with an HPM 4500 polygraph (Fukuda Denshi, Tokyo, Japan).

Because the atrial potential was biphasic in shape, conduction times were measured as the interval between stimulation (S) and each peak of the atrial potential (A1 and A2, Fig. 4), and plotted. After the experiment, a square specimen with a side length of 5 mm of coagulated right atrial wall was excised, stained with Masson trichrome, and examined microscopically.

Results

From 1st to 4th infrared application, both S-A1 conduction time and S-A2 conduction time were prolonged and incompletely reversed each time (Fig. 5).

After 4th infrared application, both S-A1 and S-A2 conduction time plateaued, and the 5th infrared application did not affect either conduction time.

S-A1 conduction time was prolonged from 7.2 ms to 10.3 ms. The conduction prolongation ratio was 10.3/7.2 = 1.43.

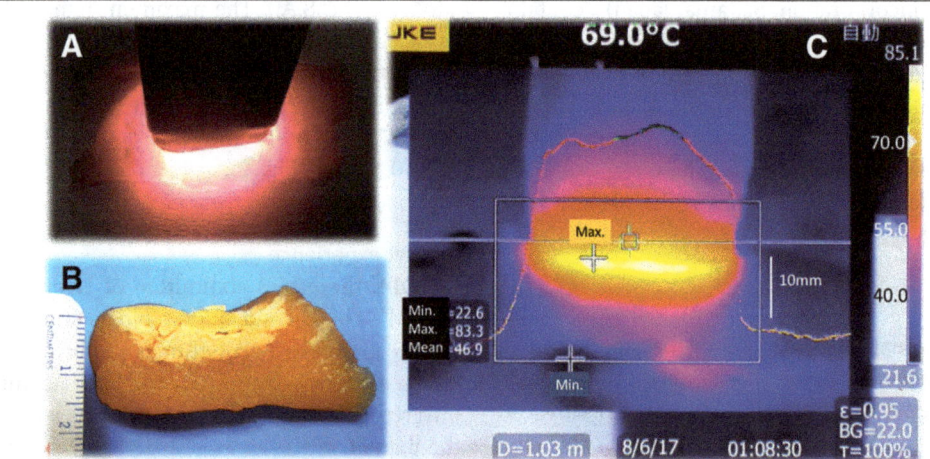

Fig. 2 Preliminary experiment on chicken muscle tissue. **a** The probe was pressed against the muscle tissue. **b** The mean depth of the lesion was 8.7 + 0.8 mm. **c** The maximum temperature was 97.9 + 2.1 °C

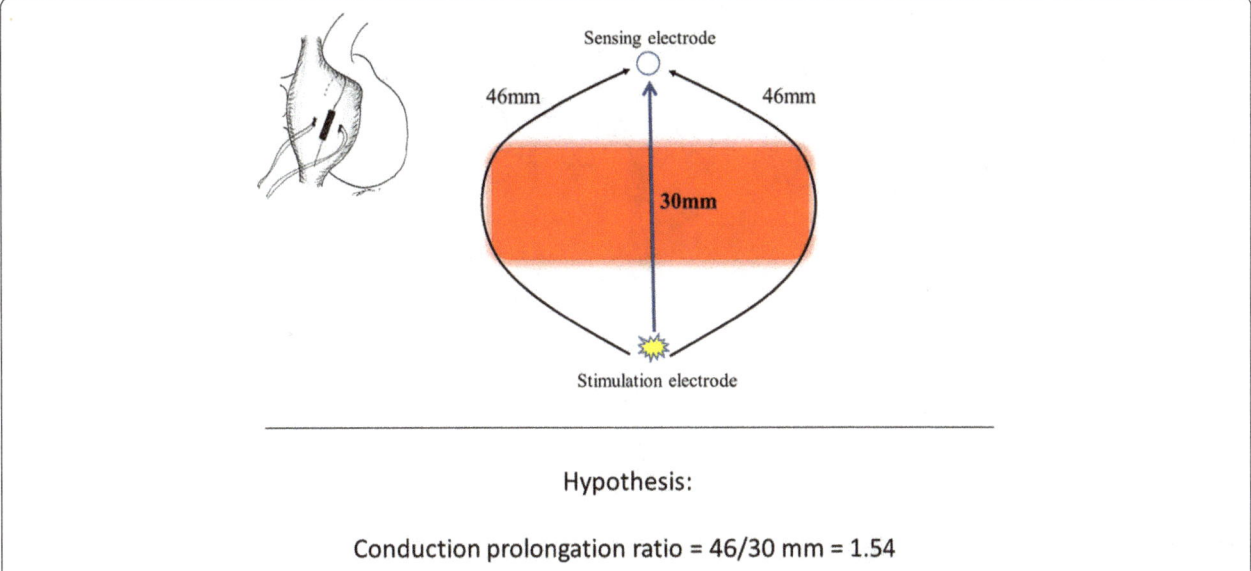

Fig. 3 Prediction. Because the conduction distance prolongation ratio is directly proportional to the conduction time prolongation ratio, when a linear transmural lesion is created in the same shape as the rectangular exit plane, the conduction time prolongation ratio is predicted to be 1.54

S-A2 conduction time was prolonged from 8.6 ms to 11.9 ms. The conduction prolongation ratio was 11.9/8.6 = 1.38.

Histopathologic examination of the ablated right atrium showed preservation of both the endocardium and epicardium of the coagulated lesion (Fig. 6). Severely degenerated myocardium was observed from the epicardial side to mid-portion of the atrial wall. Swelling and hyperchromatosis of the nuclei, acidophilic change in the cytoplasm, and deformity of the myocardium were observed in the myocardium on the endocardial side.

Discussion

To realize the epicardial maze procedure, the major drawback is how to make the transmural lesion on the beating atrial free wall under the condition of existence of inner warm blood flow which weakens heating/cooling effect of the ablation device.

Nath et al. demonstrated that hyperthermia induced by radiofrequency energy causes significant changes in the electrophysiological properties of myocardiocytes, including membrane depolarization, reversible and irreversible loss of excitability, and abnormal automaticity, in an in vitro isolated guinea pig right ventricular papillary muscle

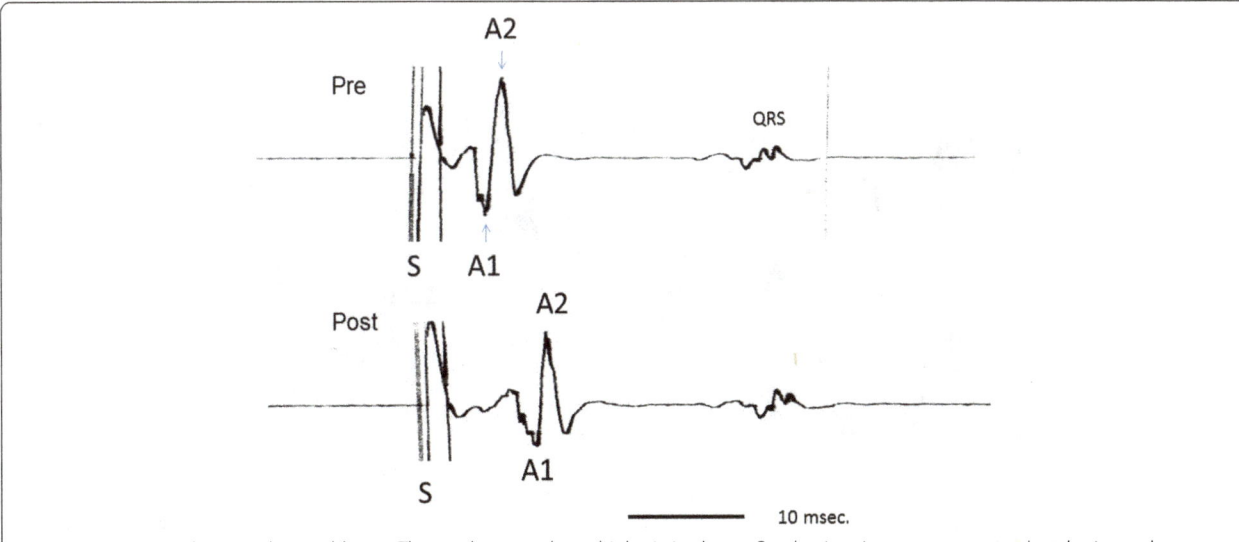

Fig. 4 Atrial potential pre- and post-ablation. The atrial potential was biphasic in shape. Conduction times were measured as the interval between stimulation (S) and each peak of the atrial potential (A1 and A2)

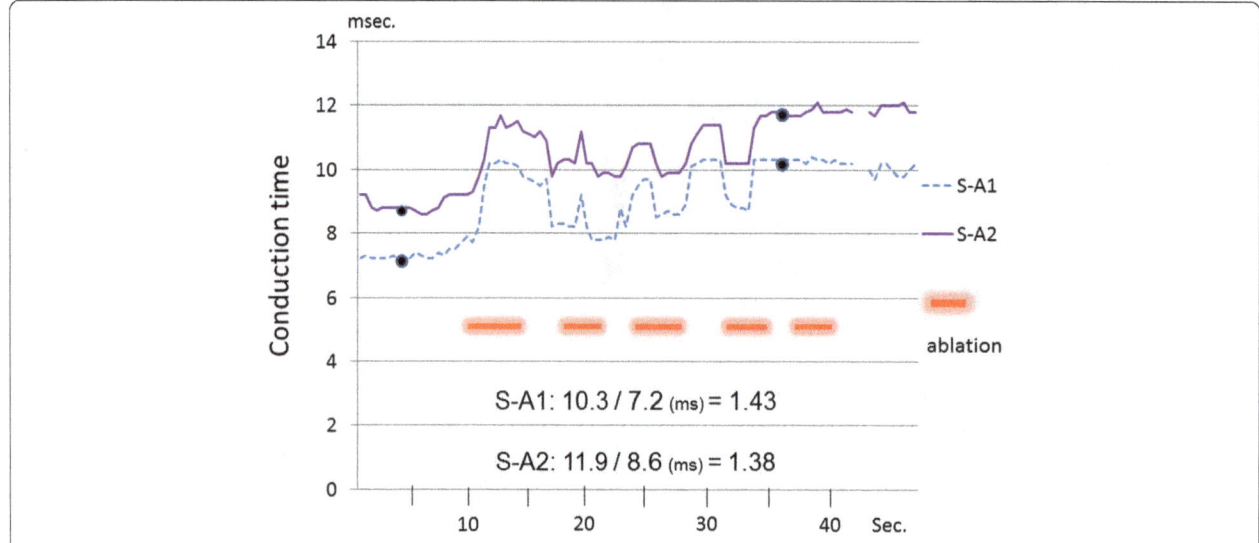

Fig. 5 Atrial potentials pre-ablation and post- ablation (S: stimulation). Biphasic atrial potentials were recorded (A1 and A2). Both S-A1 conduction time and S-A2 conduction time were prolonged after the 28 s of ablation, and the conduction prolongation ratios were 1.43 and 1.38, respectively

model. They observed reversible loss of cellular excitability and tissue injury after exposure to temperatures in the 42.7 °C to 51.3 °C range (median, 48.0 °C) for 60 s and irreversible loss of cellular excitability and tissue injury after exposure to temperatures > 50 °C for 60 seconds [1].

Bulava et al. assessed the efficacy of epicardially created lesions produced with bipolar radiofrequency (RF) energy in 70 patients who had persistent, longstanding atrial fibrillation [2] and reported achieving complete isolation of the posterior left atrial wall in only 22.9% of the patients. The success rates for creating conduction

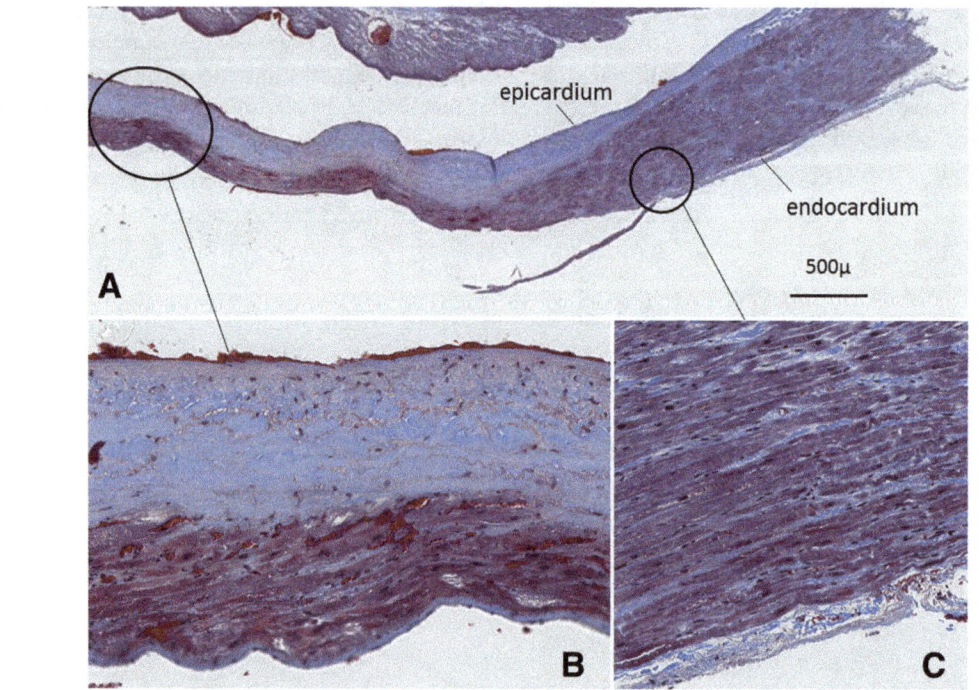

Fig. 6 Histopathologic changes in the ablated right atrium. **a** Histologic examination showed preservation of both the endocardium and epicardium of the coagulated lesion. Both the endocardium and the epicardium were intact. **b** Severely degenerated myocardium was observed from the epicardial side to the mid-portion of the atrial wall. The endocardial side showed swelling and hyperchromatosis of the nuclei, acidophilic change in the cytoplasm, and deformity of the myocardium. **c** Myocardium was intact at the endocardial side of the marginal legion

block across the inferior pulmonary veins (PVs) and across the roof line connecting the two superior PVs were only 58.0 and 24.3%, respectively. Right PVs were found to have been isolated in a significantly higher proportion of patients (91.4%) than the left PVs (75.7%) were. The low efficacy of epicardial RF ablations in creating a transmural irreversible electrophysiological block, especially on the "unclampable free wall" of the atrium, represent that heat sinking effect of the inner blood flow that weaken the thermal effect of the RF.

We previously reported the fundamental results of using an infrared coagulator in animal models [3–5]. The results of the series of experiments in animal models revealed that an infrared coagulator enables creation of a transmural lesion on the canine beating right ventricle to a maximum depth of 10.3 mm, a conduction block on an arrested heart, and a conduction block on a beating right atrium. A successful epicardial maze procedure and successful electrical isolation of the right atrial appendage with an infrared coagulator and concomitant on-pump beating coronary artery bypass grafting have been reported in a clinical case [6, 7].

A cuboid probe was newly developed to create a linear lesion and conduction block on the atrial free wall. To demonstrate the conduction block on the beating heart, encircled lesions e.g. the both atrial appendage, PV cuffs, or box lesion are easy because the ineffective overdrive pacing from inside the lesion can prove the exit block. By contrast, it is difficult to demonstrate a conduction block on a beating atrial free wall. Intraoperative epicardial mapping with multi-electrodes is in common use, but it requires a large-scaled mapping system. Furthermore, because the multi-electrodes are just placed on the epicardium, not attached to it, they slip, and it is difficult to be estimate the exact electrical conduction time. A polygraph with two channels was used in our patient, and it was possible to measure the exact conduction time in every heart beats. We hypothesized that an increase in the translesion stimulus-excitation delay indicates a continuous, transmural, linear lesion, and that the translesion stimulus-excitation delay is directly proportional to path length in the viable tissue around the lesion. Himel et al. demonstrated that complete lesions with RF in rabbit hearts increase translesion stimulus-excitation delay, whereas incomplete lesions do not increase the delay [8]. As far as we investigated, there is no report that proved the stimulus excitation delay on the ablated epicardial atrial free wall in a clinical case. The right atrial free wall was selected for examination. It is easy to apply the cuboid-shaped probe to the right atrial free wall, and it was thought that it would be more difficult to make a transmural lesion in the right atrium than in the left atrium, because the right atrium has a complicated inner structure due to its thick trabecular muscle.

In our patient the myocardium was ablated intermittently at 2-s intervals. Intermittent ablations are more effective than long continuous ablations, because the intervals prevent rapid temperature rise, and prevent to make charring that blocks the photo-energy radiation deep inside the myocardium.

The actual conduction prolongation ratios in the present study were smaller than the predicted ratios, and the main reason for the smaller ratios is thought to be that it was difficult to determine the exact distance between the ablation line and alligator clip electrodes. To determine the more acculate distance, using small bipolar needle electrodes is better. Marginal non-transmural lesions and atrial tissue shrinkage are considered to be other factors that affect conduction time; both factors may shorten the conduction distance and reduce the prolongation ratio.

Pathological examination of the tissue obtained from our patient confirmed the presence of transmural degeneration, however, it was not homogeneous. It may represent the heat sinking effect of the inner blood flow. Considering the result of the presented electrophysiologocal study, there may be a discrepancy between the histopathological transmurality of the lesion and its electrophysiological transmurality. The histopathological change may not exactly represent the electrophysiological change but instead underestimate it by overlooking the pathologically normal but electrophysiologically remodeled lesion of the myocardium. Chronic reversibility of the prolonged conduction time was not investigated in this study. However, in a previous animal study we verified hemosiderin deposition, macrophage invasion, increased capillary vessels, and increased juvenile elastic fibers in the right atrial free wall 3 months after ablation. The myocardium did not revive, the endocardium became thickened, and elastic fibers appeared.

Theoretically, same as RF, this new technology can be applied not only to the atrium but also to the ventricle. Modifying the shape and flexibility of the probe may enable safe and effective minimally invasive endoscopic ablation to create a box lesion on the beating left atrium and to treat ventricular tachycardia based on the same tissue photocoagulation principle as described above.

Conclusions
The newly developed cuboid probe of the Kyo-co infrared coagulator may have the potential to serve as a reliable device for performing the epicardial maze procedure on the beating atrial free wall clinically.

Abbreviations
ECG: Electrocardiogram; RF: Radiofrequency

Acknowledgments
The authors wish to thank Ms. Yuki Matsumoto for her assistance with the data analysis in this study.

Funding
This study was supported by funding from the "Leading-edge Industry Design Project, Medical Innovation, Saitama Prefecture, Japan, 2016."

Authors' contributions
HK designed and drafted the MS. HE, HI, HT, and YI drafted and revised the MS. YT, and KT analyzed and interpreted the measured data. All authors have approved to the submission of the MS.

Competing interests
The authors declare that they have no competing interests.

References
1. Nath S, Lynch C III, Whayne JG, Haines DE. Cellular electrophysiological effects of hyperthermia on isolated Guinea pig papillary muscle. Implications for catheter ablation. Circulation. 1993;88:1826–31.
2. Bulava A, Mokracek A, Kurfirst V. Delayed electroanatomic mapping after surgical ablation for persistent atrial fibrillation. Ann Thorac Surg. 2017; 104(6):2024–9.
3. Kubota H, Furuse A, Takeshita M, Kotsuka Y, Takamoto S. Atrial ablation with an IRK-151 infrared coagulator. Ann Thorac Surg. 1998;66:95–100.
4. Kubota H, Takamoto S, Takeshita M, Miyaji K, Kotsuka Y, Furuse A. Atrial ablation using an IRK-151 infrared coagulator in canine model. J Cardiovasc Surg. 2000;41:835–47.
5. Kubota H, Kenichi S, Takamoto S, et al. Clinical result of epicardial pulmonary vein isolation (LAVIE) by cryoablation as concomitant cardiac operation and clinical application of new device (KIRC-119 infrared coagulator) to treat atrial fibrillation. In: Choi JI, editor. Atrial fibrillation-basic research and clinical applications. Croatia: Intech; 2011. p. 267–90.
6. Kubota H, Takamoto S, Furuse A, et al. Epicardial maze procedure on the beating heart with an infrared coagulator. Ann Thorac Surg. 2005;80:1081–6.
7. Kubota H, Sudo K, Takamoto S, et al. Epicardial electrical isolation of the right atrial appendage on the beating heart with an infrared coagulator. Ann Thorac Surg. 2009;87:1592–5.
8. Himel IV, Dumas HJ III, Kiser AC, Knisley SB. Translesion stimulus-excitation delay indicates quality of linear lesions produced by radiofrequency ablation in rabbit hearts. Physiol Meas. 2007;28:611–23.

19

Thoracoscopic one-stage lobectomy and diaphragmatic plication for T3 lung cancer

Yuki Takahashi, Masahiro Miyajima, Taijiro Mishina, Ryunosuke Maki, Makoto Tada, Kodai Tsuruta and Atsushi Watanabe[*]

Abstract

Background: Combined resection of a phrenic nerve is occasionally required in T3 primary lung carcinomas invading the phrenic nerve to completely remove a malignant tumour, resulting in diaphragmatic paralysis. We describe the first case of thoracoscopic lobectomy and diaphragmatic plication as a one-stage surgery for lung cancer invading the phrenic nerve.

Case presentation: A 56-year-old woman with a T3N0M0 primary adenosquamous carcinoma in the left upper lobe presented with suspicious invasion to the anterior mediastinal fat tissue and left phrenic nerve and underwent left upper lobectomy, node dissection, and partial resection of the anterior mediastinal fat tissue with the left phrenic nerve. Furthermore, thoracoscopic diaphragmatic plication was performed as a concomitant procedure. The patient's postoperative course was favourable, without any complications, and respiratory function was preserved for 1 year postoperatively.

Conclusions: Thoracoscopic one-stage lobectomy and diaphragmatic plication for T3 lung cancer invading the phrenic nerve is effective for preservation of postoperative pulmonary function.

Keywords: Thoracoscopic lobectomy, Phrenic nerve resection, Diaphragmatic paralysis, Diaphragmatic plication, One-stage surgery

Background

Combined resection of the phrenic nerve is occasionally required in T3 primary lung carcinomas invading the nerve to completely remove a malignant tumour. This can cause diaphragmatic paralysis. Postoperative diaphragmatic paralysis leads to impaired respiratory function and pulmonary complications [1]. Diaphragmatic plication has been performed for the surgical treatment of diaphragmatic paralysis and eventration. Tokunaga et al. demonstrated the efficacy of intraoperative diaphragmatic plication by comparing postoperative vital capacity (VC) and forced expiratory volume in 1 s (FEV1) with predicted postoperative VC (ppo VC) and predicted postoperative FEV1 (ppo FEV1) for patients undergoing unilateral phrenectomy during extended surgery [2]. However, thoracoscopic one-stage pulmonary lobectomy, partial resection of the phrenic nerve, and diaphragmatic plication have seldom been performed for lung cancer invading the phrenic nerve because of technical limitations.

We report the first case of a patient in whom respiratory function was successfully preserved after performing these thoracoscopic one-stage procedures for T3 lung cancer invading the phrenic nerve.

Case presentation

A 56-year-old woman was referred to our hospital for surgical treatment of a T3N0M0 primary adenosquamous carcinoma measuring 35 × 28 mm in the anterior segment (segment 3) of the left upper lobe without mediastinal lymph node swelling in preoperative computed tomography. The ppo VC and ppo FEV1 were 2.68 L and 2.22 L, respectively. The preoperative computed tomography scan revealed that the tumour had invaded the anterior mediastinal fat tissue and phrenic nerve (Fig. 1a, b).

The patient was placed in a lateral position on the operating table under general anaesthesia with selective

* Correspondence: atsushiw@sapmed.ac.jp
Department of Thoracic Surgery, Sapporo Medical University, School of Medicine and Hospital, South 1, West 16, Chuo-ku, Sapporo, Hokkaido 060-8556, Japan

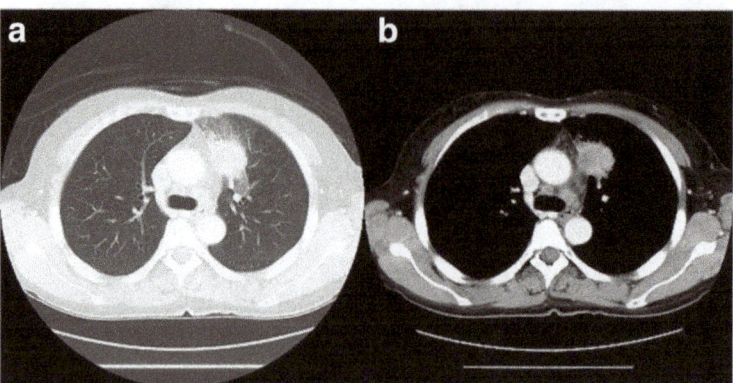

Fig. 1 Preoperative computed tomography scan showing a 35 × 28-mm tumour in the anterior segment (segment 3) of the left upper lobe (**a**) and the anterior mediastinal fat tissue invaded by the tumour (**b**)

lung ventilation. Two thoracoport trocars (15 mm) were placed in the sixth intercostal space (ICS) at the anterior axillary line and in the seventh ICS at the posterior axillary line. An anterolateral mini-thoracotomy (35 mm) was performed in the fourth ICS for left upper lobectomy (Fig. 2). We resected the phrenic nerve and pericardial fat with an optimal surgical margin and then performed left upper lobectomy and lymph node dissection. Thoracoscopic diaphragmatic plication was performed with 3–0 Prolene sutures running from the dorsolateral to ventromedial diaphragm in order to oversew the diaphragmatic tendon pars and imbricate the muscle part (Fig. 3). Dacron pledgets were only used for the first suture and the suture was retracted to the cranial side during needle stitch (Fig. 4). The thoracoscope was placed through the thoracoport trocar in the seventh ICS at the posterior axillary line and the plication was performed through the thoracoport trocar in the sixth ICS at the anterior axillary line with an endoscopic needle holder.

The pathological diagnosis was a T3N2M0 primary adenosquamous carcinoma invading the phrenic nerve with negative surgical margins. The patient's postoperative course was favourable without any complications. No clinical symptoms were observed during the follow-up. Pulmonary function testing performed 1 year after the surgery revealed VC and FEV1 values of 2.36 L and 2.08 L, respectively. The representative chest radiographs of the left hemidiaphragm showed a normal position preoperatively and only mild elevation postoperatively (Fig. 5a, b).

Discussion and conclusions

Diaphragmatic paralysis decreases VC by 20 to 30% and leads to pulmonary complications [1]. Although this does not generally cause respiratory difficulty in healthy adults, the risk of respiratory difficulty is high in most patients with lung cancer because they tend to be older and might have a history of heavy smoking inducing low pulmonary function. Tokunaga et al. reported that after surgical plication for diaphragmatic paralysis during extended surgery for pulmonary cancer, mediastinal

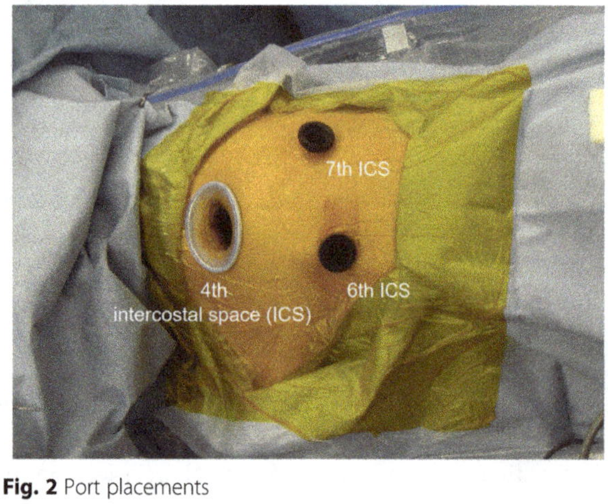

Fig. 2 Port placements

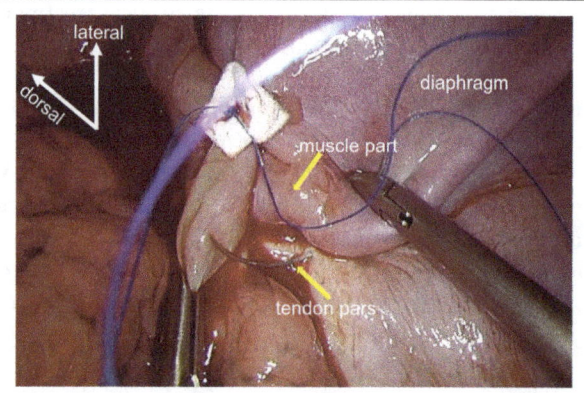

Fig. 3 Thoracoscopic view during thoracoscopic diaphragmatic plication

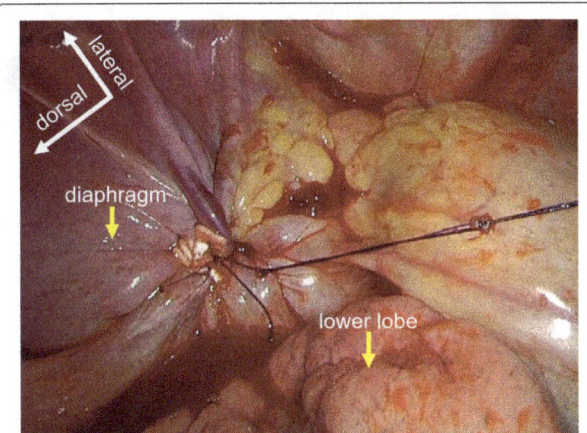

Fig. 4 Thoracoscopic view after diaphragmatic plication

tumour, and malignant pleural mesothelioma, the mean ratio of measured postoperative VC to ppo VC was 88.2% and the mean ratio of measured postoperative FEV1 to ppo FEV1 was 98.5% [2]. In the present case, the ratios of the actual postoperative VC to ppo VC and actual postoperative FEV1 to ppo FEV1 were 88 and 94%, respectively, indicating that respiratory function was preserved postoperatively. The patient did not experience any clinical symptoms 1 year postoperatively.

Previous research studies have reported on phrenic nerve reconstruction for diaphragmatic paralysis [3, 4]. Respiratory function for FEV1 in patients undergoing reconstruction of the phrenic nerve and diaphragmatic plication improved by averages of 13 and 17%, respectively. In addition, forced VC improved by an average of 14% after reconstruction of the phrenic nerve and 17% after diaphragmatic plication [3]. In our case, it was difficult to make a preoperative decision about the extent of phrenic nerve resection. Our decision to perform diaphragmatic plication was influenced by an increased likelihood that the patient would maintain her respiratory function.

Consensus was reached about performing early plication for diaphragmatic paralysis in infants and young children [5]. Çelik et al. suggested that early and timely plication for diaphragmatic paralysis improves functional status and shortens the length of hospitalization [6]. However, the timing of surgical plication remains controversial in adults. Diaphragmatic plication for phrenic nerve paralysis after surgery has been considered as a second surgery because nerve function may recover [7]. Preoperative pulmonary function testing and evaluation of phrenic nerve activity by electromyography can be performed for selecting patients in need of surgical treatment before surgical plication in two stages. However, two-stage diaphragmatic plication after ipsilateral thoracic surgery is more difficult owing to pleural adhesions, especially following lower lobectomy and posterior mediastinal lymph node dissection. In the present case, the recovery of the nerve could not be expected because nerve resection without reconstruction was performed. Therefore, a one-stage procedure of diaphragmatic plication was performed, and the patient experienced no perioperative complications.

One-stage pulmonary lobectomy and diaphragmatic plication have been reported for lung cancer in thoracotomy but not in thoracoscopic surgery. Thoracotomy transiently reduces diaphragmatic function. Demos et al. favour performing plication in a minimally invasive manner, as this deficit recovers more quickly after thoracoscopic surgery than after thoracotomy [8]. However, suturing seems to be the primary problem of diaphragmatic plication in thoracoscopic surgery, and splenic injury and/or greater omentum injury caused by blind suturing may result in abdominal bleeding. We changed the operating table to a reversed Trendelenburg position, with the patient in a lateral position during diaphragmatic plication. Furthermore, the diaphragm was sutured while staying away from the dorsal depth so as not to injure the spleen during the left side procedure.

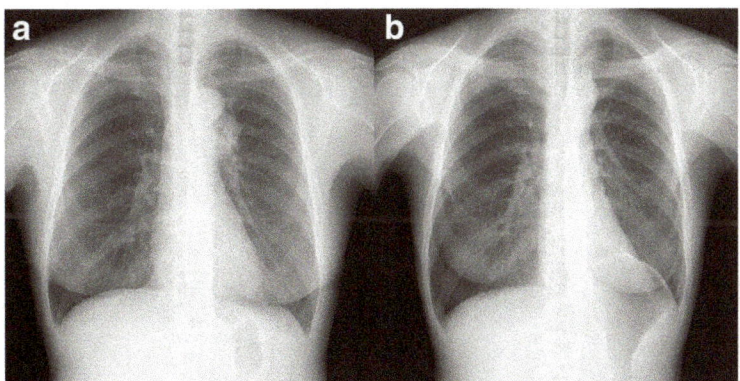

Fig. 5 a Preoperative chest radiograph and **b** postoperative chest radiograph at 1 year showing mild elevation of the left hemidiaphragm

Thoracoscopic one-stage lobectomy with phrenic nerve resection and diaphragmatic plication as a one-stage procedure is effective for preserving postoperative pulmonary function and reduces the necessity for pleurolysis due to pleural adhesion and the risks associated with additional general anaesthesia.

Abbreviations
FEV1: Forced expiratory volume in 1 second; ICS: Intercostal space; ppo FEV1: Predicted postoperative FEV1; ppo VC: Predicted postoperative VC; VC: Vital capacity

Authors' contributions
YT drafted the manuscript and collected materials. MM, TM, RM, MT and KT helped to draft the manuscript. AW helped to draft the manuscript and participated in its design. All authors contributed to revision of the manuscript. All authors read and approved the final manuscript.

Competing interests
The authors declare that they have no competing interests.

References
1. Zhao HX, D'Agostino RS, Pitlick PT, Shumway NE, Miller DC. Phrenic nerve injury complicating closed cardiovascular surgical procedures for congenital heart disease. Ann Thorac Surg. 1985;39:445–9.
2. Tokunaga T, Sawabata N, Kadota Y, Utsumi T, Minami M, Inoue M, et al. Efficacy of intra-operative unilateral diaphragm plication for patients undergoing unilateral phrenectomy during extended surgery. Eur J Cardiothorac Surg. 2010;38:600–3.
3. Kaufman MR, Elkwood AI, Colicchio AR, CeCe J, Jarrahy R, Willekes LJ, et al. Functional restoration of diaphragmatic paralysis: an evaluation of phrenic nerve reconstruction. Ann Thorac Surg. 2014;97:260–7.
4. Kawashima S, Kohno T, Fujimori S, Yokomakura N, Ikeda T, Harano T, et al. Phrenic nerve reconstruction in complete video-assisted thoracic surgery. Interact Cardiovasc Thorac Surg. 2015;20:54–9.
5. Georgiev S, Konstantinov G, Latcheva A, Mitev P, Mitev I, Lazarov S. Phrenic nerve injury after paediatric heart surgery: is aggressive plication of the diaphragm beneficial? Eur J Cardiothorac Surg. 2013;44:808–12.
6. Çelik S, Tanju S, Döngel İ, Gürer O, Toker A. Diaphragmatic plication: retrospective study with 54 patients. Open J Thorac Surg. 2013;3:87–92.
7. Tsakiridis K, Visouli AN, Zarogoulidis P, Machairiotis N, Christofis C, Stylianaki A, et al. Early hemi-diaphragmatic plication through a video assisted mini-thoracotomy in postcardiotomy phrenic nerve paresis. J Thorac Dis. 2012;4:56–68.
8. Demos DS, Berry MF, Backhus LM, Shrager JB. Video-assisted thoracoscopic diaphragm plication using a running suture technique is durable and effective. J Thorac Cardiovasc Surg. 2017;1533:1182–8.

Early hemodynamic performance of the Trifecta™ surgical bioprosthesis aortic valve in Indian patient population: 12 month outcomes of the EVEREST post-market study

Gopichand Mannam[1]*[iD], Yugal Mishra[2], Rajan Modi[3], Alla Gopala Krishna Gokhale[4], Rajan Sethuratnam[5], Kaushal Pandey[6], Rajneesh Malhotra[7], Sumit Anand[8], Anushreeta Borah[8], Sushan Mukhopadhyay[9], Dhiren Shah[10] and Tek Singh Mahant[11]

Abstract

Background: Indian patients undergoing surgical aortic valve replacement (SAVR) differ from western populations with respect to aortic annulus size and valve disease morphology. The purpose of this post-market, non-randomized observational study was to evaluate the early hemodynamic performance of the Trifecta™ bioprosthesis (Abbott, previously St. Jude Medical, Minneapolis, US) in an Indian patient population.

Methods: From January 2014 to September 2015, 100 patients (mean age 64.4 ± 7.1 years, 62% male) undergoing SAVR for valve disease (68% stenosis, 7% insufficiency, 25% mixed pathology) were enrolled across 10 centers in India. Patients implanted with a 19–27 mm Trifecta™ valve were eligible to participate and were prospectively followed for 12-months post-implantation. Echocardiographic hemodynamic performance was evaluated at pre-implant, pre-discharge and at 12-months by an independent core laboratory. Adverse events were adjudicated by the study sponsor. Functional status at 12-months was assessed according to NYHA classification. Continuous data was summarized using descriptive statistics (mean &standard deviation,) and categorical data was summarized using frequencies and percentages.

Result: Ninety patients (mean age 64.5, 62.2% male) completed the 12-month follow up. Significant improvements in hemodynamic valve performance were reported in 81 patients with available echocardiographic data at 12 months. Compared to baseline at 12-month follow up visit, mean effective orifice area increased from 0.75cm^2 to 1.61cm^2 ($p < 0.0001$), mean pressure gradient reduced to 10.42 mmHg from 51.47 mmHg ($p < 0.0001$), cardiac output increased from 4.46 l/min to 4.85 l/min (P 0.9254). Compared to baseline, functional status improved by ≥1 NYHA class in 75% of patients at 12 months (95% Clopper-Pearson (Exact) confidence limit [64.6%, 83.6%]). No instances of early mortality (< 30 days from index procedure) or structural valve dysfunction were reported.

Conclusion: In an Indian patient population, implantation of the Trifecta™ bioprosthesis is shown to be safe and associated with favorable early hemodynamic performance and improved functional status at 12 months.

(Continued on next page)

* Correspondence: gopi.mannam@gmail.com
[1]Department of cardiac surgery, Star Hospital Banjara Hills, 8-2-596/5, Road No.10, Banjara Hills, Hyderabad, Telangana 500034, India
Full list of author information is available at the end of the article

(Continued from previous page)

Keywords: Aortic valve replacement, Stented bioprosthesis, Valvular disease, Structural valve dysfunction

Background

Each year, approximately 150,000 patients undergo cardiac surgeries and 30% is the valve surgeries including both aortic and mitral valve replacement in India [1]. Compared to western populations, Indian patients indicated for SAVR tend to be younger, have a higher incidence of valve disease due to rheumatic fever and require implantation of smaller valve sizes (predominately 19 mm and 21 mm valves) [2–4]. Due to the need for implantation of smaller bioprostheses, the risk for patient-prosthetic mismatch (PPM), defined as an effective orifice area (EOA) that is too small in relation to a patient's cardiac output requirements, is high in Indian patients. PPM leads to poor hemodynamic valve performance (namely elevated transvalvular pressure gradients) despite a fully functioning prosthesis and is associated with poor clinical outcomes including late survival, freedom from heart failure, and LV mass regression [5]. Thus making selection of an appropriate bioprosthesis that maximizes EOA critical in this patient population.

The Trifecta™ bioprosthesis (Abbott, previously St. Jude Medical, Minneapolis, US) is a tri-leaflet, stented, bovine pericardial valve designed for supra-annular placement in the aortic position. The Trifecta^{TM} valve has been commercially available in India since 2012 and incorporates several novel design features to maximize valve hemodynamics while minimizing leaflet stresses [6]. Specifically, the valve features a true supra-annular polyester sewing cuff with a silicone insert that is designed to conform to the shape of the native annulus and externally-mounted bovine pericardial valve leaflets that wrap around the fatigue resistance, titanium stent frame to maximize EOA and improve hemodynamic performance. To reduce the risk of leaflet abrasion and structural valve dysfunction, the stent frame, excluding the sewing cuff, is covered with porcine pericardial tissue to allow only tissue-to-tissue contact during valve function. Linx™ AC anti-calcification technology also reduces calcification of the tissue valve.

The superior hemodynamic performance of Trifecta™ valve has been previously demonstrated in western patients with significant benefits in hemodynamic performance, EOAs and mean transvalvular pressure gradients reported in patients with different annulus sizes [7–12].

Due to the limited data available on Indian patients undergoing SAVR in rheumatic heart disease and with most of the patients having significantly smaller native aortic annuli, the EVEREST study (A clinical EValuation of hEmodynamic peRformancE of Trifecta™ valve in Indian SubjecTs), was conducted with a purpose to evaluate the early (12 months) hemodynamic performance of the Trifecta™ valve by echocardiography in Indian patients for treatment of aortic valve disease. Assessment of the early safety of the valve and changes in NYHA functional classification was also performed.

Methods

Patients

Between January 2014 to September 2015, 100 patients who had undergone SAVR with a Trifecta™ valve were recruited from 10 investigational centers in India to participate in the prospective, single-arm, post-market observational EVEREST study (CTRI/2014/02/004434). Eligibility criteria included implantation of a Trifecta™ valve within 7 days and analyzable echocardiographic data at baseline. Patients who had been previously implanted with a prosthetic valve(s) at a site other than the aortic valve, on renal dialysis, pregnant, active endocarditis or pre-existing cardiovascular abnormalities (aortic dissection or ventricular aneurysm) were excluded.

Prior to patient enrollment, appropriate institutional review board approval for protocol, patient information sheets and consent forms were obtained at each center. The study was performed in accordance with the Declaration of Helsinki and with laws and regulations of the country. A written informed consent was obtained from each patient prior to enrollment. Details on the 10 investigational centers are provided in Appendix.

Surgical technique

The study protocol permitted operative surgeon's to use any surgical technique at their discretion for implantation of the Trifecta^{TM} valve. Data on valve size, surgical approach, suture technique, cardiopulmonary bypass time and aortic cross clamp time were collected. Post-operative protocol was as per Institute's standard protocol with anticoagulant and other standard medications.

Data collection

Preoperative and procedural data was retrospectively collected from the implant centers. Perioperative data collection included patient demographics and medical history, NYHA functional class, disease valve etiology, valve dysfunction (insufficiency/incompetent/regurgitated, stenosis & mixed), echocardiographic exam and pathology.

Procedural data collection included implanted bioprosthetic valve size, suture technique, cardiopulmonary bypass time and aortic cross clamp time. All follow-up data was prospectively collected as part of routine clinical practice. At pre-discharge, 6 month and 12-month follow-up visits, subjects underwent a physical examination, echocardiographic exam (pre-discharge and 12 months only), assessment of NYHA functional class and review of relevant cardiac medication.

Echocardiography

Transthoracic echocardiographic examinations were performed on-site at baseline, pre-discharge (average 6 days of index procedure) and at 12 months by an experienced Echocardiographer. All exams were reviewed by an independent core laboratory by Department of Non-Invasive Cardiology at Fortis Escorts Heart Institute, New Delhi and evaluated for the following parameters: left ventricular function, mean transvalvular pressure gradient, mean pressure gradient, effective orifice area (EOA), cardiac output, cardiac index, and performance index (EOA/Pre-implant Interval Orifice area) [13, 14]. EOA was calculated using the continuity equation [13–15] and indexed to body surface area (indexed EOA). The incidence and severity of aortic insufficiency (paravalvular, valvular or indeterminate with clinical (visual) estimation of regurgitation as trivial, mild, moderate or severe) was assessed according to standardized VARC criteria.

Endpoints

The study's primary endpoint was valve hemodynamic performance (as measured by echocardiography) at 12 months. Secondary endpoints included change in NYHA functional class from baseline to 12 months (defined as no change, improved, or worsened), incidence of structural valve deterioration (calcification, leaflet tear and/or perforation) and cardiovascular-related adverse events at 12 months. The study sponsor (Abbott) was responsible for adjudication of adverse events and determining their seriousness and relationship to the study device and or study procedure.

Statistical analysis

Continuous data was summarized using descriptive statistics (mean &standard deviation) and categorical data was summarized using frequencies and percentages. All echocardiographic parameters were stratified according to the nominal size of the implanted Trifecta™ valve. Comparisons of change between 12-months and baseline in echocardiographic evaluation of valve performance was analysed using Student's t test (if Normal distribution assumption is met) or Wilcoxon signed-rank test (if Normal distribution assumption is not met). The 95% exact confidence interval is provided to the percentage of the patient

with improved NYHA functional between 12-months and baseline. Statistical analyses were performed using SAS™ software v9.4.

Results

Patient population and operative data

Baseline clinical and demographic data of the 100 patients enrolled in the study is presented in Table 1. Briefly,

Table 1 Baseline demographics, medical history and clinical characteristics of patients ($n = 100$)

	All ($n = 100$)
Age (years)	64.38 ± 7.05
Male n/N, (%)	62/100 (62%)
Body Mass Index (kg/m^2)	26.5 ± 4.72
Body Surface Area (m^2)	1.73 ± 0.18
NYHA functional class	
I	5/98(5.1%)
II	51/98(52.04%)
III	39/98(39.8%)
IV	3/98(3.06%)
Sinus rhythm	97/100 (97%)
Comorbidities	
Hypertension	51/100 (51%)
Coronary Artery Disease	38/100 (38%)
Non aortic Valve Disease	29/100 (29%)
Diabetes mellitus	38/100 (38%)
Hyperlipidemia	3/100 (3%)
Renal Insufficiency	2/100 (2%)
Congestive Heart Failure	2/100 (2%)
Stroke	1/100 (1%)
Transient Ischemic Attack	2/100 (2%)
Myocardial Infarction	1/100 (1%)
Previous coronary artery intervention	4/100 (4%)
Previous CABG	7/100 (7%)
Permanent pacemaker	1/100 (1%)
Aortic Valve Pathology	
Degenerative calcification	54/100 (54%)
Bicuspid	42/100 (42%)
Rheumatic	14/100 (14%)
Endocarditis	1/100 (1%)
Structural deterioration	1/100 (1%)
Other	4/100 (4%)
Aortic Valve Lesion	
Insufficiency	7/100 (7%)
Stenosis	68/100 (68%)
Mixed	25/100 (25%)

n Total number of patients, kg/m^2 Kilogram/meter^2

patients were predominately male (62%) elderly (mean age 64.38 ± 7.05 years) and had multiple comorbidities including hypertension (51%), coronary artery disease (38%) and diabetes (38%). The main indication for SAVR was valve disease due to degenerative calcification (54%); with only 14% due to rheumatic heart disease. Pre-operative NYHA functional class was distributed as 5% Class I, 52.04% Class II, 39.8% Class III and 3% Class IV. Sinus rhythm was observed in 97 patients while 3 patients had a pre-existing arrhythmia.

Procedural outcomes are summarized in Table 2. All prostheses were implanted in a supra-annular position, with the majority of surgeons using a median sternotomy surgical approach (77%) and simple interrupted suture technique (51%). Thirty-three patients underwent a concomitant surgical procedure; with 28% requiring coronary artery bypass grafting. Average cardiopulmonary bypass time was 112.1 ± 49.2 min and average aortic cross clamp time was 78.4 ± 33.8 min. Patients were predominantly implanted with a 19 mm ($n = 36$) or 21 mm ($n = 45$) Trifecta valve. For the purposes of subsequent analyses, all patients implanted with a 23 mm ($n = 13$), 25 mm ($n = 5$) and 27 mm valve ($n = 1$) have been grouped into a single cohort. There were no instances of intra-procedural mortality. A total of 90 patients completed the 12-month follow-up visit (90%; Fig. 1: Flow chart). The remaining 10 subjects either, were lost to follow-up ($n = 7$) or formally withdrew consent ($n = 2$) and died ($n = 1$). The percentage

Table 2 Procedural Characteristics

	All ($n = 100$)
Cardiopulmonary bypass time (min)	112.1 ± 49.23 (98)
Aortic cross clamp time (min)	78.35 ± 33.77 (98)
Suture technique, n (%)	
Simple interrupted	51/100 (51%)
Continuous	3/100 (3%)
Everting mattress	7/100 (7%)
Non-everting mattress	22/100 (22%)
Other	18/100 (18%)
Concomitant surgical procedure, n (%)	
Coronary artery bypass graphing	28/100 (28%)
Mitral valve repair	2/100 (2%)
Other	3/100 (3%)
Implanted valve size	
19 mm	36
21 mm	45
23 mm	13
25 mm	5
27 mm	1

n Total number of patients, *min* Minutes, *mm* Millimeter

of patients receiving anticoagulation therapy at different visits is shown in Table 3. At baseline 81%, pre-discharge 95%, 6 months 91% and 88% at 12 months were receiving anticoagulation therapy.

Valve hemodynamic performance

Analyzable echocardiographic data was available for 81 patients (90%; echocardiographic images for 9 patients were not as per the Core Laboratory requirements) at 12 months follow-up.

A consistent low mean pressure gradient across the prosthesis was observed, which was maintained till 12 months of follow-up. Baseline, pre-discharge and 12 month's echocardiographic parameters according to valve size are summarized in Table 4. The average mean pressure gradients were 51.47 ± 18.34, 10.44 ± 4.40 and 10.42 ± 4.77 at baseline, pre-discharge & 12 months respectively. Results for effective orifice area and effective orifice area index are shown in Table 4. The average effective orifice area was 0.75 ± 0.42, 1.59 ± 0.37 and 1.61 ± 0.30 at baseline, pre-discharge & 12 months respectively The average cardiac was 4.46 ± 2.39 at the time of baseline, 4.45 ± 2.03 at pre-discharge and between 4.85 ± 1.69 at 12 months. (Table 4). Performance Index was calculated at baseline and pre-discharge and at 12 month and is depicted in Table 4. The average performance index was 0.22 ± 0.11 at the time of baseline, 0.47 ± 0.11 at pre-discharge and 0.48 ± 0.08 at 12 months. The average indexed EOAI for all the valves is 0.91 ± 0.19 cm^2/m^2 which is above the PPM threshold of ≤ 0.85 cm^2/m^2 with a significance p-value of < 0.0001. Hence, no prosthetic patient mismatch was observed (Table 4).

Aortic regurgitation was observed at baseline in 36 patients (Mild to Severe), at pre-discharge in 4 patients (mild) and at 12 month in 1 patient (mild); none of the patients had moderate or severe aortic regurgitation at pre-discharge and 12 month. (Fig. 2: Summary Statistics for incidence/severity of aortic insufficiency Measurements).

Clinical events

At 12 months, no incidence of structural valve deterioration, valve thrombosis, or hemolysis was observed. Nine subjects reported 9 separate SAEs events including: hepatic encephalopathy, post pericardiotomy effusion, cerebrovascular accident/intracerebral hemorrhage, complete heart block, metastatic lymph nodes, peripheral vertigo, ventricular arrhythmias, decreased sodium levels and increased total white blood cells and low tract respiratory infection. No SAEs were deemed to be valve related. A single patient death (1%) was reported 37 days post-implant, and was deemed related to a low sodium level (no valvular/para valvular leak was observed in pre-discharge echocardiographic images and had a well- functioning prosthetic aortic valve).

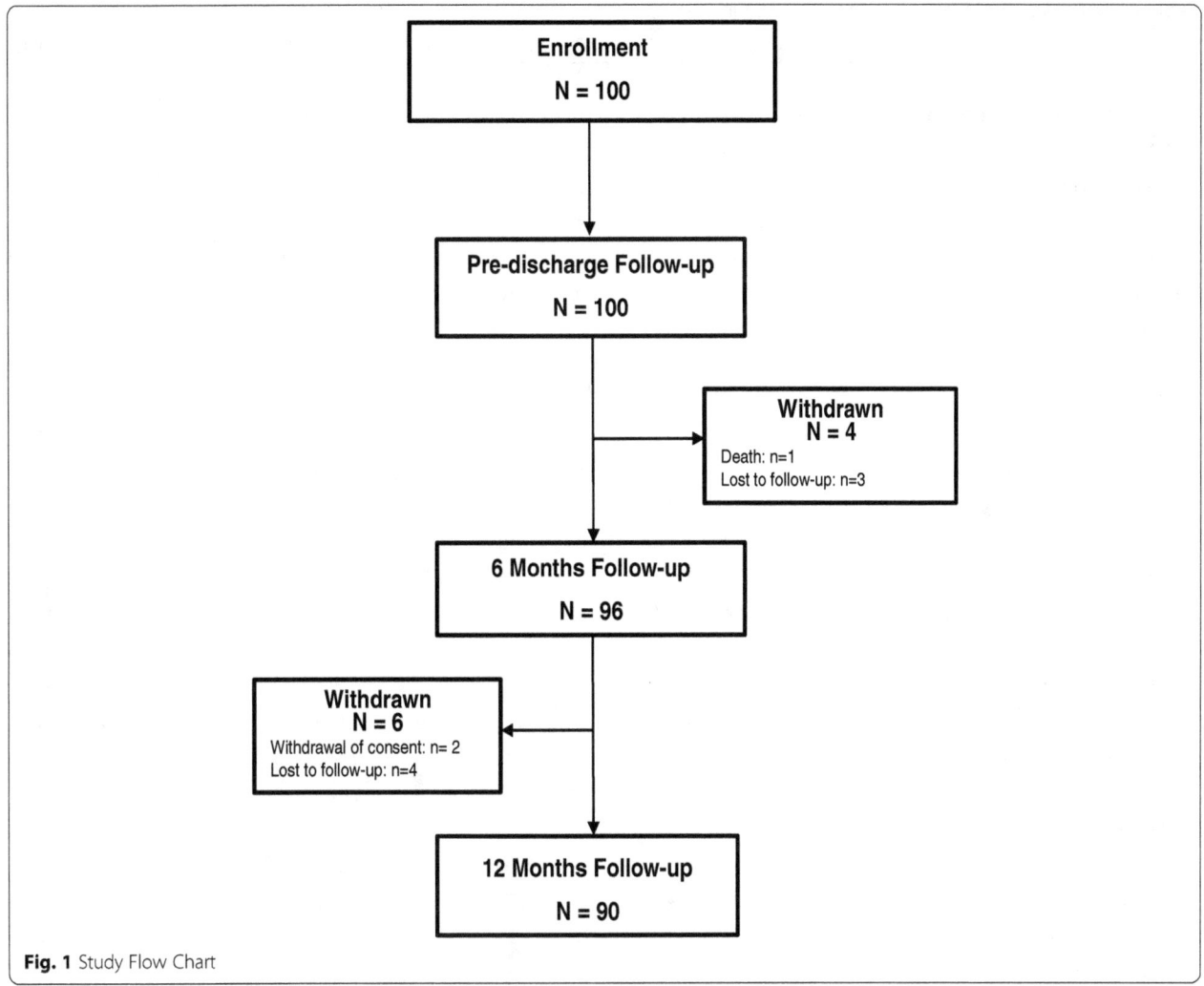

Fig. 1 Study Flow Chart

Change in NYHA functional status

In 88 (NYHA data not available for 2 patients) patients with available data at 12 months, NYHA functional status improved by ≥1 class in 75% of patients (66/88) compared to baseline. Only 1 patient reported a worsening in NYHA function class at 12 months compared to baseline (mild AR was observed at 12 months); the remaining 23.9% of patients experienced no change. (Fig. 3: Changes in NYHA functional status at pre-discharge, 6 months and 12 months compared to baseline) summarizes the proportion of patients that improved, did not change, or worsened in NYHA functional status at pre-discharge, 6 months and 12 months compared to baseline.

Discussion

According to the guidelines of the American Heart Association/American College of Cardiology (AHA/ACC), bioprostheses have been chosen as the most appropriate aortic valve treatment for patients older than 65 years with severe valve stenosis [16]. It is predictable that the number of AVRs with bioprosthesis will become more frequent in future owing to growth of aging population. This is further relevant for developing countries like India where majority of the population cannot afford Transcatheter aortic valve replacement therapy and would rely on surgical approach for treatment of aortic valve disease.

The present prospective, multicenter study evaluated the safety and hemodynamic performance of the Trifecta™

Table 3 Anticoagulants regimen

Visits	Anticoagulant regimen n (%)
Baseline	81/100 (81%)
Pre-discharge	95/100 (95%)
6 Month	87/96 (91%)
12 Month	79/90 (88%)

n = Total number of patients

Table 4 Pre-Implant and Pre-Discharge Echocardiographic Parameters

Parameters	Baseline	Pre-Discharge	12 Months Follow-Up	p-value
19 mm				
Mean Pressure Gradient (mmHg)	53.07 ± 20.21	10.39 ± 3.94	10.89 ± 5.76	< 0.0001
EOA (cm²)	0.67 ± 0.24	1.53 ± 0.28	1.58 ± 0.14	< 0.0001
EOA Index (cm²/m²)	0.4 ± 0.14	0.93 ± 0.20	0.95 ± 0.14	< 0.0001
Cardiac Output (l/min)	4.00 ± 1.98	4.42 ± 2.05	5.12 ± 1.64	0.2698
Cardiac Index (l/min/m²)	2.42 ± 1.17	2.7 ± 1.35	3.05 ± 1.05	0.4247
Performance Index	0.24 ± 0.09	0.54 ± 0.10	0.56 ± 0.05	< 0.0001
21 mm				
Mean Pressure Gradient (mmHg)	51.26 ± 16.91	11.4 ± 5.00	10.71 ± 4.41	< 0.0001
EOA (cm²)	0.75 ± 0.37	1.55 ± 0.35	1.56 ± 0.13	< 0.0001
EOA Index (cm²/m²)	0.43 ± 0.24	0.87 ± 0.24	0.87 ± 0.13	< 0.0001
Cardiac Output (l/min)	4.71 ± 2.64	4.29 ± 2.23	4.83 ± 1.57	0.1918
Cardiac Index (l/min/m²)	2.88 ± 2.06	2.44 ± 1.32	2.67 ± 0.79	0.1067
Performance Index	0.22 ± 0.11	0.45 ± 0.10	0.45 ± 0.04	< 0.0001
23/25/27 mm				
Mean Pressure Gradient (mmHg)	48.95 ± 18.57	8.25 ± 2.76	8.96 ± 3.75	< 0.0001
EOA (cm²)	0.9 ± 0.68	1.78 ± 0.52	1.76 ± 0.60	< 0.0001
EOA Index (cm²/m²)	0.49 ± 0.35	0.99 ± 0.52	0.96 ± 0.32	< 0.0001
Cardiac Output (l/min)	4.74 ± 2.50	4.9 ± 1.43	4.48 ± 2.08	0.806
Cardiac Index (l/min/m²)	2.64 ± 1.35	2.73 ± 0.83	2.47 ± 1.13	0.810
Performance Index	0.2 ± 0.13	0.41 ± 0.10	0.41 ± 0.10	< 0.0001
Total (All Valves)				
Mean Pressure Gradient (mmHg)	51.47 ± 18.34	10.44 ± 4.40	10.42 ± 4.77	< 0.0001
EOA (cm²)	0.75 ± 0.42	1.59 ± 0.37	1.61 ± 0.30	< 0.0001
EOA Index (cm²/m²)	0.43 ± 0.24	0.91 ± 0.24	0.91 ± 0.19	< 0.0001
Cardiac Output (l/min)	4.46 ± 2.39	4.45 ± 2.03	4.85 ± 1.69	0.9254
Cardiac Index (l/min/m²)	2.67 ± 1.66	2.59 ± 1.25	2.75 ± 0.97	0.6921
Performance Index	0.22 ± 0.11	0.47 ± 0.11	0.48 ± 0.08	< 0.0001

mmHg Millimeter of Mercury, *cm²* Centimeter², *cm²/m²* Centimeter²/Meter², *l/min* Liter/Minute, *l/min/m²* Liter/Minute/Meter²

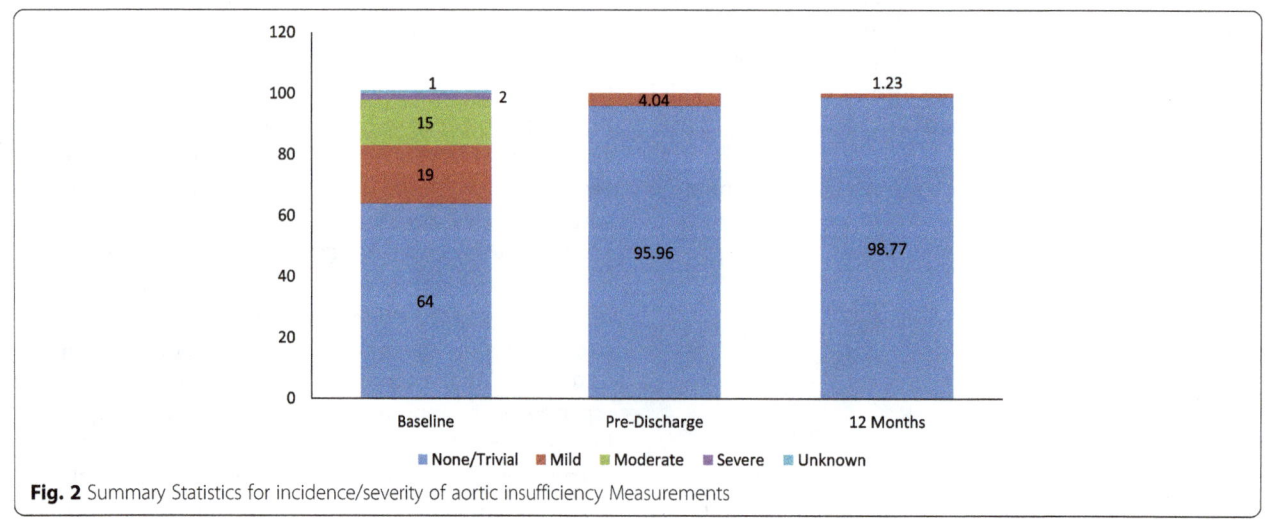

Fig. 2 Summary Statistics for incidence/severity of aortic insufficiency Measurements

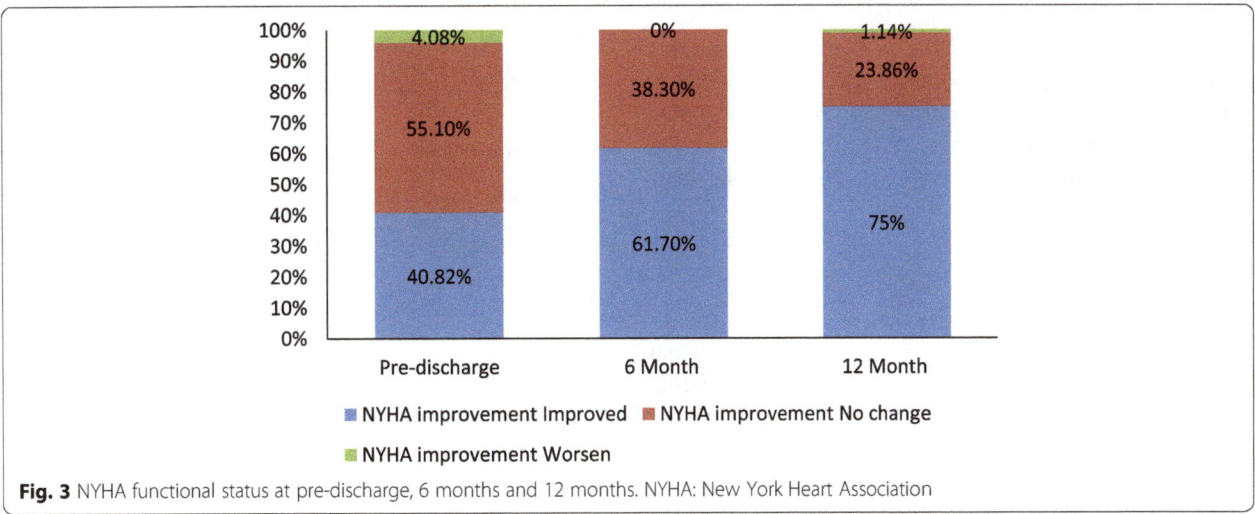

Fig. 3 NYHA functional status at pre-discharge, 6 months and 12 months. NYHA: New York Heart Association

valve across 10 centers in India over a 12 month follow-up duration. The study showed significant portion of patients within smaller age group (mean age of 64 years), 81% had smaller valve size of 19 & 21 mm. The patients with rheumatic heart disease were relatively smaller (14%) owing to study being conducted at big cities across India with relatively better hygiene conditions. The data was in line with previously reported literature [2, 3, 7, 8, 11, 12].

The Trifecta valve was associated with a good safety profile with no incidences of valve thrombosis, clinically significant hemolysis or structural deterioration reported during the 12-month follow-up period. No patient reported any valve-related perioperative complications and overall survival at 12 months was 99% (One death), which is in line with previous reported data [7–10] for patients implanted with the Trifecta valve.

The data from present study establishes acute safety of Trifecta™ Valve in Indian patients.

In previous studies, it has been demonstrated that the external mounting of leaflets in Trifecta™ valve allow for a wider opening, and the expansible stent could limit impedance to flow during high flow conditions as during exercise [17]. The present study demonstrated excellent early hemodynamic performance of the Trifecta™ valve across 12 month follow-up. In the study, the mean pressure gradient for each sized valve was 10.89, 10.71 and 8.96 mmHg for the 19, 21, and (23 + 25) mm valve sizes respectively which compares favourable with previously published data in 1022 patients implanted with a Trifecta valve [18]. Similar results were also reported by Dell'aquila and colleagues [19] who studied 70 patients undergoing SAVR with the Trifecta™ valve. Echocardiographic data at discharge showed that the mean pressure gradient was 14.4, 11.1, and 10.9 mmHg for the 19, 21, and 23 mm valve sizes respectively. The results of a multi-center study by Bavaria and colleagues [7] evaluating

1014 patients undergoing AVR with the Trifecta™ valve were recently reported. In that report, echocardiographic data at discharge and at 12 month showed that mean PG was 9.3/10.7, 7.8/8.1, and 7.3/7.2 mmHg for the 19, 21, and 23 mm valve sizes respectively [7].

In our study, EOA for each size valve was 1.58, 1.56, and 1.76 cm^2 for the 19, 21, and 23 mm valve sizes, respectively. These data suggest that Trifecta™ valve has a large EOA, similar to previous data (1.41, 1.63, and 1.81 cm^2 for the 19, 21, and 23 mm valve sizes, respectively) and multicenter study by Bavaria and colleagues (1.58, 1.77, and 1.94 cm^2 for the 19, 21, and 23 mm valve sizes, respectively) [7].

Currently, the importance of avoiding prosthesis patient mismatch (PPM) (i.e. effective prosthetic valve area, after implantation, which is less than that of a normal human valve) is widely accepted [20–23]. The best variable for defining PPM is ratio of prosthetic EOA to BSA i.e. EOAI< 0.85 cm^2/m^2 which is the common cut-off value for all types of prosthetic valves. In our study the average EOAI observed for 19 mm valve size is 0.95 ± 0.14 cm^2/m^2, 21 mm valve size is 0.87 ± 0.13 cm^2/m^2 and 23/25/27 mm is 0.96 ± 0.32 cm^2/m^2. The Trifecta™ valve demonstrates excellent hemodynamic performance on this point and no PPM observed in our study in patients with smaller annulus which is in line with the previous studies' result.

The study also showed patients had significant improvement with respect to functional class over period of 12 months (75% showed improvement).

With the availability of the Trifecta™ valve, several bioprostheses, options are now available, Carpentier-Edwards Perimount (CEP, Edwards Lifesciences, Irvine, CA, USA); CEP Magna (CEPM, Edwards Lifesciences); Mosaic (Medtronic, Minneapolis, MN, USA); Mosaic Ultra (Mosaic U, Medtronic). However, the performance of these valves in Indian scenario over a long term follow-up study is still warranted.

Limitations

There are few limitations of the present study including limited number of patients' enrolled and short follow-up duration without any comparator arm. In the study, fractional shortening was used to evaluate left ventricular function instead of ejection fraction. Left ventricular mass regression was also not assessed.

Conclusion

This study reports excellent early clinical and hemodynamic performance of the Trifecta™ valve in an Indian patient population. Importantly, no procedural mortality or structural valve deterioration was reported.

Endnotes

The current study evaluated 12 months follow-up data of hemodynamic performance of Trifecta™ valve however a long term follow-up study is required in India.

Appendix

Table 5 Subject Enrollment according to Investigational Site ($n = 10$)

Investigational site	Principal Investigator	Subject Enrollment
Star Hospital	Mannam, Gopichand	26
Yashoda Hospital	Gokhale, Alla Gopala	14
Escorts Heart Institute and Research Centre	Mishra, Yugal	13
The Madras Medical Mission	Sethuratnam, Rajan	12
SAL Hospital	Modi, Rajan	11
P D Hinduja Hospital and Medical Research Center	Pandey, Kaushal	10
Max Super Specialty Hospital	Malhotra, Rajneesh	5
Apollo Gleneagles Hospitals	Mukhopadhyay, Sushan	4
Care Institute of Medical Sciences	Shah, Dhiren	4
Fortis Hospital	Mahant, Tek Singh	1
Total		100

Abbreviations

ACC: American College of Cardiology; AHA: American Heart Association; AR: Aortic Regurgitation; AVR: Aortic valve replacement; BSA: Body surface area; CAD: Coronary Artery Disease; CEP: Carpentier- Edwards Perimount; CEPM: Carpentier- Edwards Perimount Magna; EOA: Effective orifice area; EOAI: Effective orifice area index; IEC: Institutional Ethics Committee; IRB: Institutional Review Board; LVM: Left ventricular mass; NYHA: New York Heart Association; PG: Pressure Gradient; PPM: Prosthesis patient mismatch; RHD: Rheumatic Heart Disease; SVD: Structural Valve Deterioration; TIA: Transient Ischemic Attack; TPG: Trans pulmonary pressure gradient; VARC: Valve Academic Research Consortium

Acknowledgments

The author's thank to Sameer Srivastava & Arif Mustaqueem for echocardiographic data collection.

Funding

The study was funded by Abbott Pvt. Ltd.

Authors' contributions

The number of the authors is justified by the multicenter design of the study. All authors participated in data collection and/ or interpretation of the data, drafting of the manuscript or revising it critically for important intellectual content. All authors provided final approval to submit the manuscript.

Competing interests

The authors declare that they have no competing interests.

Author details

[1]Department of cardiac surgery, Star Hospital Banjara Hills, 8-2-596/5, Road No.10, Banjara Hills, Hyderabad, Telangana 500034, India. [2]Department of cardiac surgery, Escorts Heart Institute and Research Centre, New Delhi, India. [3]Department of cardiac surgery, SAL Hospital, Ahmedabad, India. [4]Department of cardiac surgery, Yashoda Hospital, Secunderabad, India. [5]Department of cardiac surgery, The Madras Medical Mission, Chennai, India. [6]Department of cardiac surgery, P. D. Hinduja National Hospital & Medical Research Center, Mumbai, India. [7]Department of cardiac surgery, Max Super Speciality Hospital, New Delhi, India. [8]Abbott Pvt. Ltd, New Delhi, India. [9]Department of cardiac surgery, Apollo Gleneagles Hospitals , Kolkata, India. [10]Department of cardiac surgery, Care Institute of Medical Sciences, Ahmedabad, India. [11]Department of cardiac surgery, Fortis Hospital, Mohali, India.

References

1. Hosain N, Amin F, Rehman S, Koirala B. Know thy neighbors: the status of cardiac surgery in the south Asian countries around India. Indian Heart J. 2017;69:790–6.
2. Talwar S, Sharma AK, Kumar AS. Tissue heart valve implantation in India; Indications, results and impact on quality of life. IJTCVS. Tissue valves. 2008; 24:10–4.
3. Joshi K, et al. Aortic valve replacement in predominant aortic stenosis: what is an appropriate size valve? IJTCVS. 2007;23:141–5.
4. Rajendran HSR, Seshayyan S, Victor A, Rajapandian G. Aortic valve annular dimension in Indian population. J Clin Diagn Res. 2013;7:1842–5.
5. Dumesnil JG, Pibarot P. Prosthesis–patient mismatch and clinical outcomes: the evidence continues to accumulate. J Thorac Cardiovasc Surg. 2006;131:952–5.
6. St. Jude Medical. Trifecta valve, pre-market approval application summary of safety and effectiveness data. P100029. 2011.
7. Bavaria JE, Desai ND, Cheung A, Petracek MR, Groh MA, et al. The St Jude medical trifecta aortic pericardial valve: results from a global, multicenter, prospective clinical study. Am Assoc Thorac Surg. 2014;147:590–7.
8. Seo H, Tsutsumi Y, Monta O, Numata S, Yamazaki S, et al. Early outcomes and hemodynamics after implantation of the trifecta aortic bioprosthesis. Gen Thorac Cardiovasc Surg. 2014;62:422–7.
9. Goldman S, Cheung A, Bavaria JE, Petracek MR, Groh MA, et al. Midterm, multicenter clinical and hemodynamic results for the trifecta aortic pericardial valve. J Thorac Cardiovasc Surg. 2017;153:561–9.
10. Phan K, Ha H, Phan S, Misfeld M, Di Eusanio M, et al. Early hemodynamic performance of the third generation St Jude trifecta aortic prosthesis: a systematic review and meta-analysis. J Thorac Cardiovasc Surg. 2015;149:1567–75.
11. Ruggieri VG, Anselmi A, Chabanne C, Lelong B, Flecher E, et al. Three-year haemodynamic performance of the St Jude trifecta bioprosthesis. Eur J Cardiothorac Surg. 2016;49:972–7.
12. St. Jude Medical. The trifecta valve, in vitro hydrodynamic and durability comparisons of aortic bioprostheses; IDE10CVD1858EN1 2010.
13. Izzat MB, Birdi I, Wilde P, Bryan AJ, Angelini GD. Comparison of hemodynamic performances of St. Jude Medical and Carbomedics 21mm

aortic prostheses by means of dobutamine stress echocardiography. J Thorac Cardiovasc Surg. 1996;111:408–15.

14. Chafizadeh ER, Zoghbi WA. Doppler echocardiographic assessment of the St. Jude Medical prosthetic valve in the aortic position using the continuity equation. Circulation. 1991;83:213–23.

15. Otto CM, Pearlman AS, Comess KA, Reamer RP, Janko CL, et al. Determination of the stenotic valve area in adults using Doppler echocardiography. J Am Coll Cardiol. 1986;7:509–17.

16. Bonow RO, Carabello BA, Chatterjee K, de Leon AC, Faxon DP, et al. ACC/ AHA 2006 guidelines for the management of patients with valvular heart disease: a report of the American College of Cardiology/American Heart Association Task Force on Practice Guidelines (writing Committee to Revise the 1998 guidelines for the management of patients with valvular Gen Thorac Cardiovasc Surg (2014) 62:422–427 heart disease) developed in collaboration with the Society of Cardiovascular Anesthesiologists endorsed by the Society for Cardiovascular Angiography and Interventions and the Society of Thoracic Surgeons. J Am Coll Cardiol. 2006;48:1–148.

17. Hanke T, Charitos EI, Paarmann H, Stierle U. Hans-H. Sievers. Haemodynamic performance of a new pericardial aortic bioprosthesis during exercise and recovery: comparison with pulmonary autograft, stentless aortic bioprosthesis and healthy control groups. Eur J Cardiothorac Surg. 2013;44:295–301.

18. Draft Guidance for Industry and FDA Staff. Heart Valves - Investigational Device Exemption (IDE) and Premarket Approval (PMA) Applications. Federal Register. 2010;75:12.

19. Dell' Aquila AM, Schlarb D, Schneider SRB, Sindermann JR, Hoffmeier A, et al. Clinical and echocardiographic outcomes after implantation of the trifecta aortic bioprosthesis: an initial single-Centre experience. Interact Cardiovasc Thorac Surg. 2013;16:112–5.

20. Pibarot P, Dumesnil JG. Hemodynamic and clinical impact of prosthesis– patient mismatch in the aortic valve position and its prevention. J Am Coll Cardiol. 2000;36:1131–41.

21. Cotoni DA, Palac RT, Dacey LJ, O'Rourke DJ. Defining patient–prosthesis mismatch and its effect on survival in patients with impaired ejection fraction. Ann Thorac Surg. 2011;91:692–9.

22. Yadlapati A, Diep J, Barnes MJ, Grogan T, Bethencourt DM, et al. Comprehensive hemodynamic performance and frequency of patient- prosthesis mismatch of the St. Jude Medical trifecta bioprosthetic aortic valve. J Heart Valve Dis. 2014;23:516–23.

23. Vicchio M, Corte AD, De Santo LS, De Feo M, Caianiello G, et al. Prosthesis– patient mismatch in the elderly: survival, ventricular mass regression and quality of life. Ann Thorac Surg. 2008;86:1791–7.

21

Prosthesis-patient mismatch after mitral valve replacement

Armah M Akuffu, Haige Zhao, Junnan Zheng[*] and Yiming Ni

Abstract

Background: Prosthesis–patient mismatch (PPM) may affect the clinical outcomes of patients undergoing mitral valve replacement (MVR) surgery. We aimed to investigate the incidence of PPM of the mitral position in our center and analyze the possible predictors of PPM as well as its effect on short-term outcomes.

Methods: We retrospectively examined all consecutive patients with isolated or concomitant MVR at our center from 2013 to 2015. PPM was defined as an indexed effective orifice area (iEOA) of ≤1.2 cm2/m2. After inclusion and exclusion, a total of 1067 patients were analyzed. The baseline information were collected and compared between the two groups. Multivariate logistic regression analysis was conducted to determine the preoperative predictors of PPM as well as the effect of PPM on early mortality.

Results: A total of 1067 patients were included in the study. PPM was detected in 15.9% of the patients while 12 patients (1.12%) met the criteria for severe PPM. Patients with PPM compared to the non-PPM patients had higher age, larger body surface area and were more likely to be male and obese. Logistic regression analysis showed that higher age, larger BSA, bioprosthesis and smaller left ventricle end-diastolic diameter were predictors of PPM. There were no significant differences between the PPM and non-PPM groups regarding post-operative complications. Logistic regression analysis showed that PPM was not a risk factor of short-term mortality ($P = 0.654$). Also, there were no significant differences regarding short–/mid-term heart function between the PPM and non PPM groups ($P = 0.902$).

Conclusions: Our results demonstrated that higher age, bioprosthesis, larger BSA and smaller left ventricle size were associated with mitral PPM. However, PPM was not associated with poorer early outcomes after MVR surgery. In eastern of China, the prevalence of mitral valve stenosis is high; therefore, whether the standard PPM criteria are suitable for patients of this district needs to be further verified.

Keywords: Prosthesis-patient mismatch, Mitral valve replacement, Effective orifice area, Short-term mortality

Background

The phenomenon of prosthesis-patient mismatch (PPM) was initially described by Rahimtoola and Murphy about 40 years ago [1, 2]. Currently, PPM is considered a condition in which the effective orifice area (EOA) of the implanted valve prosthesis does not match the patient's body size.

PPM of the aortic position has been proved to be associated with poorer outcomes including long- and short-term cardiac death [3–5]. However, PPM following mitral valve replacement (MVR) has still been less investigated.

In recent years, PPM after MVR has attracted more and more attention from researchers. Researches has shown that the EOA of mitral valve prosthesis is often too small in relation to body size, thus, normally functioning mitral prosthesis often has relatively high transvalvular gradients similar to those found in mild to moderate mitral valve stenosis patients [6–10].

In East Asia, where rheumatic mitral valve stenosis is very common, the mitral valve annulus in patients is

* Correspondence: zhengjunnan@zju.edu.cn
Department of Cardiothoracic Surgery, the First Affiliated Hospital of Zhejiang University, No.79 Qingchun Road, Hangzhou 310003, China

relatively small; therefore more patients meet the standard of mitral PPM [11]. We aim to investigate the incidence of PPM of the mitral position in our center and analyze the possible predictors of PPM as well as its effect on short-term outcomes. We will also discuss the eligibility of the current PPM standard for this population.

Methods

Patient population and data collection

We retrospectively reviewed all consecutive patients who underwent elective isolated or concomitant MVR at our center, the Department of Cardiothoracic Surgery, the First Affiliated Hospital, Zhejiang University, School of Medicine, from January 2013 to December 2015. Written informed consent waivers obtained from the Hospital Review Board were completed by all patients.

We analyzed all consecutive patients aged more than 18 years undergoing isolated MVR or MVR concomitant with other non-valve-replacement procedures. Patients with incomplete clinical data or patients who received MVR due to failed mitral valvuloplasty were excluded (Fig. 1).

In total, 1067 patients were included in this study. Baseline, intraoperative and outcome data were prospectively collected and validated, which were queried retrospectively. 30-month postoperative follow-up was conducted for discharged patients at the outpatient clinic. Patients who did not show up at the visit were contacted by telephone.

PPM definition and EOA index (EOAi) calculation

Body surface area (BSA) of the patients was calculated using the Dubois formula. The EOA of the mitral valve prosthesis was derived from in vitro measurements provided by the manufacturers and from scientific publications, as outlined in Table 1.

EOAi (also called indexed effective orifice area, iEOA) was obtained with EOA divided by BSA. Mitral PPM was defined as EOAi ≤ 1.2 cm^2/m^2. EOAi ≤ 0.9 cm^2/m^2 was considered severe mitral PPM.

Other definitions were listed as follows. Chronic renal insufficiency: serum creatinine ≥ 2 mg/dl. Peripheral arterial disease: claudication, carotid stenosis > 50% or previous/planned intervention on the abdominal aorta, limb arteries or carotids. Coronary artery disease: $\geq$ 50% reduction in one or more coronary vessels in single or multiple plane angiographic images. Emergency surgery: operation required within 24 h of onset of symptoms. Postoperative renal failure: increase in baseline creatinine greater than 2 mg/dl.

Surgical technique and prosthesis application

The operation records of all patients were reviewed. A total of 868 mechanical valve prostheses and 199 bioprostheses were implanted. The following prostheses were used in as followings:

Mechanical prosthesis: CarboMedics Orbis Universal (CarboMedics, Inc., Austin, TX, USA) ($n = 679$); St Jude Master (St Jude Medical, Inc., St Paul, MN, USA) ($n = 154$); ATS open pivot (ATS Medical, Inc., Minneapolis,

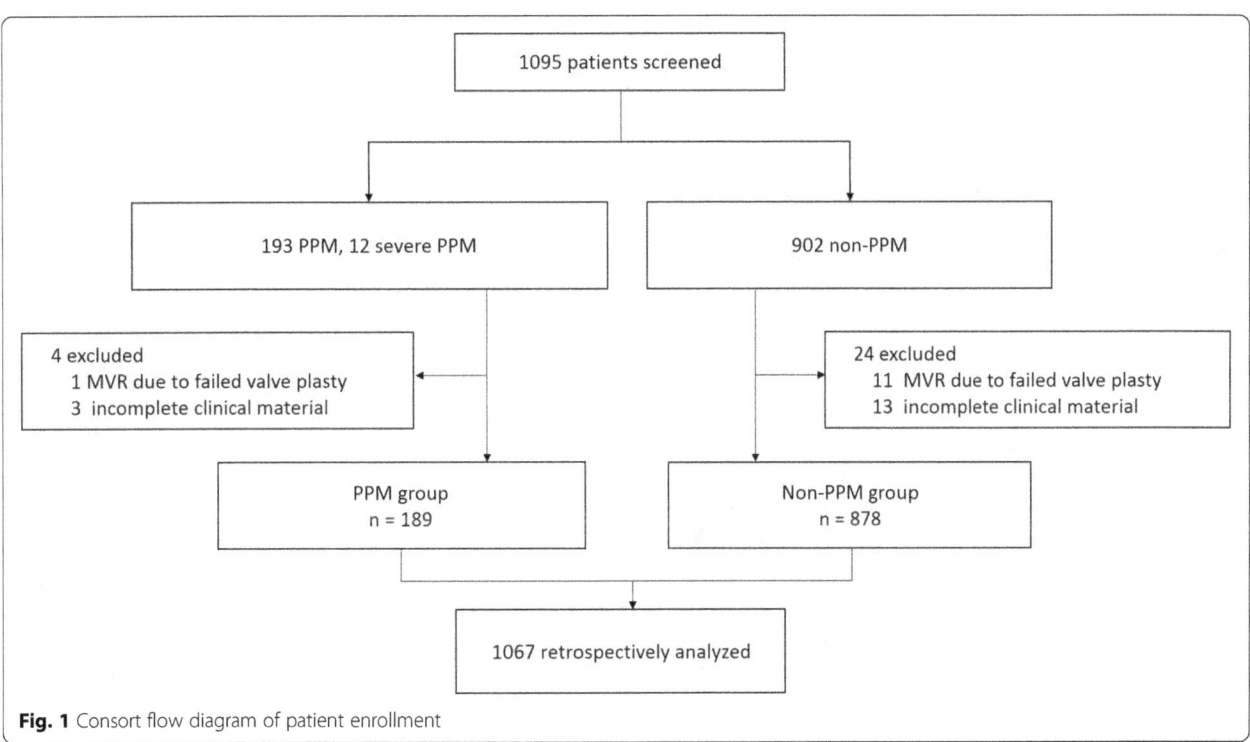

Fig. 1 Consort flow diagram of patient enrollment

Table 1 In vivo effective orifice area values (cm^2) corresponding to each valve

Valve prosthesis	patients	23 mm	25 mm	27 mm	29 mm	31 mm	33 mm	Ref
Mechanical	868							
CarboMedics Orbis Universal	680	1.8	2.2	2.2	2.4	2.4	2.3	[12]
St.Jude Master series	154	1.0	1.5	1.8	1.8	2.0	2.0	[13, 21]
ATS open pivot	33	–	1.8	2.8	2.8	2.9	2.9	[22]
Bioprosthesis	199							
Medtronics Hancock II	110	–	1.5	1.8	1.9	2.6	2.6	[12]
Medtronics Mosaic	5	–	1.5	1.7	1.9	1.9	–	[13]
St. Jude Bicor Stented	45	–	1.4	1.5	2.3	2.2	2.3	[23]
Carpentier-Edwards perimount	39	–	1.7	1.9	2.3	2.8	2.7	[12]

Ref: reference

MN, USA) ($n = 33$); Bioprosthesis: Hancock II Porcine Bioprosthesis (Medtronic, Inc., Minneapolis, MN, USA) ($n = 110$); Mosaic Porcine Bioprosthetic Valves (Medtronic, Inc., Minneapolis, MN, USA) ($n = 5$); Bicor Stented Bioprosthesis (St Jude Medical, Inc., St Paul, MN, USA) ($n = 45$); Carpentier-Edwards perimount (Baxter Healthcare Corp., Edwards Division, Santa Ana, CA, USA) ($n = 39$).

An isolated or concomitant MVR was performed in all patients. Concomitant procedures included tricuspid valvuloplasty, coronary artery bypass grafting, atrial septum defect repair and/or other procedures. Standard anesthesia and cardiopulmonary bypass methods were implemented. Most of the patients were approached through a full median sternotomy followed by an antegrade 4:1 cold blood cardioplegia for myocardial protection. Antegrade plus retrograde cardioplegia was applied for patients with coronary stenosis. Intermittent perfusion of cold blood cardioplegia was maintained at a frequency of once every 20 min.

After consulting with the patients preoperatively, the final decision of the type of prosthesis was made by the surgeons during operation, taking into consideration the preoperative information and intraoperative findings. When performing the MVR, sub-valvular structures were preserved as much as possible.

Statistical analysis

The Kolmogorov-Smirnov test was used to verify the distribution of all the quantitative variables. Gaussian distributed continuous variables were presented as mean ± standard deviation (SD), while non-Gaussian distributed variables were presented as medians (interquartile range). Categorical variables were expressed as an absolute number (percentage). Pearson's χ2 test was used for descriptive, univariate statistics, such as the comparison of portions, while the Student's unpaired *t*-test was used for normally distributed data comparisons. Otherwise, the Mann-Whitney *U* test was otherwise used for comparison of non-Gaussian distributed variables. Two-tailed

P-values were derived from the calculated test statistics, and $P \leq 0.05$ was considered statistically significant. Binary multivariate logistic regression analysis was performed to study the factors affecting PPM as well as mortality. IBM SPSS Statistics 20.0 software (IBM, Armonk, NY, USA) was used to analyze the data.

Results

Preoperative data and baseline information

A total of 1067 patients were included in this study. Mitral PPM was detected in 17.71% (189/1067) of the patients and only 12 (1.12%) patients met the criteria for severe PPM.

Compared with the non-PPM group, patients with PPM were older, taller and heavier and had a higher prevalence of male gender, hypertension, smoking history, coronary heart disease, and had a lower prevalence of mitral stenosis (Table 2).

Patient characterize, PPM and valve prosthesis size

We analyzed the association among age, weight, height, BSA and valve size (Fig. 2). Krusal-Wallis analysis showed that weight, height and BSA are significantly associated with valve size ($P < 0.01$). In summary, larger mitral bioprosthetic valves were implanted in the taller and more obese patients.

Also, the PPM rate of each size of the prostheses was analyzed (Fig. 3). The results showed that the PPM rate of mechanical valve prostheses was considerably lower compared with bioprostheses (10.6% vs 48.5%, respectively, $P < 0.001$). As for the mechanical prostheses, there were no significant differences regarding the PPM occurrence of each valve size, whereas, the PPM rate of the 25 mm bioprosthesis was higher than that of the 27 mm and 29 mm bioprostheses ($P < 0.01$).

On the other hand, the PPM rate also differed among different brands of prostheses. As for mechanical prostheses, according to our data, PPM rate was highest (55.8%, 86/154) in patients underwent MVR with

Table 2 Preoperative patient baseline information

preoperative information	total (n = 1067)	PPM group (n = 189)	non-PPM group (n = 878)	P value
Age, y	56(48–62)	63(55–67)	54(46–61)	< 0.001
Male	379(35.5%)	89(47.1%)	290(33.0%)	< 0.001
Height, cm	160.72 ± 7.82	163.26 ± 7.87	160.17 ± 7.71	< 0.001
Weight, kg	57.72 ± 10.33	62.42 ± 10.23	56.70 ± 10.07	< 0.001
BMI, kg/m^2	22.29 ± 3.67	23.34 ± 2.86	22.07 ± 3.79	< 0.001
BSA, m^2	1.57 ± 0.16	1.64 ± 0.17	1.55 ± 0.16	< 0.001
Smoking history	123(11.5%)	32(16.9%)	91(10.4%)	0.016
Diabetes	102(9.6%)	22(11.6%)	80(9.2%)	NS
Hypertention	192(18.0%)	47(24.9%)	145(16.5%)	0.009
Cerebrovascular accident	34(3.2%)	6(3.2%)	28(3.2%)	NS
Coronary heart disease	22(2.1%)	9(4.8%)	13(1.5%)	0.009
NYHA functional class (≥ III)	400(37.5%)	77(40.7%)	323(36.8%)	NS
Atrial fibrillation	533(50.0%)	92(48.7%)	441(50.2%)	NS
Previous cardiac surgery	54(5.1%)	8(4.2%)	46(5.2%)	NS
Previous MI	1(0.1%)	0(0.0%)	1(0.1%)	NS
Mitral stenosis	786(76.7%)	128(67.7%)	658(74.9%)	0.036
MR (moderate to severe)	470(44.0%)	88(46.5%)	382(43.5%)	NS
LVEF	62.11 ± 8.48	62.23 ± 8.95	62.09 ± 8.38	NS
LVdD, mm	50(45–56)	51(46–58)	50(45–56)	NS
LAD, mm	51.36 ± 12.04	51.36 ± 11.93	51.36 ± 12.07	NS
Emergency surgery	2(0.2%)	0(0.0%)	0(0.0%)	NS
Aspirin within 5 days	29(2.7%)	9(4.8%)	20(2.3%)	NS
Clopidogrel within 5 days	19(1.8%)	6(3.2%)	13(1.5%)	NS

BMI body mass index, BSA body surface area, NYHA New York Heart Association, MI myocardial infarction, MR mitral valve regurgitation, LVEF left ventricular ejection fraction, LVdD left ventricular diastolic diameter, LAD left atrial diameter, NS not significant

St. Jude Master Mechanical prostheses. And PPM rate was considerably low regarding CarboMedics mechanical prosthesis (0.9%, 6/679) and ATS open pivot mechanical prostheses (0.0%, 0/33). As for bioprosthesis, our results showed that PPM rate was high in patients using Medtronic Mosaic porcine bioprosthesis (80.0%, 4/5) or St. Jude Bicor bioprosthesis (82.2%, 37/45), whereas patients underwent MVR with Carpentier-Edwards Perimount bioprosthesis (17.7%, 5/38) and Medtronic Hancock II (45.4%, 50/110) showed lower rate of PPM.

Operative data

As shown in Table 3, there were no significant differences between PPM and non-PPM patients regarding cardiopulmonary bypass (CPB) time. However, we found that there is an average five-minute cross-clamp time reduction in the PPM group.

Not surprisingly, remarkably more patients with a PPM were implanted with a bioprosthetic mitral valve. And as for patients who received a bioprosthesis, the prevalence of mitral stenosis was higher for mismatch

patients (58.3% vs 41.7%, P = 0.019), whereas patients of mechanical prostheses did not differ in the prevalence of mitral stenosis, whether PPM or not (77.4% vs 79.4%, P > 0.05).

As for combined procedures, there were more combined coronary artery bypass grafting (CABG) and surgical ablation for atrial fibrillation in the PPM group.

Factors affecting PPM

According to a multivariate binary logistic regression analysis including all preoperative and intraoperative variables, higher age (P = 0.011), larger BSA (P < 0.001), smaller left ventricular diastolic diameter (LVDd) (P < 0.001) and bioprosthesis (P < 0.001) were factors affecting mitral PPM (Table 4).

Postoperative outcomes and factors affecting postoperative mortality

There were no obvious differences between the two groups regarding early post-operative complications including blood transfusion, ventilation time, reintubation, intensive care unit (ICU) time, postop stroke, postop

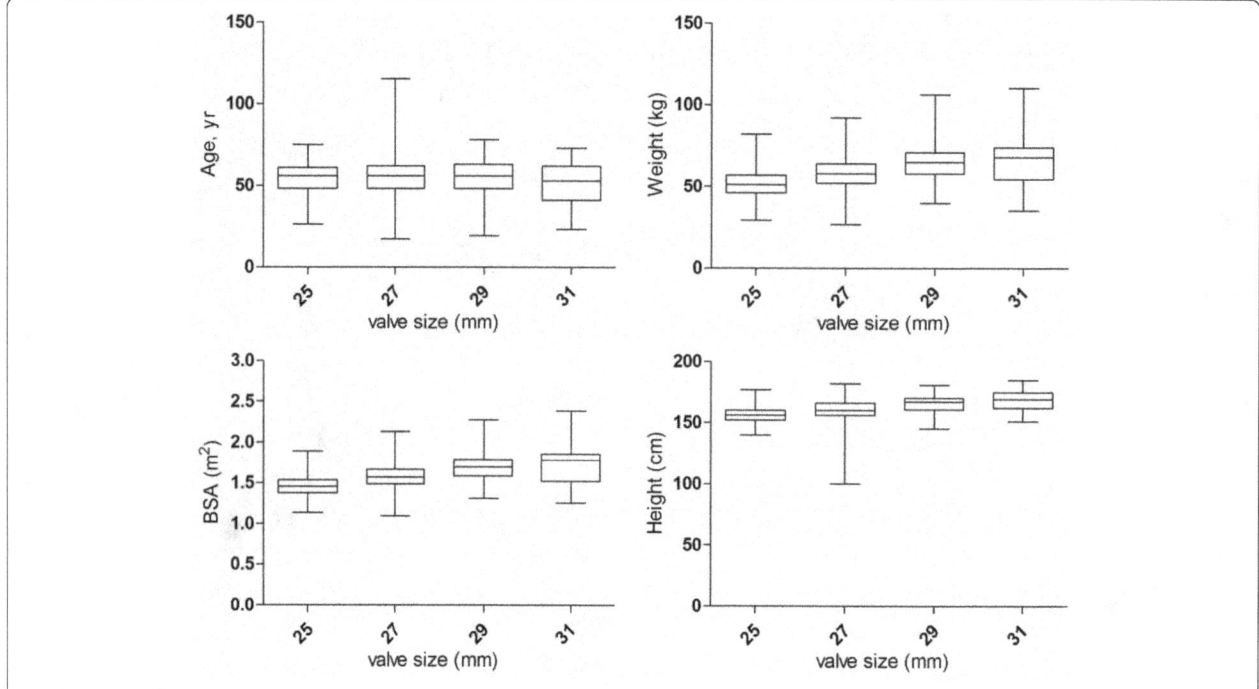

Fig. 2 Boxplot showing distribution of age (NS), weight ($P < 0.01$), height ($P < 0.01$), and body surface area ($P < 0.01$), respectively, according to aortic valve size implanted

atrial fibrillation and short-term mortality. Also, there were no other reoperation for valve-rated complications including PPM or other cardiac disease during hospital-stay except that two patients underwent emergency percutaneous coronary intervention for acute myocardium ischemia. Interestingly, we found that there was a small increase in hospitalization expense as well as a slightly prolonged hospital stay for the PPM patients (Table 5).

Altogether there were nine patients died within 30 days after surgery. Among them, five patients died due to malignant arrhythmia or cardiac arrest, two patient died of sever systematic infection, one patient died of uncontrollable bleeding and one patient died because of stroke. Among these short-term deaths, 2 patients underwent

MVR with Hancock II bioprostheses, whereas 7 patients were replaced with CarboMedics mechanical prostheses.

Logistic regression analysis showed that smoking history and preoperative low left ventricular ejection fraction (LVEF) were independent factors predicting post-operative short-term all-cause mortality. However, PPM was not a risk factor for short-term mortality (Table 6).

Mid-term follow-up

During mid-term follow-up, two patients underwent re-operative for stuck of the mechanical prostheses (both CarboMedics Mechanical prostheses). Both of the patients had an irregular medication history of Warfarin.

Mid-term deaths occurred in eight patients who all underwent MVR with a mechanical prosthesis, adding to the previously mentioned nine short-term deaths. Cumulative mid-term overall survival is 0.986 for both PPM and non-PPM patients (Fig. 4), and there were no significant difference regarding mid-term mortality for the two groups (SE 0.037, Log-rank $p = 0.847$). All the later occurring eight deaths were coagulation-related death. The overall mortality at 30 months was approximately 1.6% (Table 7). During follow-up, about 9.2% of the patients presented compromised cardiac functions with New York Heart Association (NYHA) functional classes III to IV. However, there were no significant differences between the PPM and non-PPM patients.

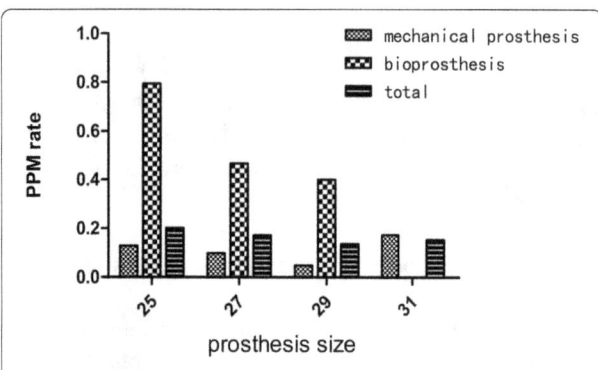

Fig. 3 The PPM rate of each valve size for bioprostheses and mechanical prostheses respectively

Table 3 Intraoperative data

	total	PPM group $n = 189$	non-PPM group $n = 878$	P value
First time surgery	1013(94.9%)	181(95.8%)	832(94.7%)	NS
CPB time (min)	83(70–92)	83(70–89)	83(70–93)	NS
Cross-clamp time (min)	50(41–62)	45(40–55)	50(41–63)	< 0.001
Bioprosthesis	199(18.7%)	96(50.8%)	103(11.7%)	< 0.001
Combined procedure				
Tricuspid valve plasty	277(26.0%)	38(20.1%)	239(27.2%)	NS
CABG	28(2.6%)	11(5.8%)	17(1.9%)	0.005
AFRA or Maze surgery	106(9.9%)	30(15.9%)	76(8.7%)	0.005
Others	139(13.0%)	30(15.9%)	109(12.4%)	NS

CPB cardiopulmonary bypass, *CABG* coronary artery bypass grafting surgery, *AFRA* atrial fibrillation radio frequency surgery, *NS* not significant

Discussion

PPM occurrence and its risk factors

Although highly variable, PPM rates for mitral position in most of the literature ranged from 20 to 70% [11–16]. However, the incidence of PPM after MVR in our single-centered cohort was 17.7% and only 1.2% of the cases met the criteria for severe PPM.

We performed logistic regression analysis and found that larger BSA, higher age, implantation of bioprosthesis and smaller LVDd were risk factors for PPM. Besides BSA, EOA was the only variable defining the EOAi which determined the occurrence of PPM. Bioprosthesis possessed smaller EOA compared with mechanical prosthesis of the same valve size, leading to an increased rate of PPM. Also, bioprostheses were more prone to late degenerative calcification, which may further decrease its EOA. Thus, the more common use of bioprosthesis for degenerative mitral regurgitation might explain the lower prevalence of mitral stenosis of the PPM group in the preoperative data. As for LVDd, it was an indirect reflection of the mitral annulus diameter, which was another decisive factor in choosing prosthesis size, affecting the EOA of the prosthesis implanted. Higher age was then associated with more bioprosthesis implantation, thus leading to the increase in PPM occurrence. Hence, the difference of patient baseline characteristics between the PPM and non-PPM patients in hypertension and coronary heart disease could be explained by the higher age and obesity of the PPM patients.

Table 4 Logistic regression analysis for prosthesis-patient mismatch

Factors	mean or %	OR	95% CI	P value
Age	54	1.029	1.006–1.051	0.011
BSA (m²)	1.57	152.111	45.261–511.208	< 0.001
LVDd (mm)	51.26	0.964	0.944–0.984	< 0.001
bioprosthesis	18.7%	7.539	4.632–12.273	< 0.001

OR odds ratio, *CI* confidence interval, *BSA* body surface area, *LVDd* left ventricular diastolic diameter

In the Asian population, especially the eastern Chinese population, mitral stenosis and small size mitral prosthesis implantation might generally be considered to occur more frequently than in Western populations due to rheumatic causes associated with a small annulus. However, due to rheumatic etiology, the episode age of these patients was considerably younger than patients with valvular degeneration as predominant causes in Western countries. Thus, a larger ratio of patients of this population were implanted with mechanical mitral prostheses which possessed larger EOA than bioprosthesis. Also, patients of this population had a smaller body surface area than those in Western populations, leading to a further reduction in PPM occurrence. The aforementioned factors altogether help explain the low PPM rate in our study population.

PPM and patient outcomes

Since its first description in 1978 by Rahimtoola [1], PPM after MVR has been suggested to potentially correlate with poor clinical outcomes including late tricuspid regurgitation and persistent pulmonary hypertension [11, 14, 17], similar to the outcomes of residual mitral stenosis. However, there were also reports suggesting that PPM did not affect survival after MVR [18, 19].

In our analysis, no impact of PPM on patient mortality was detected either in the postoperative short-term period or in the mid-term follow-up. Our findings are consistent with several large sample multi-centered analyses [15, 19]. Our results showed that smoking history and low preoperative LVEF were associated with higher short-term mortality, but not PPM.

Interestingly, our study showed that cross-clamp times were shorter in patients with PPM, with an average shortened time of 5 min. This might be explained because less time was spent suturing the mitral prosthesis due to the smaller mitral annulus diameter of the PPM patients. The longer hospitalization time of the PPM patients shown in the results might be due to the their

Table 5 Postoperative outcomes

	total	PPM group	non-PPM group	P
Perioperative transfusion	269(25.2%)	47(24.9%)	222(25.3%)	NS
Ventilation time (hr)	21(20–23)	21(20–23)	21(20–23)	NS
Reintubation	3(0.3%)	0(0.0%)	3(0.3%)	NS
Duration of first time ICU	72(72–96)	72(72–96)	72(72–96)	NS
Reentering ICU	2(0.2%)	2(1.1%)	0(0.0%)	NS
Chest tube output (ml)	545.88 ± 365.82	555.15 ± 295.51	543.87 ± 379.47	NS
Reoperation for bleeding	18(1.7%)	1(0.5%)	17(1.9%)	NS
Sternal wound infection	3(0.3%)	0(0.0%)	3(0.3%)	NS
Cerebral infarction	5(0.5%)	0(0.0%)	5(0.6%)	NS
Postoperative stroke	1(0.1%)	0(0.0%)	1(0.1%)	NS
Newly onset AF	3(0.3%)	0(0.0%)	3(0.3%)	NS
Mortality within 30 days	9(0.8%)	2(1.1%)	7(0.8%)	NS
Hospitalization expense (USD)	13,726 (11632–16,030)	14,446 (12538–17,010)	13,628 (11509–15,775)	0.032
Length of stay (d)	14(12–18)	15(13–19)	14(12–18)	0.011

ICU intensive care unit, *AF* atrial fibrillation, *NS* not significant

higher average age and because their recovery time might be longer than in younger patients. Also, the elevated hospitalization expense could be explained by higher price of the bioprosthesis which was more common in the PPM group.

Clinical implication for east Asian population

Currently, the most precise parameter in characterizing PPM is the EOAi [20], which is defined as the EOA of the prosthesis divided by the patient's BSA. EOAi is in fact the only parameter found to consistently correlate with the postoperative gradient; therefore it is the most widely used. In Western countries, the predominant cause of mitral valve disease is degenerative mitral valve regurgitation. For this population, patients with mitral valve diseases usually have a larger left ventricle volume (left ventricular diastolic diameter) than the eastern Asian population; therefore, implantation of a large size prosthesis to avoid PPM will not have an obvious effect on left ventricular function. Hence, the parameter of EOAi has high feasibility in characterizing PPM for Western populations.

However, in a rheumatic population such as the eastern Asian population, the incidence of mitral valve stenosis is

much higher than mitral valve regurgitation [11]. A larger proportion of this population has small left ventricle size, with part of the patients' LVDd even smaller than the mitral annulus diameter. For these patients, implantation of a large sized prosthesis might compromise the effective cardiac muscular contraction of the left ventricle, causing

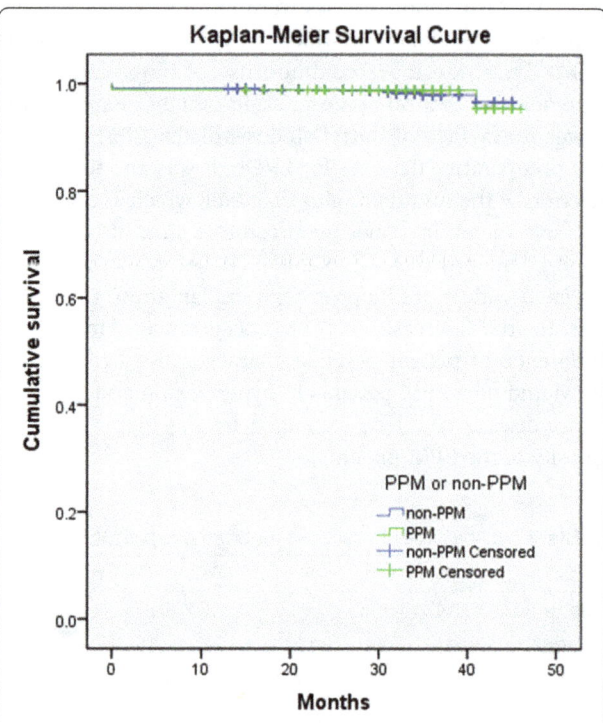

Fig. 4 Kaplan-Meier cumulative mid-term survival, Prosthesis-patient mismatch (PPM) vs non prosthesis-patient mismatch

Table 6 Logistic regression model for postoperative 30-day global mortaliy

Factors	mean or %	Odds ratio	95% CI	P value
smoking history	11.5%	3.199	0.729–14.041	0.004
preoperative LVEF	62.11	0.955	0.887–1.029	0.001
PPM	17.7%	1.138	0.226–5.743	0.654

CI confidence interval, *LVEF* left ventricular ejection fraction

Table 7 Mid-term follow-up information

	Total	PPM group	non-PPM group	P value
Follow-up time (months)	31(23–35)	32(24–35)	31(23–33)	$P = 0.362$
NYHA functional class (III-IV)	9.2%	9.0%	9.6%	$P = 0.902$
Mortality	17(1.6%)	3(1.6%)	14(1.6%)	$P = 0.994$

NYHA New York Heart Association

left ventricular systolic dysfunction or, even worse, increase the risk of left ventricular rupture.

In our opinion, whether the current PPM standard is suitable for a rheumatic population such as the eastern Chinese is worth further exploration. Our results showed that there were no differences regarding the PPM occurrence of each valve size in the mechanical prosthesis. In our future study, we hope that we can explore a more precise parameter in predicting PPM then the current one, hence providing a more accurate prediction of patient outcomes for patients who underwent MVR in our population.

Limitations of the study

There are limitations of the study which must be recognized. First, this is a retrospective analysis, and, as an inherent disadvantage, the recorded differences in patient outcomes could have originated from smaller recorded or unrecorded differences between PPM and non-PPM patients. Second, in our study, EOA was predicted by reference tables, which might not reflect the actual in vivo values of the EOAi. Moreover, this is a single-centered short/mid-term study, and sample size and follow-up time were limited. Therefore, a randomized prospective multi-centered clinical trial with a long follow-up time is needed to study the effect of mitral PPM on longer-term patient outcomes.

Conclusions

Our results demonstrated that higher age, bioprosthesis, larger BSA and smaller left ventricle were associated with mitral PPM. However, PPM was not associated with poorer early outcomes after MVR surgery. In eastern China, the prevalence of mitral valve stenosis is high; therefore, whether the standard PPM criteria are suitable for patients of this district needs to be further verified.

Abbreviations

AF: Atrial fibrillation; AFRA: Atrial fibrillation radio frequency surgery; BMI: Body mass index; BSA: Body surface are; CABG: Coronary artery bypass grafting; CABG: Coronary artery bypass grafting; CI: Confidence interval; CPB: Cardiopulmonary bypass; EOA: Effective orifice area; EOAi (iEOA): Effective orifice area index; ICU: Intensive care unit; LAD: Left atrial diameter; LVDd: Left ventricular diastolic diameter; LVEF: Left ventricular

ejection fracture; LVESV: Left ventricular end-systolic volume; MR: Mitral valve regurgitation; MVR: mitral valve replacement; NS: Not significant; NYHA: New York Heart Association; OR: Odd ratio; PHM: Prosthesis-patient mismatch; PPM: Prosthesis-patient mismatch; SD: Standard deviation

Acknowledgements
The authors would like to thank the anesthetists, intensivists, heart surgeons, nursing staff, perfusionists and the laboratory department at the First Affiliated Hospital, Zhejiang University for the collection and management of the data presented in this report.

Authors' contributions
AA and JZ analyzed and interpreted the patient data, and wrote the paper. HZ and YN prepared the tables and figure, and were major contributors in writing the manuscript. JZ drafted the final manuscript. All authors read and approved the final manuscript.

Competing interests
The authors declare that they have no competing interests.

References
1. Rahimtoola SH. The problem of valve prosthesis-patient mismatch. Circulation. 1978;58(1):20–4.
2. Rahimtoola SH, Murphy E. Valve prosthesis--patient mismatch. A long-term sequela. Br Heart J. 1981;45(3):331–5.
3. Hong S, Yi GJ, Youn YN, Lee S, Yoo KJ, Chang BC. Effect of the prosthesis-patient mismatch on long-term clinical outcomes after isolated aortic valve replacement for aortic stenosis: a prospective observational study. J Thorac Cardiov Sur. 2013;146(5):1098–104.
4. Fuster RG, Montero Argudo JA, Albarova OG, et al. Patient-prosthesis mismatch in aortic valve replacement: really tolerable? Eur J Cardiothorac Surg. 2005;27(3):441–9 discussion 9.
5. Guo L, Zheng J, Chen L, et al. Impact of prosthesis-patient mismatch on short-term outcomes after aortic valve replacement: a retrospective analysis in East China. J Cardiothorac Surg. 2017;12(1):42.
6. Dumesnil JG, Honos GN, Lemieux M, Beauchemin J. Validation and applications of mitral prosthetic valvular areas calculated by Doppler echocardiography. Am J Cardiol. 1990;65(22):1443–8.
7. Dumesnil JG, Yoganathan AP. Valve prosthesis hemodynamics and the problem of high transprosthetic pressure gradients. Eur J Cardiothorac Surg. 1992;6(Suppl 1):S34–7 discussion S8.
8. Leavitt JI, Coats MH, Falk RH. Effects of exercise on transmitral gradient and pulmonary artery pressure in patients with mitral stenosis or a prosthetic mitral valve: a Doppler echocardiographic study. J Am Coll Cardiol. 1991;17(7):1520–6.
9. Rosenhek R, Binder T, Maurer G, Baumgartner H. Normal values for Doppler echocardiographic assessment of heart valve prostheses. J Am Soc Echocardiogr. 2003;16(11):1116–27.
10. Dumesnil JG, Pibarot P. Prosthesis-patient mismatch: an update. Curr Cardiol Rep. 2011;13(3):250–7.
11. Lee SH, Chang BC, Youn YN, Joo HC, Yoo KJ, Lee S. Impact of prosthesis-patient mismatch after mitral valve replacement in rheumatic population: does mitral position prosthesis-patient mismatch really exist? J Cardiothorac Surg. 2017;12(1):88.
12. Lam BK, Chan V, Hendry P, et al. The impact of patient-prosthesis mismatch on late outcomes after mitral valve replacement. J Thorac Cardiovasc Surg. 2007;133(6):1464–73.

13. Magne J, Mathieu P, Dumesnil JG, et al. Impact of prosthesis-patient mismatch on survival after mitral valve replacement. Circulation. 2007; 115(11):1417–25.

14. Li M, Dumesnil JG, Mathieu P, Pibarot P. Impact of valve prosthesis-patient mismatch on pulmonary arterial pressure after mitral valve replacement. J Am Coll Cardiol. 2005;45(7):1034–40.

15. Jamieson WR, Germann E, Ye J, et al. Effect of prosthesis-patient mismatch on long-term survival with mitral valve replacement: assessment to 15 years. Ann Thorac Surg. 2009;87(4):1135–41 discussion 42.

16. Aziz A, Lawton JS, Maniar HS, Pasque MK, Damiano RJ Jr, Moon MR. Factors affecting survival after mitral valve replacement in patients with prosthesis-patient mismatch. Ann Thorac Surg. 2010;90(4):1202–10 discussion 10-1.

17. Angeloni E, Melina G, Pibarot P, et al. Impact of prosthesis-patient mismatch on the regression of secondary mitral regurgitation after isolated aortic valve replacement with a bioprosthetic valve in patients with severe aortic stenosis. Circ Cardiovasc Imaging. 2012;5(1):36–42.

18. Sakamoto H, Watanabe Y. Does patient-prosthesis mismatch affect long-term results after mitral valve replacement? Ann Thorac Cardiovasc Surg. 2010;16(3):163–7.

19. Shi WY, Yap CH, Hayward PA, et al. Impact of prosthesis--patient mismatch after mitral valve replacement: a multicentre analysis of early outcomes and mid-term survival. Heart. 2011;97(13):1074–81.

20. Pibarot P, Dumesnil JG. Prosthesis-patient mismatch: definition, clinical impact, and prevention. Heart. 2006;92(8):1022–9.

21. Bitar JN, Lechin ME, Salazar G, Zoghbi WA. Doppler echocardiographic assessment with the continuity equation of St. Jude Medical mechanical prostheses in the mitral valve position. Am J Cardiol. 1995;76(4):287–93.

22. Cohn LH, Edmunds LH. Cardiac surgery in the adult. 3rd ed. New York: McGraw-Hill Medical; 2008.

23. Borracci RA, Rubio M, Sestito ML, Ingino CA, Barrero C, Rapallo CA. Incidence of prosthesis-patient mismatch in patients receiving mitral Biocor(R) porcine prosthetic valves. Cardiol J. 2016;23(2):178–83.

Congenital aortic stenosis due to unicuspid unicommissural aortic valve

Arnar B. Ingason[1]* ⓘ, Gunnlaugur Sigfusson[2] and Bjarni Torfason[1,3]

Abstract

Background: Unicuspid unicommissural aortic valve is an extremely rare congenital anomaly that usually presents in adulthood but can rarely present in infancy. We report a 17-year-old patient with congenital aortic stenosis secondary to unicuspid unicommissural aortic valve that was successfully treated with aortic valve replacement.

Case presentation: The patient was diagnosed with aortic stenosis after a murmur was heard in the newborn nursery and subsequently underwent aortic balloon valvuloplasty 6 weeks after birth. He had been regularly followed up since and underwent numerous cardiac catheterizations, including another aortic balloon valvuloplasty at age 13. During follow-up at age 17, the patient presented with symptomatic severe aortic stenosis and mild left ventricular hypertrophy. Aortic valve replacement was planned since the patient was nearly adult-sized and to reduce the risk of cardiac decompensation. During the operation an unicuspid unicommissural aortic valve was revealed. The patient recovered well post-operatively. He was discharged 5 days after the surgery in good condition and was completely symptom-free at follow-up 6 weeks later.

Conclusions: Unicuspid aortic valve is a rare congenital anomaly that can cause congenital aortic stenosis. It is seldom diagnosed pre-operatively but should be suspected in infants presenting with aortic stenosis.

Keywords: Unicuspid aortic valve, Congenital aortic stenosis, Aortic valve replacement, Case report

Background

Unicuspid aortic valve (UAV) is an extremely rare congenital malformation with an estimated prevalence of 0.02% in adults [1]. UAVs share many characteristics with bicuspid valves, such as premature valvular calcifications, aortic root dilations, and aortic dissection [2]. In unicuspid valves, these changes occur even more rapidly. UAVs most often present with aortic stenosis, either isolated or with concomitant aortic regurgitation [2, 3].

UAVs are divided into two subtypes; unicommissural and acommissural UAVs. Since acommissural UAVs have smaller aortic orifice compared to unicommissural valves, they have a more aggressive presentation and are usually symptomatic at birth [3]. Unicommissural UAVs generally present in the 4th to 6th decade of life [2, 4], but can rarely present at infancy [5]. We report a case of 17-year-old male with congenital aortic stenosis secondary

to a unicommissural UAV that was successfully treated with aortic valve replacement (AVR).

Case report

A 17-year-old male with congenital aortic stenosis presented to his pediatric cardiologist for follow-up. He had been diagnosed with aortic stenosis after a murmur was heard in the newborn nursery, and subsequently underwent aortic balloon valvuloplasty 6 weeks after birth. He had been regularly followed up since and underwent numerous cardiac catheterizations, including another aortic balloon valvuloplasty at age 13.

Upon presentation, echocardiography was performed and revealed a mean gradient of 54 mmHg, maximum gradient of 119 mmHg through the aortic valve orifice, aortic valve area of 0.4 cm^2/m^2, and septal diameter of 1.6 cm^2 (Fig. 1). Subsequently, the patient was scheduled for AVR 3 weeks later. A CT angiography was obtained before surgery and revealed a mild ascending aortic dilation of 34.4×42.2 mm in maximal diameter, without increased annular size (Fig. 2).

* Correspondence: abi12@hi.is
[1]Department of Medicine, University of Iceland, Vatnsmyrarvegur 16, 101 Reykjavik, Reykjavik, Iceland
Full list of author information is available at the end of the article

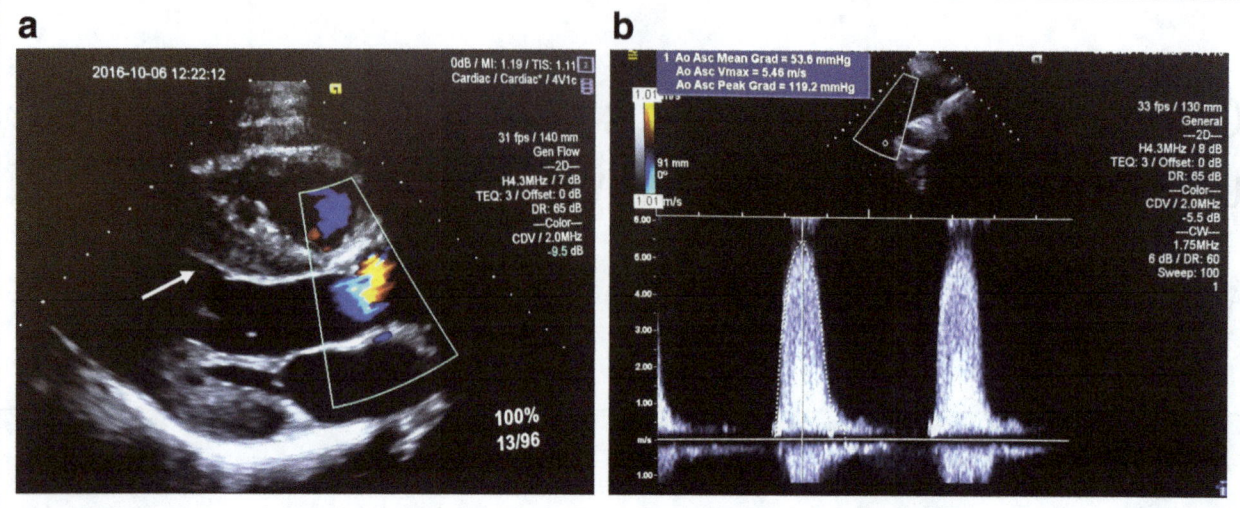

Fig. 1 a Echocardiography demonstrating an increased septal diameter (arrow). **b** Echocardiography measurements demonstrating a mean gradient of 54 mmHg, maximal gradient of 119 mmHg, and peak flow of 5.5 m/s through the aortic valve orifice

During pre-operative examination, the patient admitted having dyspnea during exertion but had never experienced angina, palpations, or syncope. He reported being very physically active. A 4/6 crescendo/decrescendo systolic murmur was auscultated over the whole precordium, with the murmur radiating to the neck. Lung auscultation was clear and jugular venous distension was absent. His chest X-ray was normal with cardiac index within referral range. The patient and his parents expressed their desire for biologic valve implantation.

AVR was performed under normothermic cardiopulmonary bypass. Following aortotomy an unicuspid unicommissural aortic valve was revealed, with a single commissure located just right of the left coronary ostium. The valve was thickened and extremely stenotic with mild calcification underneath the right coronary ostium (Fig. 3). The valve was removed in one piece using scissors and knife, and replaced with a 27 mm biologic Freestyle valve (Medtronic Inc., Minneapolis, Minnesota) using continuous 4–0 Prolene sutures. The stentless valve was implanted subcoronally to allow for a nonobstructive position for the right and left coronary ostia between the commissures of the newly implanted bioprosthesis. Finally, the ascending aorta was closed using continuous 4–0 Prolene sutures.

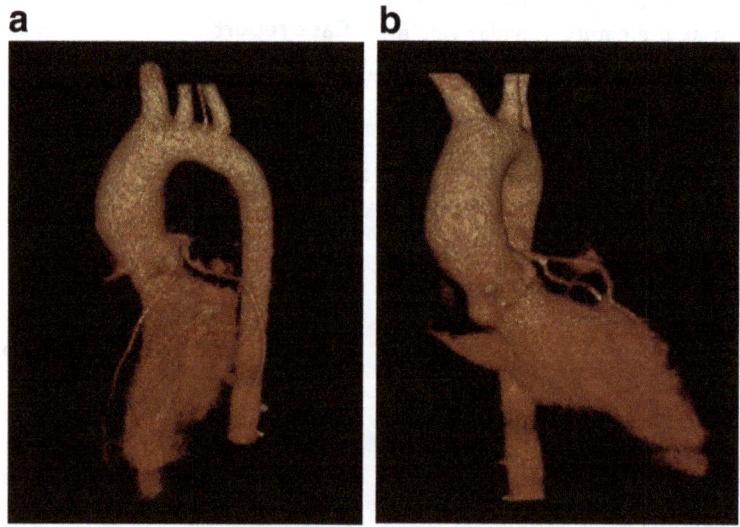

Fig. 2 a Lateral and **b** anterior projection of a three-dimensional reconstructed CT angiography demonstrating a slightly dilated ascending aorta and normal sized aortic annulus

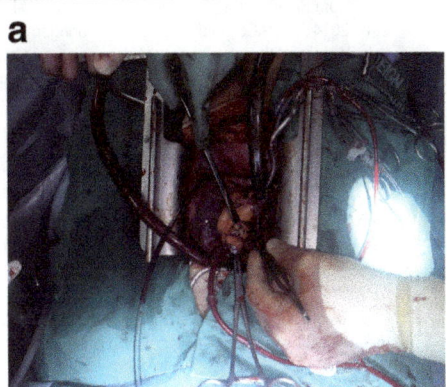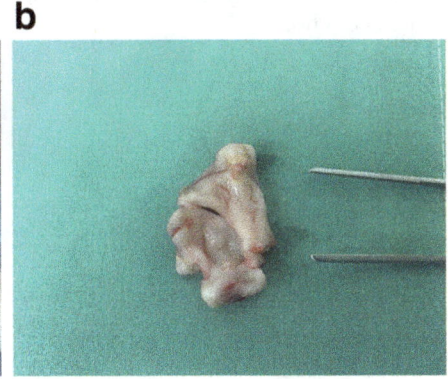

Fig. 3 a The aortic valve revealed during surgery. **b** Macroscopic view of the resected unicommissural unicuspid aortic valve

Post-operatively, there were no adverse events and the patient recovered well. He was discharged 5 days after surgery in good condition. At follow up 6 weeks later, the patient had returned to his daily activities and was completely symptom-free. An echocardiography revealed a functional valve with no regurgitation and insignificant gradient across the valve. The left ventricular hypertrophy was receding with a measured septal diameter of 1.2–1.4 mm. Left ventricular function was considered normal and no pericardial effusion was noted.

Discussion and conclusions

UAV is a rare cause of aortic stenosis. Unicommissural UAVs are usually asymptomatic early in life, although they can rarely present at infancy, as in the previously described case. In a case series of 21 patients with unicommissural UAV, only 2 patients presented during the first year of life [5]. Even though the patient was diagnosed with aortic stenosis shortly after birth, the diagnosis of UAV was not made until open heart surgery was performed 17 years later. This is common, indeed the majority of UAVs are diagnosed peri-operatively [2, 6]. Transesophageal echocardiography (TEE) is the gold standard for diagnosis of UAV with a sensitivity and specificity of 75 and 86% respectively [7]. With evolving imaging technology, such as three-dimensional TEE, a higher frequency of pre-operative diagnosis is anticipated.

Congenital aortic stenosis due to UAV is most often treated with balloon valvuloplasty, surgical valvotomy, or commissurotomy [3]. AVR is generally not recommended until the patient has reached full size. This is due to higher mortality rates compared to adults as well as higher frequency of re-operation due to patient-prosthesis mismatch and structural valve degeneration [8]. If AVR is needed in infancy or early childhood, a Ross surgery is often recommended [9, 10]. In a Ross procedure, the aortic valve is replaced with the patient's own pulmonary valve. The autograft has some capacity to grow along with the patient's heart thereby reducing the risk of patient-prosthesis mismatch in a growing child. The main problem with the Ross procedure is that a simultaneous pulmonary valve replacement is required, thus converting a single valve disease into a double valve pathology [11]. The Ross procedure is more technically difficult than other valve replacement alternatives, with relatively high mortality, but has been shown to be safe in experienced hands [8].

When the patient presented pre-operatively, he had symptomatic severe aortic stenosis and mild left ventricular hypertrophy. AVR was planned since the patient was nearly adult-sized and to reduce the risk of cardiac decompensation due to further cardiac hypertrophy. In preparation for the AVR, the patient and his guardians expressed their desire for bioprosthetic valve replacement. Although mechanical valves have generally been recommended for patients younger than 60 years old, multiple factors have led to increased use of bioprosthetic valves in younger populations, including high re-operative survival rate, lifestyle expectations, and recent advances in transcatheter valve replacements. AHA/ACC guidelines for managing valvular heart diseases state that the choice of prosthetic valve type should be a shared decision and bioprosthetic valves should be recommended if anticoagulation is not desired [12]. Lifelong anticoagulation following mechanical valve replacement can be debilitating for physically active individuals and reduce quality of life. Additionally, the annual risk of major bleeding is about 3% for oral anticoagulants [13, 14] but has been reported as high as 4.4% following mechanical valve replacement [15]. The benefit of lower re-operative rates in mechanical valve replacements must be carefully weighed to the risk of bleeding complications and reduction in quality of life on a case-by-case basis.

In conclusion, UAV is a rare cause of aortic stenosis, but should be suspected in infants presenting with aortic stenosis. Although rarely diagnosed pre-operatively, TEE has relatively high sensitivity and specificity for the condition. AVR is generally not recommended until patients have reached full-size due to higher mortality and re-operation rates compared to adults. Instead, balloon valvuloplasty, surgical valvotomy, or commissurotomy are the initial treatments of choice.

Abbreviations

AVR: Aortic valve replacement; CT: Computer Tomography; TEE: Transesophageal echocardiography; UAV: Unicuspid aortic valve

Authors' contributions

AB Ingason collected the case data, drafted the manuscript, and did the literature search. G Sigfusson and B Torfason treated the patient and critically reviewed the manuscript. All authors contributed to the design of the case report, and read and approved the final version of the manuscript.

Competing interests

The authors declare that they have no competing interests.

Author details

[1]Department of Medicine, University of Iceland, Vatnsmyrarvegur 16, 101 Reykjavik, Reykjavik, Iceland. [2]Children's Hospital, Landspitali University Hospital, Reykjavik, Iceland. [3]Department of Cardiothoracic Surgery, Landspitali University Hospital, Reykjavik, Iceland.

References

1. Novaro GM, Mishra M, Griffin BP. Incidence and echocardiographic features of congenital unicuspid aortic valve in an adult population. J Heart Valve Dis. 2003;12(6):674–8.
2. Mookadam F, Thota VR, Garcia-Lopez AM, Emani UR, Alharthi MS, Zamorano J, et al. Unicuspid aortic valve in adults: a systematic review. J Heart Valve Dis. 2010;19(1):79–85.
3. Mookadam F, Thota VR, Lopez AM, Emani UR, Tajik AJ. Unicuspid aortic valve in children: a systematic review spanning four decades. J Heart Valve Dis. 2010;19(6):678–83.
4. Roberts WC, Ko JM. Frequency by decades of unicuspid, bicuspid, and tricuspid aortic valves in adults having isolated aortic valve replacement for aortic stenosis, with or without associated aortic regurgitation. Circulation. 2005;111(7):920–5.
5. Falcone MW, Roberts WC, Morrow AG, Perloff JK. Congenital aortic stenosis resulting from a unicommisssural valve. Clinical and anatomic features in twenty-one adult patients. Circulation. 1971;44(2):272–80.
6. Noly PE, Basmadjian L, Bouhout I, Viet Le VH, Poirier N, El-Hamamsy I. New insights into Unicuspid aortic valve disease in adults: not just a subtype of bicuspid aortic valves. Can J Cardiol. 2016;32(1):110–6.
7. Chu JW, Picard MH, Agnihotri AK, Fitzsimons MG. Diagnosis of congenital unicuspid aortic valve in adult population: the value and limitation of transesophageal echocardiography. Echocardiography. 2010;27(9):1107–12.
8. Alsoufi B. Aortic valve replacement in children: options and outcomes. J Saudi Heart Assoc. 2014;26(1):33–41.
9. Sharabiani MT, Dorobantu DM, Mahani AS, Turner M, Peter Tometzki AJ, Angelini GD, et al. Aortic valve replacement and the Ross operation in children and young adults. J Am Coll Cardiol. 2016;67(24):2858–70.
10. Svensson LG, Adams DH, Bonow RO, Kouchoukos NT, Miller DC. P.T. O'Gara, et al., *Aortic valve and ascending aorta guidelines for management and quality measures.* Ann Thorac Surg. 2013;95(6):S1–66.
11. Brancaccio G, Polito A, Hoxha S, Gandolfo F, Giannico S, Amodeo A, et al. The Ross procedure in patients aged less than 18 years: the midterm results. J Thorac Cardiovasc Surg. 2014;147(1):383–8.
12. Nishimura RA, Otto CM, Bonow RO, Carabello BA, Erwin JP 3rd, Guyton RA, et al. 2014 AHA/ACC guideline for the Management of Patients with Valvular Heart Disease: a report of the American College of Cardiology/ American Heart Association task force on practice guidelines. Circulation. 2014;129:23.
13. Miller CS, Grandi SM, Shimony A, Filion KB, Eisenberg MJ. Meta-analysis of efficacy and safety of new oral anticoagulants (dabigatran, rivaroxaban, apixaban) versus warfarin in patients with atrial fibrillation. Am J Cardiol. 2012;110(3):453–60.
14. Torn M, van der Meer FJ, Rosendaal FR. Lowering the intensity of oral anticoagulant therapy: effects on the risk of hemorrhage and thromboembolism. Arch Intern Med. 2004;164(6):668–73.
15. Labaf A, Grzymala-Lubanski B, Stagmo M, Lovdahl S, Wieloch M, Sjalander A, et al. Thromboembolism, major bleeding and mortality in patients with mechanical heart valves- a population-based cohort study. Thromb Res. 2014;134(2):354–9.

23

Intraoperative transit-time flowmetry in patients undergoing coronary surgery to determine relationships between graft flow and patency and prior coronary interventions and flow demand

Hiroyuki Nakajima*⬭, Akitoshi Takazawa, Akihiro Yoshitake, Masato Tochii, Chiho Tokunaga, Jun Hayashi, Hiroaki Izumida, Daisuke Kaneyuki, Toshihisa Asakura and Atsushi Iguchi

Abstract

Background: The aim of this study was to delineate impacts of percutaneous coronary intervention (PCI), flow demand, and status of myocardium on graft flow.

Methods: We retrospectively assessed 736 individual coronary artery bypass grafts that had been created as the sole bypass graft for a vascular region in 405 patients. The grafts comprised 334 internal thoracic artery (ITA) to left anterior descending (LAD), 129 ITA and 65 saphenous vein grafts (SVG) to left circumflex (LCX), and 142 gastroepiploic artery (GEA) and 66 SVG to right coronary artery (RCA). Minimal luminal diameter, size of revascularized area, history of myocardial infarction, and PCI in the relevant area were examined to determine whether these factors are associated with flow insufficiency (FI), which was defined as ≤ 20 mL/min.

Results: FI developed in 123/736 grafts (16.7%) and correlated significantly with stenosis in the distal portion (23.0% vs. 12.8%, $p = 0.0003$). Prior myocardial infarction significantly correlated with FI in GEA–RCA ($p = 0.002$) and ITA–LCX grafts ($p = 0.04$). There was a history of PCI to the LAD (PCI group) in 54 ITA to LAD bypass grafts (16.2%), whereas the remaining 280 had no history of PCI to the LAD (no-PCI group). Graft flow was significantly greater in the no-PCI than in the PCI group (53 ± 29 vs. 42 ± 27; $p = 0.006$). The incidences of FI and graft failure were significantly higher in the PCI than the no-PCI group (22.2%, vs. 8.2%; $p = 0.003$; 9.2% vs. 1.8%; $p = 0.003$, respectively).

Conclusions: Prior PCI has a negative impact on graft flow. The influences of small revascularized area, myocardial infarction, and PCI are greater, necessitating consideration of factors associated with flow demand or microvasculature when planning revascularization.

Keywords: Off-pump, Coronary artery bypass graft, Transit-time flowmetry, Graft flow, Flow demand, Percutaneous coronary intervention

* Correspondence: hn00504@ybb.ne.jp
Department of Cardiovascular Surgery, Saitama Medical University,
International Medical Center, 1397-1 Yamane Hidaka, Saitama 350-1298,
Japan

Background

After coronary artery bypass grafting (CABG), flow to the relevant myocardial area comprises the sum of graft flow and native coronary flow. Prediction of native coronary flow has been improved by evaluating the severity of stenosis in the native coronary artery, for example, by measuring fractional flow reserve (FFR). FFR, which is calculated by measurement of intraluminal pressure, represents the ratio of maximal blood flow through the stenosis to theoretically normal maximal flow, and reportedly reliably detects myocardial ischemia. If myocardial flow demand in the relevant area is smaller than a certain amount, graft flow may be insufficient to achieve long-term patency, irrespective of FFR value. The impact of flow demand has not yet been fully delineated.

Graft flow is commonly measured by transit-time flowmetry (TTFM) intraoperatively. Several recent retrospective observational studies have found that TTFM correlates significantly with graft patency in the early [1] and mid-term [2–4]. We have previously reported that the risk of graft failure increases fourfold or more when graft flow as measured by TTFM is insufficient [5].

In the present study, we examined the characteristics of target coronary lesions and status of revascularized areas to determine the mechanisms underlying graft flow insufficiency and the impacts of flow demand and peripheral vasculature on graft flow and patency.

Methods

We reviewed the clinical records and angiograms of 405 patients with 1284 bypass grafts who had undergone off-pump CABG and had postoperative coronary angiograms between 2007 and May 2015. They comprised 315 men and 90 women with a mean age of 67 ± 9 years. Postoperative coronary angiography had been performed in all 405 patients (Table 1).

Table 1 Baseline patients' characteristics

No. of patients	405
Age (yrs)	67 ± 9
Male/Female	315 / 90
Hypertension	244 (64%)
Hyperlipidemia	218 (58%)
Diabetes	201 (50%)
Atrial Fibrillation	21 (7%)
Intraaortic balloon pump	55 (17%)
Ejection fraction of LV (%)	55 ± 16
Ejection fraction of LV < 40%	65 (15%)
Total distal anastomoses	1284
Targets per patient	3.2 ± 1.0

LV; left ventricle

To minimize bias, we selected the 736 of these patients' bypass grafts that were individual and created as the sole bypass graft for the relevant vascular region. These patients were consecutive after exclusion of those without eligible bypass grafts. The selected grafts comprised 334 in situ internal thoracic artery (ITA) to left anterior descending (LAD), 129 in situ ITA and 65 aorto-coronary saphenous vein grafts (SVG) to the left circumflex (LCX), and 142 in situ gastroepiploic artery (GEA) and 66 aorto-coronary SVG to the right coronary artery (RCA). This retrospective study was approved by our Institutional Review Board, which waived the requirement for written informed consent because this was a retrospective observational study.

Our standard procedure has been off-pump CABG using the ITA and GEA. At the beginning of the study period, we preferred to use arterial grafts irrespective of the severity of stenosis. However, we have increasingly used aorto-coronary vein grafts for the LCX and RCA when the stenosis seems to be moderate. We performed preoperative quantitative coronary angiography for all targets of the 736 bypass grafts, measuring the minimal luminal diameter (MLD; measured at the narrowest stenotic lesion proximal to the anastomotic site) and its reference diameter. We categorized the location of stenosis as proximal or distal to indicate the size of myocardial flow demand in the revascularized area. We defined proximal lesions as stenosis at #1–3, 5, 6 and 11, and distal lesions as stenosis at #4, 7 and 12–14. We defined a history of percutaneous coronary intervention (PCI) as any catheter procedure for treating coronary artery disease, even it had been unsuccessful. We defined myocardial infarction (MI) as diagnosis by a cardiologist or the presence of Q-wave on an electrocardiogram and asynergy on echocardiography in the relevant area. PCI and MI were recorded for each vascular region.

After completion of anastomosis, we measured graft flow by using a transit time flow meter (Medi-Stim AS, Oslo, Norway) at approximately 100 to 120 mmHg of systolic arterial pressure with minimal or no inotropic support. We usually administered papaverine or another vasodilator. We defined flow insufficiency (FI) as 20 mL/min or less as measured by intraoperative TTFM and graft failure as occlusion or string sign on postoperative angiography. When we identified significant difference in the incidence of FI between higher and lower values, we defined the value with lowest p as the cuff-off MLD. As we have previously reported, FI correlates significantly with future failure of ITA, GEA, and SV grafts [5].

Statistical analysis

We have expressed continuous variables as mean ± standard deviation and compared them by unpaired Student's *t*-test. We compared data of two independent groups by the χ^2 test. The mean duration of follow-up was 10 ± 14 months. We considered differences in outcomes statistically significant when the p value was less than 0.05.

Results

FI developed in 123/736 (16.7%) grafts and there were 47/736 (6.4%) graft failures. The incidence of FI according to characteristics of the target vessel, bypass graft, revascularized area, and prior MI and PCI is shown in Table 2. For ITA to LAD bypass grafts, the incidence of FI in ITA to LAD with prior PCI was 22.2% (12/54), which is significantly higher than the 8.2% (23/280) in patients without prior PCI ($p = 0.002$). The incidence of FI for distal lesions was 15.0% (20/133), which is significantly higher than that for proximal lesions, namely 7.5% (15/201) ($p = 0.03$). Presence of prior MI did not correlate with FI in LAD.

For ITA to LCX and GEA to RCA grafts, the incidence of FI was significantly higher in patients with prior MI in the revascularized area ($p = 0.04$ and $p = 0.002$, respectively). The incidence of FI was significantly higher when the stenosis was located in the distal portion than that when it was in the proximal portion ($p = 0.0003$).

Reference diameters and cut-off MLDs are shown in Table 3. For ITA to LAD grafts, the cut-off MLD was 1.29 for proximal and 0.95 for distal lesions; for ITA to

LCX, 1.26 for proximal and 0.80 for distal lesions; for GEA to RCA, 1.27 for proximal lesions. No cut-off value was identified for GEA to RCA distal lesions. The incidence of FI was 50.0% for GEA-RCA distal lesions, irrespective of severity of stenosis. We were unable to identify a significant cut-off value for SVG to LCX or to RCA grafts. Compared with proximal lesions, cut-off values for MLD and % stenosis were lower by 0.34 mm and 3%, respectively, for the LAD, and by 0.46 mm and 6%, respectively, for the LCX (Fig. 1).

As shown in Table 4, for 54/334 ITA to LAD bypass grafts (16.2%) there was a history of PCI to the LAD (PCI group), whereas for the remaining 280 ITA to LAD grafts there was no history of PCI to the LAD (no-PCI group). Stents had been implanted in 28 of the 54 in the PCI group (51.8%) and PCI had been unsuccessful in 15/54 (27.8%). Graft flow was significantly greater in the no-PCI than in the PCI group (53 ± 29 vs. 42 ± 27; $p = 0.006$). The incidences of FI and graft failure were significantly higher in the PCI than the no-PCI group (22.2%, vs. 8.2%; $p = 0.003$; 9.2% vs. 1.8%; $p = 0.003$, respectively). Of 54 ITA–LAD bypass grafts in the PCI group, 25 were for distal and 29 for proximal lesions. In the PCI group, graft flow and incidence of FI and graft failure were 35 ± 24, 8/25 (32.0%), and 3/25 (12.0%), respectively, for distal lesions, whereas they were 49 ± 29

Table 2 Flow insufficiency according to characteristics of target vessel, bypass graft and stenosis location

Target vessel	Bypass graft	(n)	Flow insufficiency	MI (+)	MI (−)	PCI (+)	PCI (−)	Distal lesion	Proximal lesion
LAD	in-situ ITA	334	10.5%(35/334) *	7.0%(3/43)	11.0%(32/291)	22.2%(12/54)	8.2%(23/280)	15.0%(20/133)	7.5%(15/201)
				$p = 0.42$		$p = 0.002$		$p = 0.03$	
LCX		194	18.0%(35/194) **	28.6%(4/14)	17.2%(31/180)	15.0%(3/20)	18.4%(32/174)	27.7%(26/94)	9.0%(9/100)
				$p = 0.29$		$p = 0.71$		$p = 0.0007$	
	in-situ ITA	129	24.0%(31/129)	36.4%(4/11)	22.9%(27/118)	18.8%(3/16)	24.8%(28/113)	37.1%(23/62)	11.9%(8/67)
				$p = 0.04$		$p = 0.60$		$p = 0.0008$	
	aorto-coronary SVG	65	6.2%(4/65)	0%(0/3)	6.5%(4/62)	0%(0/4)	6.6%(4/61)	9.4%(3/32)	3.0%(1/33)
				$p = 0.65$		$p = 0.60$		$p = 0.29$	
RCA		208	25.5%(53/208) ***	45.1%(23/51)	19.1%(30/157)	26.3%(5/19)	25.4%(48/189)	48.7%(19/39)	20.1%(34/169)
				$p = 0.0002$		$p = 0.93$		$p = 0.0002$	
	in-situ GEA	142	26.8%(38/142)	45.9%(17/37)	20.0%(21/105)	30.0%(3/10)	26.5%(35/132)	50.0%(11/22)	22.5%(27/120)
				$p = 0.002$		$p = 0.81$		$p = 0.007$	
	aorto-coronary SVG	66	22.7%(15/66)	42.9%(6/14)	17.3%(9/52)	22.2%(2/9)	22.8%(13/57)	47.1%(8/17)	14.3%(7/49)
				$p = 0.04$		$p = 0.97$		$p = 0.006$	
Overall		736	16.7%(123/736)	28.0%(30/107)	14.8%(93/629)	21.5%(20/93)	16.0%(103/643)	23.0%(65/283)	12.8%(58/453)
				$p = 0.0007$		$p = 0.19$		$p = 0.0003$	

GEA; gastroepiploic artery ITA; internal thoracic artery LAD; left anterior descending artery LCX; left circumflex artery
MI; myocardial infarction PCI; percutaneous coronary intervention RCA; right coronary artery SVG; saphenous vein graft; * vs. **; $p = 0.01$; * vs. ***; $p < .0001$

Table 3 Flow insufficiency according to MLD higher and lower than cut-off value and stenosis location

Bypass graft	Stenosis location	Reference diameter (mm)	MLD < cutt-off value	Cut-off value (mm)	calculated % stenosis	MLD ≥ cut-off value
in-situ ITA	Proximal	3.07 ± 0.75	8/159	1.29	58%	7/42
			(5.0%)	*p = 0.01		(16.7%)
	Distal	2.42 ± 0.53	10/100	0.95	61%	10/33
			(10.0%)	*p = 0.005		(30.3%)
in-situ ITA	Proximal	3.21 ± 0.84	1/46	1.26	61%	7/21
			(2.2%)	*p = 0.0003		(33.3%)
	Distal	2.40 ± 0.53	7/35	0.80	67%	16/27
			(20.0%)	*p = 0.0005		(59.3%)
in-situ GEA	Proximal	3.00 ± 0.73	22/110	1.27	58%	5/10
			(20.0%)	*p = 0.03		(50.0%)
	Distal	2.79 ± 0.77		N/A		

GEA; gastroepiploic artery ITA; internal thoracic artery LAD; left anterior descending artery LCX; left circumflex artery
MLD; minimalluminal diameter RCA; right coronary artery *; comparison of higher versus lower than MLD

($p = 0.03$), 4/29 (13.8%) ($p = 0.10$), and 2/29(6.9%) ($p = 0.51$), respectively, for proximal lesions.

Discussion

Flow demand and peripheral vascular resistance in revascularized areas are the fundamental factors that influence graft flow and patency; however, they have not yet been fully explored, probably because vascular resistance varies as a result of continuously being adjusted according to oxygen consumption and left ventricular work. Thus, vascular resistance cannot be reliably quantified in clinical studies. In an attempt to circumvent these difficulties, we examined location of stenosis (distal vs. proximal) and history of MI and PCI in the relevant area, all of which are presumably associated with the status and size of revascularized myocardial areas and flow demand, to determine how these factors influence graft flow and patency.

Competitive flow can be avoided by appropriate target assessment, graft selection, and configuration [6, 7]. Functional assessment of native coronary stenosis, such as by assessing FFR or coronary flow velocity reserve (CFVR), has raised some issues. Van de Hoef and colleagues reported that results of FFR and CFVR were discordant in 31% or 37% of target vessels at cut-off FFR values of 0.75 or 0.80, respectively [8]. This discordance is characteristic of microvascular disease (MVD); adverse cardiac events and deaths were significantly associated with normal FFR and abnormal CFVR in that study [8]. Additionally, in patients with multivessel disease, including chronic total occlusion (CTO), FFR in collateral donating branches can be overestimated [9].

In the present study, we assessed native coronary stenosis by using quantitative coronary angiography to ascertain the MLD and reference diameter, both of which are

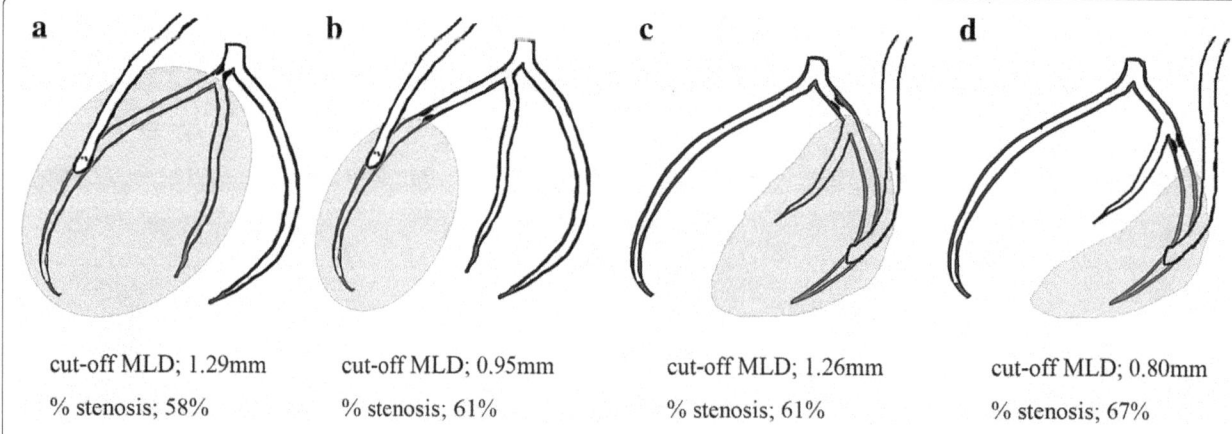

cut-off MLD; 1.29mm   cut-off MLD; 0.95mm   cut-off MLD; 1.26mm   cut-off MLD; 0.80mm

% stenosis; 58%   % stenosis; 61%   % stenosis; 61%   % stenosis; 67%

Fig. 1 Cut-off values for minimal luminal diameter and calculated % stenosis. The cut-off values for minimal luminal diameter and calculated % stenosis were (**a**) 1.29 mm and 58% for proximal LAD stenosis; (**b**) 0.95 mm and 61% for distal LAD stenosis; (**c**) 1.26 mm and 58% for proximal LCX stenosis; and (**d**) 0.80 mm and 67% for distal LCX stenosis. The smaller the revascularized area, the more severe stenosis is necessary to avoid flow insufficiency. LAD; left anterior descending artery, LCX; left circumflex artery

Table 4 Graft flow and angiographic results according to prior history of percutaneous coronary intervention

		PCI (+)	PCI (−)	p value
Number of patients		54	280	–
Age		67 ± 9	67 ± 10	0.44
Female		12 (22.2%)	68 (24.3%)	0.75
DM		25 (46.3%)	149 (53.2%)	0.35
Stenosis location and severity	Stenosis at distal portion #7 or #8	25 (46.3%)	107 (38.2%)	0.27
	Minimal luminal diameter (mm)	0.82 ± 0.53	0.73 ± 0.52	0.12
	Reference diameter (mm)	2.76 ± 0.57	2.82 ± 0.78	0.29
	Calculated severity of stenosis (%)	70 ± 19	74 ± 17	0.07
Prior coronary intervention	Stent implantation	28 (51.8%)	–	–
	Drug-eluting	18	–	–
	Bare metal / unknown stent	6 / 4	–	–
	Balloon angioplasty	3 (5.6%)	–	–
	Unsuccessful	15 (27.8%)	–	–
	No detailed information about old PCI	5 (9.2%)	–	–
	PCI complications, such as dissection, perforation, etc.	3 (5.6%)	–	–
Graft flow and angiographic results	Graft flow (ml/min)	42 ± 27	53 ± 29	0.006
	Fow insufficiency (≤ 20 ml/min)	12 (22.2%)	23 (8.2%)	0.002
	Angiographic competitive flow	5 (9.2%)	3 (1.1%)	< 0.001
	Graft failure	5 (9.2%)	5 (1.8%)	0.003

PCI; percutaneous coronary intervention

traditional but standard measures. Additionally, off-pump CABG favours use of TTFM [10] because cardiopulmonary bypass can reduce systemic vascular resistance and increase graft flow by inducing a hyperaemic state, thus creating a major bias in flow measurements [11]. Moreover, to minimize any bias caused by bypass grafts or targets, we excluded all sequential and composite graft and bypass grafts that were not the sole bypass grafts in the relevant vascular region. For example, when there was a bypass graft to a diagonal branch, we excluded ITA to LAD bypasses in case of any negative interactions [12].

We found that FI was significantly associated with distal lesions, history of MI in the LCX and RCA areas, and history of PCI in the LAD. The cut-off values were higher by 3% for LAD and 6% for LCX for distal lesions than for proximal lesions. These findings suggest that severity of stenosis and CABG strategy should be modified according to whether the stenosis is located distally or proximally and the size of the area to be revascularized. Competitive flow that is attributable simply to moderately stenotic native targets does not remain the primary mechanism for FI at later stages.

We were unable to determine cut-off values for SVG to LCX and RCA grafts, in the case of SVG to LCX possibly because SVG patency is not influenced by the severity of stenosis and there were too few grafts with FI to demonstrate a significant difference. In comparison, as shown in Table 2, for distal RCA, the incidence of FI in SVGs was as high as 47.1%, which is comparable to that for GEA, irrespective of MLD. SVGs have been widely accepted as providing high pressure capacity and being more reliable than arterial grafts for targets with moderate stenosis. The results of this study suggest that SVG is reliable irrespective of stenosis severity provided that flow demand in the grafted area is adequate.

PCI had a negative impact on graft flow only in ITA to LAD grafts, likely because PCI is indicated for LCX and RCA only when the vessel is sufficiently large. Possible mechanisms for reduced graft flow, higher rate of FI, and graft failure after PCI include the following. First, stenosis in the LAD may have been less severe in patients who had undergone PCI than in those who had not. Although, there was not a statistically significant difference in severity of stenosis and MLD, the incidence of angiographic competitive flow was higher in the PCI than in the no-PCI group. Second, revascularized areas were sometimes made smaller by sacrificing epicardial coronary vessels, such as the LAD, diagonal or septal branch (Fig. 2). A third possible mechanism is microvascular disease (MVD) distal to a PCI. It is widely accepted that PCI can cause microembolization of atherosclerotic debris or thrombus to distal myocardial tissue. Additionally, drug-eluting stents may adversely affect peripheral vascular function. Shin and colleagues reported that coronary segments distal to drug-eluting

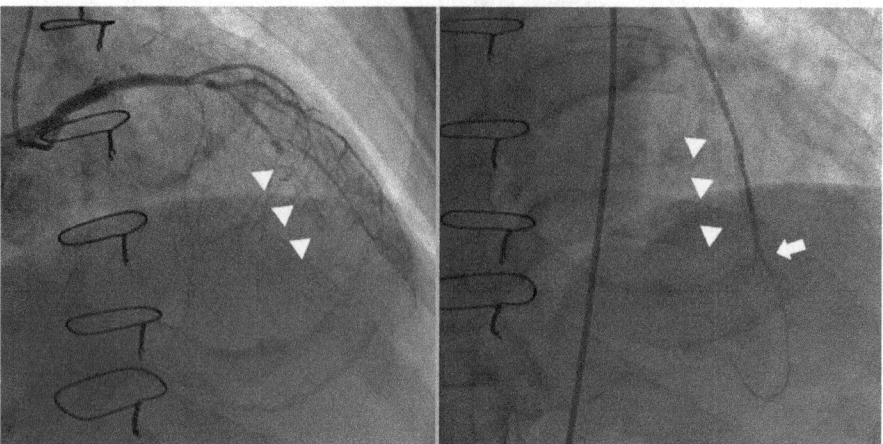

Fig. 2 Illustrative case. A 71-year old man with three stents in the LAD underwent coronary artery bypass grafting including ITA to LAD. Two years later, the LAD had totally occluded at the stent that had been implanted distally (arrow heads, left image), limiting the revascularized area to the apical area (right image). A broad area of anterior ischemia had redeveloped. An arrow indicates the site of anastomosis of the ITA and LAD. ITA; internal thoracic artery, LAD; left anterior descending artery

stents have more severe vasoconstriction than those distal to bare metal stents. These researchers suspected endothelial dysfunction in the myocardium distal to the treated vessel [13]. De Villa and colleagues have proposed normalized perfusion pressure, secondary inflammation, and platelet activation as possible mechanisms for MVD [14]. Fourth, patients who present with MVD are vulnerable to developing restenosis after PCI and therefore tend to be referred for CABG. De Villa and colleagues reported that lower coronary flow responses to adenosine and cold pressor tests are associated with restenosis after PCI [14]. Guidelines for revascularization recommend CABG only for proximal lesions of the LAD in patients with multivessel disease [15]. However, in our experience, graft flow is significantly reduced in ITA to LAD distal lesions with prior PCI and the incidence of FI and graft failure are as high as 32 and 12%, respectively. Both proximal and distal LAD stenosis should be carefully managed by the cardiovascular team, otherwise PCI to LAD distal lesions may cause MVD and compromise the efficacy of future CABG.

Recently, hybrid procedures comprising in situ ITA to LAD bypass grafting with drug-eluting stents for non-LAD vessels have been increasingly performed on patients at high risk of sternotomy [16, 17]. Rosenblum and colleagues reported finding no significant differences between such hybrid procedures and CABG using bilateral ITA over a mean duration of follow-up of 2.83 years and concluded that hybrid revascularization is effective in appropriately selected patients [18]. Patients are usually selected for hybrid revascularization when the morphology of LAD lesions contraindicates PCI [15, 19]. However, CABG is not necessarily appropriate in patients with morphology that contraindicates PCI, except

for those with CTO. Even in vessels with CTO, small revascularized areas and a history of PCI have negative impacts on ITA to LAD grafts. Inversely, ITA grafting may be more beneficial than PCI in some patients with LAD in whom PCI would be appropriate. Moreover, the latest randomized study found no significant advantage of bilateral ITA over single ITA over a 5 year follow-up [20]. Detailed assessment of the suitability of coronary lesions for ITA or CABG and precise prediction of graft patency would contribute to improving outcomes of both hybrid revascularization and CABG using multiple arteries or both ITAs.

This study has the following limitations. First, it was retrospective and therefore not randomized. Second, we were unable to reliably examine FFR because it cannot be measured in target vessels with CTO and was not performed in other patients in some of the referral hospitals during the study period. Especially for in stent stenosis, FFR or intravascular ultrasonography may be more reliable than angiography. However, these investigations had been performed only for selected vessels or patients, such as those with moderate stenosis or who were candidates for re-stenting. Difficulty in assessment or overestimation of in-stent stenosis may have introduced bias. Third, there may have been too few patients, especially for examining the effects of PCI in the LCX and RCA. We speculate that prior PCI in the LCX and RCA would show a statistically significant negative impact with greater numbers of patients and bypass grafts. Fourth, indications for PCI were not precisely defined because these procedures were performed using several different devices and techniques over more than a decade in a number of different hospitals. Of note, PCI has been performed more aggressively by cardiologists in

Intraoperative transit-time flowmetry in patients undergoing coronary surgery to determine relationships...

157

Japan than in other countries. Fifth, myocardial flow demand in an area with a history of MI correlates with the extent of remaining viability. Unfortunately, viability had not been assessed by the appropriate specific preoperative investigations. Sixth, blood pressure or dose of catecholamine may have introduced biases in flow measurements. However, we could not precisely define these factors because this study was retrospective and the measurements had been taken intraoperatively. Finally, the most important limitation is the lack of a standard protocol for preoperative assessment and resultant uncertainty about all aspects of assessment and previous treatment.

Conclusions

In conclusion, flow demand and myocardial status significantly influence graft flow and patency. The smaller the revascularized area, the more severe the stenosis must be to avoid FI. Moreover, too small a revascularized area or MVD, associated with PCI, can reduce the benefits of surgical coronary revascularization. When planning revascularization strategies, it is necessary to establish a logical and optimal way of taking into account factors associated with flow demand and microvasculature.

Abbreviations

CABG: Coronary artery bypass grafting; FFR: Fractional flow reserve; FI: Flow insufficiency; GEA: Gastroepiploic artery; ITA: Internal thoracic artery; LAD: Left anterior descending artery; LCX: Left circumflex artery; MLD: Minimal luminal diameter; MVD: Microvascular disease; PCI: Percutaneous coronary intervention; RCA: Right coronary artery; SVG: Saphenous vein graft; TTFM: Transit-time flowmetry

Acknowledgements
None.

Funding
None.

Authors' contributions
HN carried out data analysis and wrote the manuscript. AT and TA participated in the design of the study. AY supported writing of the manuscript. MT participated in collection of data. CT and AI participated in the design of the study and performed the statistical analysis. JH carried out data collection. HI and DK conceived of the study, participated in its design and coordination, and helped to draft the manuscript. All authors read and approved the final manuscript.

Competing interests
The authors declare that they have no competing interests.

References
1. Di Giammarco G, Pano M, Cirmeni S, Pelini P, Vitolla G, Di Mauro M. Predictive value of intraoperative transit-time flow measurement for short-term graft patency in coronary surgery. J Thorac Cardiovasc Surg. 2006;132:468–74.
2. Lehnert P, Moller CH, Damgaard S, Gerds TA, Steinbruchel DA. Transit-time flow measurement as a predictor of coronary bypass graft failure at one year angiographic follow-up. J Card Surg. 2015;30:47–52.
3. Amin S, Pinho-Gomes AC, Taggart DP. Relationship of intraoperative transit time Flowmetry findings to angiographic graft patency at follow-up. Ann Thorac Surg. 2016;101(5):1996–2006.
4. Tokuda Y, Song MH, Oshima H, Usui A, Ueda Y. Predicting midterm coronary artery bypass graft failure by intraoperative transit time flow measurement. Ann Thorac Surg. 2008;86:532–6.
5. Nakajima H, Iguchi A, Tabata M, Koike H, Morita K, Takahashi K, Asakura T, Nishimura S, Niinami H. Predictors and prevention of flow insufficiency due to limited flow demand. J Cardiothorac Surg. 2014;9:188.
6. Nakajima H, Kobayashi J, Toda K, Fujita T, Shimahara Y, Kasahara Y, Kitamura S. A 10-year angiographic follow-up of competitive flow in sequential and composite arterial grafts. Eur J Cardiothorac Surg. 2011;40(2):399–404.
7. Glineur D, Boodhwani M, Hanet C, de Kerchove L, Navarra E, Astarci P, Noirhomme P, El Khoury G. Bilateral internal thoracic artery configuration for coronary artery bypass surgery: a prospective randomized trial. Circ Cardiovasc Interv. 2016;9:e003518.
8. van de Hoef TP, van Lavieren MA, Damman P, Delewi R, Piek MA, Chamuleau SA, Voskuil M, Henriques JP, Koch KT, de Winter RJ, Spaan JA, Siebes M, Tijssen JG, Meuwissen M, Piek JJ. Physiological basis and long-term clinical outcome of discordance between fractional flow reserve and coronary flow velocity reserve in coronary stenoses of intermediate severity. Circ Cardiovasc Interv. 2014;7(3):301–11.
9. Iqbal MB, Shah N, Khan M, Wallis W. Reduction in myocardial perfusion territory and its effect on the physiological severity of a coronary stenosis. Circ Cardiovasc Interv. 2010;3:89–90.
10. Nakajima H, Iguchi A, Tabata M, Kambe M, Ikeda M, Uwabe K, Asakura T, Niinami H. Preserved autoregulation of coronary flow after off-pump coronary artery bypass grafting: retrospective assessment of intraoperative transit time flowmetry with and without intra-aortic balloon counterpulsation. J Cardiothorac Surg. 2016;11(1):156.
11. Balacumaraswami L, Abu-Omar Y, Selvanayagam J, Pigott D, Taggart DP. The effects of on-pump and off-pump coronary artery bypass grafting on intraoperative graft flow in arterial and venous conduits defined by a flow/pressure ratio. J Thorac Cardiovasc Surg. 2008;135(3):533–9.
12. Harskamp RE, Alexander JH, Ferguson TB Jr, Hager R, Mack MJ, Englum B, Wojdyla D, Schulte PJ, Kouchoukos NT, de Winter RJ, Gibson CM, Peterson ED, Harrington RA, Smith PK, Lopes RD. Frequency and Predictors of internal mammary artery graft failure and subsequent clinical outcomes insights from the project of ex-vivo vein graft engineering via transfection (PREVENT) IV trial. Circulation. 2016;133:131–8.
13. Shin DI, Kim PJ, Seung KB, Kim DB, Kim MJ, Chang K, Lim SM, Jeon DS, Chung WS, Baek SH, Lee MY. Drug-eluting stent implantation could be associated with long-term coronary endothelial dysfunction. Int Heart J. 2007;48(5):553–67.
14. De Vita A, Milo M, Sestito A, Lamendola P, Lanza GA, Crea F. Association of coronary microvascular dysfunction with restenosis of left anterior descending coronary artery disease treated by percutaneous intervention. Int J Cardiol. 2016;219:322–5.
15. Fihn SD, Gardin JM, Abrams J, Berra K, Blankenship JC, Dallas AP, Douglas PS, Foody JM, Gerber TC, Hinderliter AL, King SB 3rd, Kligfield PD, Krumholz HM, Kwong RY, Lim MJ, Linderbaum JA, Mack MJ, Munger MA, Prager RL, Sabik JF, Shaw LJ, Sikkema JD, Smith CR Jr, Smith SC Jr, Spertus JA, Williams SV, American College of Cardiology Foundation.; American Heart Association Task Force on Practice Guidelines.; American College of Physicians.; American Association for Thoracic Surgery.; Preventive Cardiovascular Nurses Association.; Society for Cardiovascular Angiography and Interventions. Society of Thoracic Surgeons. 2012 ACCF/AHA/ACP/AATS/PCNA/SCAI/STS guideline for the diagnosis and management of patients with stable ischemic heart disease: a report of the American

College of Cardiology Foundation/American Heart Association task force on practice guidelines, and the American College of Physicians, American Association for Thoracic Surgery, preventive cardiovascular nurses association, Society for Cardiovascular Angiography and Interventions, and Society of Thoracic Surgeons. J Am Coll Cardiol. 2012;60(24):e44–e164.

16. Puskas JD, Halkos ME, DeRose JJ, Bagiella E, Miller MA, Overbey J, Bonatti J, Srinivas VS, Vesely M, Sutter F, Lynch J, Kirkwood K, Shapiro TA, Boudoulas KD, Crestanello J, Gehrig T, Smith P, Ragosta M, Hoff SJ, Zhao D, Gelijns AC, Szeto WY, Weisz G, Argenziano M, Vassiliades T, Liberman H, Matthai W, Ascheim DD. Hybrid coronary revascularization for the treatment of multivessel coronary artery disease: A Multicenter Observational Study. J Am Coll Cardiol. 2016;68(4):356–65.

17. Adams C, Burns DJ, Chu MW, Jones PM, Shridar K, Teefy P, Kostuk WJ, Dobkowski WB, Romsa J, Kiaii B. Single-stage hybrid coronary revascularization with long-term follow-up. Eur J Cardiothorac Surg. 2014;45(3):438–42.

18. Rosenblum JM, Harskamp RE, Hoedemaker N, Walker P, Liberman HA, de Winter RJ, Vassiliades TA, Puskas JD, Halkos ME. Hybrid coronary revascularization versus coronary artery bypass surgery with bilateral or single internal mammary artery grafts. J Thorac Cardiovasc Surg. 2016;151(4):1081–9.

19. Bonatti J, Lehr E, Vesely MR, Friedrich G, Bonaros N, Zimrin D. Hybrid coronary revascularization: which patients? When? How? Curr Opin Cardiol. 2010;25(6):568–74.

20. Taggart DP, Altman DG, Gray AM, Lees B, Gerry S, Benedetto U, Flather M, Investigators ART. Randomized trial of bilateral versus single internal-thoracic-artery grafts. N Engl J Med. 2016;375(26):2540–9.

Cost-effectiveness analysis of single use negative pressure wound therapy dressings (sNPWT) compared to standard of care in reducing surgical site complications (SSC) in patients undergoing coronary artery bypass grafting surgery

Leo M Nherera[1]* [iD], Paul Trueman[1], Michael Schmoeckel[2] and Francis A Fatoye[3]

Abstract

Background: There is a growing interest in using negative pressure wound therapy in closed surgical incision to prevent wound complications which continue to persist following surgery despite advances in infection measures.

Objectives: To estimate the cost-effectiveness of single use negative pressure wound therapy (sNPWT) compared to standard of care in patients following coronary artery bypass grafting surgery (CABG) procedure to reduce surgical site complications (SSC) defined as dehiscence and sternotomy infections.

Method: A decision analytic model was developed from the Germany Statutory Health Insurance payer's perspective over a 12-week time horizon. Baseline data on SSC, revision operations, length of stay, and readmissions were obtained from a prospective observational study of 2621 CABG patients in Germany. Effectiveness data for sNPWT was taken from a randomised open label trial conducted in Poland which randomised 80 patients to treatment with either sNPWT or standard care. Cost data (in Euros) were taken from the relevant diagnostic related groups and published literature.

Results: The clinical study reported an increase in wounds that healed without complications 37/40 (92.5%) in the sNPWT compared to 30/40 (75%) patients in the SC group $p = 0.03$. The model estimated sNPWT resulted in 0.989 complications avoided compared to 0.952 and the estimated quality adjusted life years were 0.8904 and 0.8593 per patient compared to standard care. The estimated mean cost per patient was €19,986 for sNPWT compared to €20,572 for SC resulting in cost-saving of €586. The findings were robust to a range of sensitivity analyses.

Conclusion: The sNPWT can be considered a cost saving intervention that reduces surgical site complications following CABG surgery compared to standard care. We however recommend that additional economic studies should be conducted as new evidence on the use of sNPWT in CABG patients becomes available to validate the results of this economic analysis.

Keywords: Single use negative pressure wound therapy; cost-effectiveness, Surgical site complications, CABG

* Correspondence: leo.nherera@smith-nephew.com
[1]Smith & Nephew Advanced Wound Management, Global Market Access, 101 Hessle Road, Hull HU3 2BN, UK
Full list of author information is available at the end of the article

Background

There has been advances in infection control practices and wound dressings yet surgical site infections (SSI) remains common in patients undergoing surgery [1–4]. European Centre for Disease Prevention and Control (ECDC) reports that SSI are among the most common healthcare-associated infections (HAIs) which occur after surgery in the area of the body where the surgery took place. European-wide SSI incidence rates range from 0.7% in knee prosthesis to 9.7% in colon surgery [2]. Reddy et al. [3], reported that approximately 0.3–5% of median sternotomy incisions are affected by complications, such as infection and dehiscence.

Surgical site infections impacts on morbidity, health-related quality of life, longer post-operative hospital stays, additional surgical procedures, mortality and increased costs [4–10]. Graf et al. [6] estimated the financial loss to a hospital due to deep sternal wound infection following coronary artery by-pass surgery to be $12,482 (€9154) in Germany. In the United Kingdom, attributable median hospital length of stay (LOS) due to SSI for cardiac patients is estimated to be 23 days and the attributable median costs due to SSI are £11,003 ($8517- $15,395) respectively [10].

Many strategies have been introduced to control SSI, ranging from antibiotics prophylaxis, dressings and new protocols including the use of single use negative pressure wound therapy (sNPWT). Evidence on the clinical effectiveness of sNPWT is accumulating rapidly [11, 14, 15] and has been shown to be effective in reducing SSI in closed incisions such as in caesarean-section, orthopaedic and cardiac surgery. Cost-effectiveness studies have been performed in patients undergoing caesarean-section [13] and Orthopaedic surgery [12], however the cost-effectiveness of sNPWT following cardiothoracic surgery has not been reported.

This study therefore examined the cost-effectiveness of sNPWT PICO$^\lozenge$ (Smith & Nephew, Hull, UK) compared with standard care dressing (standard post-operative dressings) in preventing surgical site complications defined as dehiscence and sternotomy infections in patients undergoing coronary artery by-pass (CABG) surgery from a Germany Insurance payer's perspective.

Methods

To describe the clinical problem, we constructed a decision analytic model in Microsoft Excel 2016 (Microsoft Corporation, Redmond, WA, US) to simulate the expected outcomes and costs of patients undergoing CABG surgery. The mean age of patients that were modelled is 65 years, which represents the mean age of the majority of patients included in the studies were baseline and effectiveness data were drawn from [16, 17]. Following skin closure, one

group would be managed by sNPWT while the other group would receive standard of care dressings. The modeled patients may develop complications of sternotomy wounds which in this model was defined as SSI (superficial and deep wound infections) or dehiscence. The complications are assumed to result in readmissions and revision surgery in some cases as shown in Fig. 1. The model assumed a proportion of patients could die from natural causes and also die due to surgery. The perspective adopted was that of the Statutory Health Insurance payers in Germany. The economic model adopted a 12 week time horizon to enable the both superficial and deep infection to manifest themselves. Superficial SSI usually occurs within 30 days after surgery while deep SSI normally occurs within 30 to 90 days following surgery [1]. No discounting was done for both costs and outcomes due to a shorter time horizon (12 weeks). The schematic representation of the model is shown below in Fig. 1, showing the branches of the complications node, there are similar branches for the no complications node not shown in the figure.

Baseline clinical data

Data for this economic analysis were derived from published clinical studies. In particular the baseline data was obtained from a single centre prospective observational study that followed patients who underwent CABG for 36 months in Germany [16]. The study collected information on the following outcomes; revision operations, patients' length of stay, and readmissions to the hospital from 2621 patients. Twenty-seven patients (4.85%) were diagnosed SSI according to the Centres for Disease Control and Prevention criteria. Data on length of stay, readmission, revision surgery and mortality due to surgery was taken from the same source [16].

Effectiveness data for sNPWT was taken from a randomised open label trial conducted in Poland [17]. The study evaluated sNPWT use in patients after an off-pump CABG procedure, using the internal mammary artery in 80 patients. There were 40 patients in each arm with similar patient characteristics ie, 40 in sNPWT and 40 in the standard care arm in whom conventional dressings were applied in the postoperative period. The ECDC definition of SSI was used in this study. The endpoint of the study was wound healing defined as absence of SSI and wound dehiscence of wound margins without clinical or microbiological signs of infections. 37/40 (92.5%) patients had their wounds healed without complications in the sNPWT compared to 30/40 (75%) patients in the standard care group $p = 0.03$ [17]. We calculated the Odds ratio (OR) from this data to be, OR;0.22, 95% confidence interval 0.06 to 0.81, $p = 0.002$ We are also aware of an ongoing study in Spain which is comparing sNPWT with standard

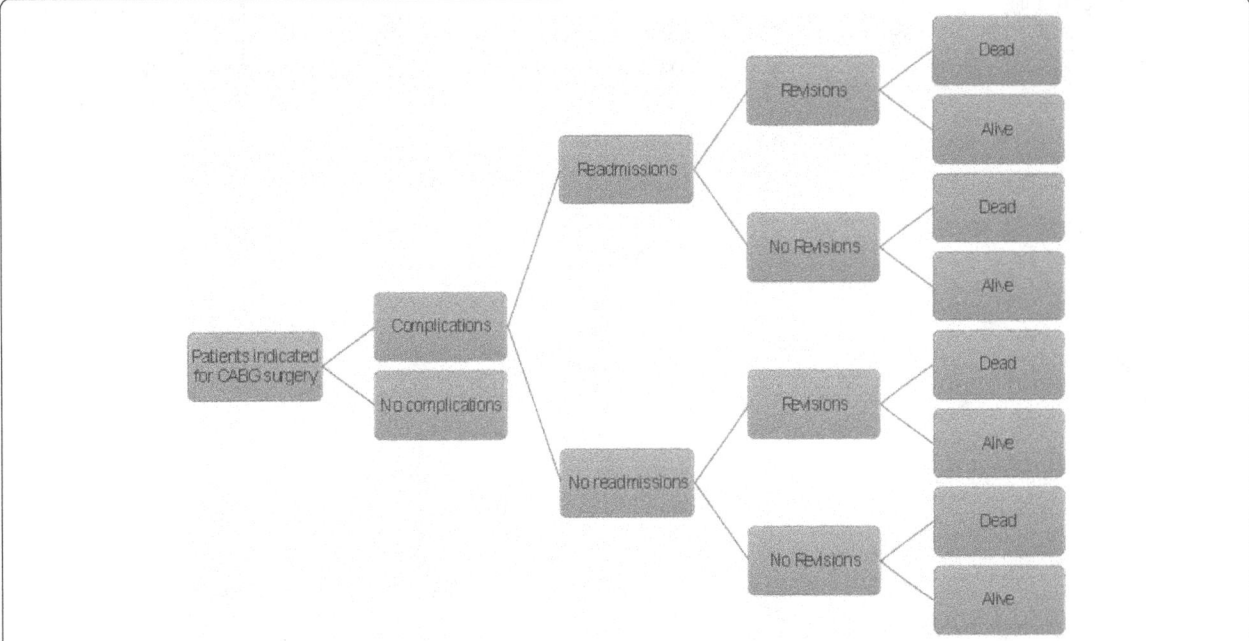

Fig. 1 Model structure for sNPWT compared to SC in patients following CABG surgery. The decision tree model used to predict cost and outcome of sNPWT and standard of care. The tree maps the outcomes (health states) modelled following a complication or no complication. The branches for no complication are not shown in the figure

of care in patients undergoing CABG with preliminary results expected in 2019 (Dr Carlos Velasco, Hospital Juan Canalejo, Spain; – personal communication).

Strugala and Martin found that sNPWT reduced length of stay on average by 0.5 days [14] in a meta-analysis that assessed the prophylactic use of PICO negative pressure wound therapy on surgical site complications. We applied this reduction in the base case model and assessed the assumption that there was no difference in sensitivity analysis. All-cause mortality was obtained from the Germany Federal Statistical Office [18]. We made a further assumption that mortality following revision surgery will be 30% higher than that of patients who did not have revision surgery in accordance to published literature [19]. The clinical data used in the model is shown in Table 1.

Health state utilities

The health state utilities in the model were sourced from published literature. The utility scores for patients undergoing CABG and discharged without complications were set at 0.91 and for those discharged with complications was set at 0.71 obtained from a study by Tuffaha 2015. The study by Tuffaha et al. considered the cost-utility analysis of negative pressure wound therapy in high-risk caesarean section wounds [13]. Currently there is no evidence that utility values differ by type of dressing used, we therefore assumed that utility was independent of the type of dressing in the model. The utility data parameters used in the model is shown in Table 1.

Cost data

Costs were derived from standard cost references with resource utilisation valued in Euros (2017). For inpatient care we used data from Cristofolini who identified length of stay in different hospital wards from intensive care unit to the general ward before discharge for patients with or without infections. We calculated the mean cost for a patient with or without infection and applied it in the model. The cost for the stay in each ward were obtained from the hospital management website [20]. For procedure costs, we used the average reimbursement costs from the relevant Germany Diagnosis Related Group Report Browser 2017 of the procedure code 5–361 "Application of an aortocoronary bypass", and Procedure code 5–363.1: "Revision of an aortocoronary bypass" see Table 2. The mean cost for the main procedure was estimated to be €15,135.58, while for revision it was estimated to be €24,740.45. We assumed that costs of standard of care dressings and nursing costs were all included in the DRG costs while the cost of the intervention (sNPWT) was obtained from the manufacturer. The model applied the cost of one sNPWT device, which is designed to last for 7 days and is supplied with two dressings. In the sensitivity analysis we assumed patients received two sNPWT dressings to assess changes in expected total costs.

For post discharge outpatient consultations, we assumed patients would be seen in an outpatient rehabilitation facilities for 3 weeks. Rehabilitation costs were

Table 1 Clinical and utility data used in the model for sNPWT compared to standard care in patients following CABG surgery. The table shows the baseline data, effectiveness of sNPWT and health related quality of life (utility) data that was applied in the model

Outcome	Mean	Number of patients	Events	Distribution	Reference
Baseline SSC rate	0.048	2621	127	Beta	Cristofolini [16]
Mortality with SSC	0.017	118	2	Beta	ibid
Mortality without SSC	0.007	2503	18	Beta	
Readmission SSC	0.034	118	4	Beta	
Readmission No SSC	0.000	2503	1	Beta	
Revision SSC	0.068	118	8	Beta	
Revision No SSC	0.005	2503	12	Beta	
All-cause mortality	0.003				[18]
Multiplier for revision mortality	1.300				Wu [19]
Length of stay data					
Length of stay with surgical site complications	Mean	Lower CI	Upper CI		
Intensive care unit	15.2	1	87.2	Log normal	Cristofolini [16]
Intermediate care	4.8	0.5	25.2	Log normal	
General ward	22.3	0.5	68.4	Log normal	
Length of stay without surgical site complications					
Intensive care unit	3.8	1	26	Log normal	Cristofolini [16]
Intermediate care	2.4	0.5	10	Log normal	
General ward	8.3	0.5	19	Log normal	
Utility data used in the model					
Parameter	Mean	Alpha	Beta	Distribution	Source
Disutility with SSI	0.2	8	41	Beta	Tuffaha [13]
Utility with no SSI	0.91	185	18	Beta	
Effectiveness data (Odds ratio and 95% CI)					
Outcome	Mean	Lower CI	Upper CI	Distribution	Source
Odds ratio for SSC	0.220	0.060	0.810	Log normal	Witt-Majchrzak [17]
Reduction in LOS (days)	0.500	0.020	0.70	Log normal	Strugala [14]

Abbreviations: *sNPWT* single use negative pressure wound therapy, *SSC* surgical site complications, *CI* confidence interval, *LOS* length of stay

Table 2 Cost data used in the model for sNPWT compared to standard care in patients following CABG surgery

Cost component	Mean cost	Lower value	Upper value	Source
Cost of hospital stay in ICU ward (inclusive of all done inpatient)	€1400.00	€1050.00	€1750.00	[20]
Intermediate ward	€850.00	€637.50	€1062.50	ibid
General ward cost/day	€200.00	€150.00	€250.00	
CABG procedure (code 5–361.[a]: "Application of an aortocoronary bypass")	€15,135.58	€11,351.69	€18,919.48	ibid
Cost of revision CABG procedure	€24,740.45	€18,555.34	€30,925.56	ibid
Outpatient rehabilitation	€1726.46	€1294.85	€2158.08	[21]
Community doctor consultation fee per quarter	€16.53	€12.40	€20.66	[22]
Electrocardiography	€16.53	€12.40	€20.66	ibid
Community Cardiologist	€21.06	€15.80	€26.33	ibid
Duplex-Electrocardiography	€71.50	€53.63	€89.38	ibid
Home visits	€11.53	€8.65	€14.41	ibid
sNPWT unit cost	€153.00	€114.75	€191.25	[a]

Abbreviations: *CABG* coronary artery bypass grafting, *sNPWT* single use negative pressure wound therapy, Gamma distribution was used for costs, we assumed the cost values will be 25% above and below the mean value to calculate the lower and upper values. [a]Data obtained from manufacturer

obtained from a study by Zeidler et al. [21] which considered cost of outpatient and inpatient rehabilitation for cardiac diseases in Germany. Mean costs were inflated to 2018 using the Germany consumer price index and were estimated to be €1726.47 for outpatient rehabilitation which included the costs of 25–30 min of physiotherapy once per week for 3 weeks. In addition, we included the costs of one community doctor and community cardiologist visit where an electrocardiography a duplex-electrocardiography would be done respectively. Furthermore, the cost of once a week visit by a community nurse for 6 weeks was also estimated [22]. Cost of post-surgery medication was assumed to be the same ie, patients were all prescribed antiplatelet, statins, betablockers, ACE inhibitors and was therefore not explicitly costed. The relevant costs and their sources are presented in Table 2.

Cost-effectiveness and sensitivity analysis

The incremental cost-effectiveness ratio is the added cost per additional unit of health, in this model measured in quality adjusted life years (QALYs) and complications avoided. This was calculated as the difference between the expected costs divided by the expected difference between the QALYs or complications avoided of sNPWT and standard care over the modelled time horizon.

Sensitivity analysis was done to assess the uncertainty around the model inputs and their impact on the main conclusions of the model. One-way sensitivity analyses were conducted by varying some of the critical model parameters, each key parameter was alternately assigned a low and high value then re-evaluate the cost-effectiveness results. Furthermore, we implemented a probabilistic sensitivity analysis where we assigned prior distributions to model parameter and then simultaneously selecting values at random from those distributions using Monte Carlo simulation to estimate the expected costs and effects associated with each intervention. The lognormal distribution was implemented to capture the uncertainty surrounding the treatment effect; the gamma and beta distributions were used to capture the uncertainty in cost and utility values respectively.

Results

The total mean costs per patient in the sNPWT group were lower than the total mean costs per patient in the standard care group. The use of sNPWT was associated with more QALYs and fewer wound related complications compared to the use of standard care. Overall, the use of sNPWT is a dominant strategy (cost-saving) compared to standard care as it costs less and results in better clinical outcomes as shown in Table 3.

Sensitivity analysis

One-way sensitivity analyses was performed and the results are displayed in Table 4 showing the mean incremental costs of sNPWT compared to standard care. Negative costs shows that sNPWT is cost-saving compared to standard care, hence model's conclusions were not changed by changes in input parameters tested as shown in Table 4 where all the cost differences are below €0.

We also performed a probabilistic sensitivity analysis, and presented the results as cost-effectiveness acceptability curves and the cost-effectiveness plane. The cost-effectiveness acceptability curves illustrate the probability that an intervention is cost-effective compared with the alternative, for a range of maximum monetary values that a decision-maker is willing to pay for a unit change in outcome in this case measured in QALYs. In our model, the cost-effectiveness acceptability curves demonstrates that sNPWT is 100% cost-effective for the willingness-to-pay threshold figure of €50,000 as shown in Fig. 2. The cost-effectiveness plane shows that both incremental cost and incremental QALY estimates are associated with little uncertainty as 99% of samples (red dots) are located in the South East (SE) quadrant where sNPWT is associated with less costs and better clinical outcomes as shown in Fig. 3.

Subgroup analysis

A study by Olsen 2002 et al. [23] which considered the risk factors for deep and superficial SSI after CABG surgery indicates that the risk of deep chest SSI was associated with a combination of obesity and diabetes, whereas increased risk of superficial chest SSI was associated primarily with obesity. In our analysis we considered the sub-group of patients with obesity, diabetes and smoking. The risk of SSI was increased by more than threefold for patients with BMI > 30 while for diabetes and smoking it's more than 2.5 fold. In these high risk patients, sNPWT was shown result in greater savings when compared to standard care in patients following CABG surgery. Table 5 shows the results of the subgroup analysis. Bigger savings are observed when

Table 3 Base case results for sNPWT compared to standard care in patients following CABG surgery

Intervention	Costs	Complications avoided	QALYs	Cost difference	Complication difference	QALY difference
Standard of care	€ 20,572	0.952	0.8593			
sNPWT	€ 19,986	0.989	0.8904	-€ 586	0.0374	0.0311

Abbreviations: *sNPWT* single use negative pressure wound therapy, *QALY* quality adjusted life years

Table 4 Results of one way-sensitivity analysis for sNPWT compared to standard care in patients following CABG surgery

Parameter, mean value (lower and upper value)	Savings with lower value	Savings with upper value
Baseline Risk 4.8% (2.5% and 7.8%)	€ 428	€ 793
Treatment effect complications 0.22 (0.06 and 0.81)	€ 654	€ 337
Cost of sNPWT €153 (€114.75 and €191.25)	€ 624	€ 548
Number of sNPWT 1 (2)	€ 433	
Length of stay difference 0.5 (0)	€ 178	

Abbreviations: *sNPWT* single use negative pressure wound therapy

patients with BMI ≥ 30 are prophylactically treated with sNPWT than with standard care dressings.

Discussion

This study examined the cost-effectiveness analysis of sNPWT compared to standard of care dressings in preventing SSI for patients undergoing CABG. The results of the study suggest that treating patients undergoing CABG with sNPWT is cost-saving resulting better clinical outcomes (0.311 more QALYs) and cheaper overall, with cost savings of €586 per patient. The probability of sNPWT being cost-effective is 100%, indicating decision certainty and little chance of error in a decision based on this cost-effectiveness analysis.

A limited number of cost-effectiveness studies evaluating the use of sNPWT in closed incisions have been published [12, 13] and they conclude that negative pressure wound therapy is cost-effective. However, to our knowledge, there is no published data on cost-effectiveness analysis of sNPWT in preventing wound complications following CABG surgery. This may be explained by lack of clinical evidence to support sNPWT as we found out during the literature search. As noted earlier, we are aware of an ongoing clinical trial comparing sNPWT with standard care following CABG surgery (Dr Carlos Velasco; Hospital Juan Canalejo, Spain; personal communication).

The model adopted a number of conservative assumptions so the projected savings may actually underestimate the true financial impact. For instance, we only captured SSI as an outcome and did not include other outcomes such as healing. Potentially infected wounds will take longer to heal and might develop into chronic wounds which are costly to treat [24]. Equally, dressing changes was not captured as an outcome, however we know based on previous studies that infected wounds would require more dressing changes making the model conservative favoring the strategy with more SSIs. For instance there were few dressing changes in the sNPWT group (*p* = 0.002) compared to standard care after hip and knee surgery, while there were more wounds with superficial infections in the standard care arm [11].

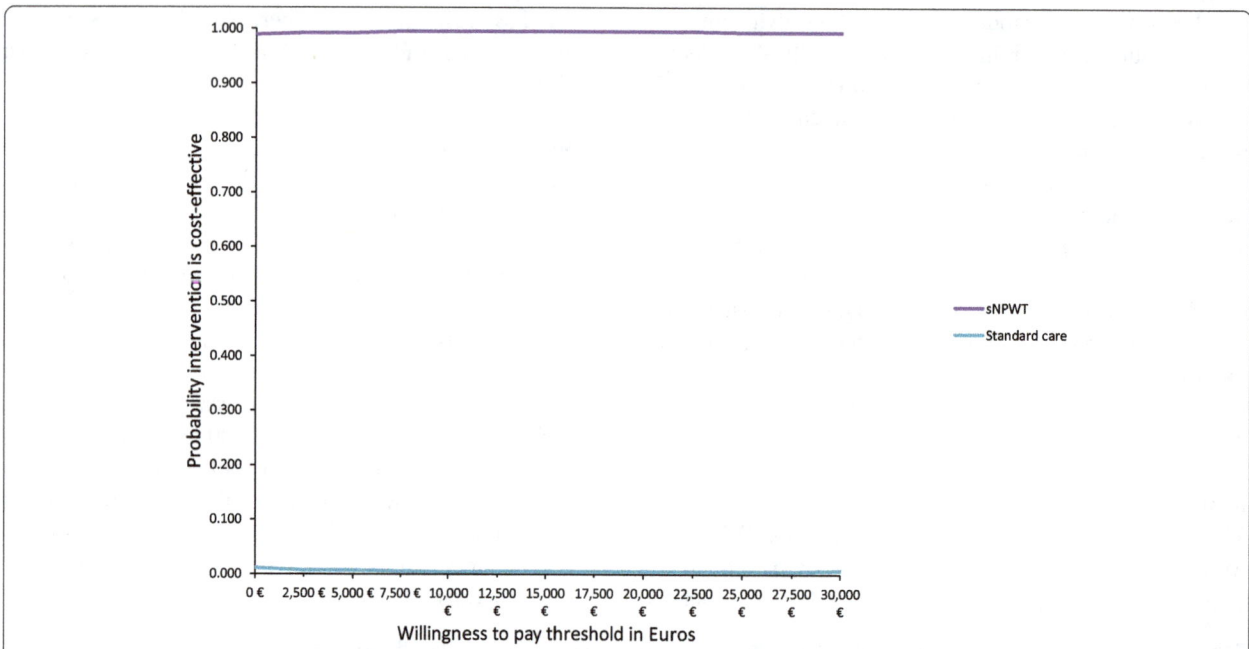

Fig. 2 Cost effectiveness acceptability curves for sNPWT compared to standard care in patients following CABG surgery. Cost-effectiveness acceptability curves depicting results of the probabilistic sensitivity analysis for the two interventions sNPWT and SC. The y-axis gives the probability that each intervention is cost effective as a function of willingness to pay shown on the x-axis. A willingness to pay of €50,000/QALY is within the bounds of accepted cost-effectiveness thresholds. The figure suggests there is little uncertainty regarding the cost-effectiveness of sNPWT compared to SC (100% probability that sNPWT is cost-effective)

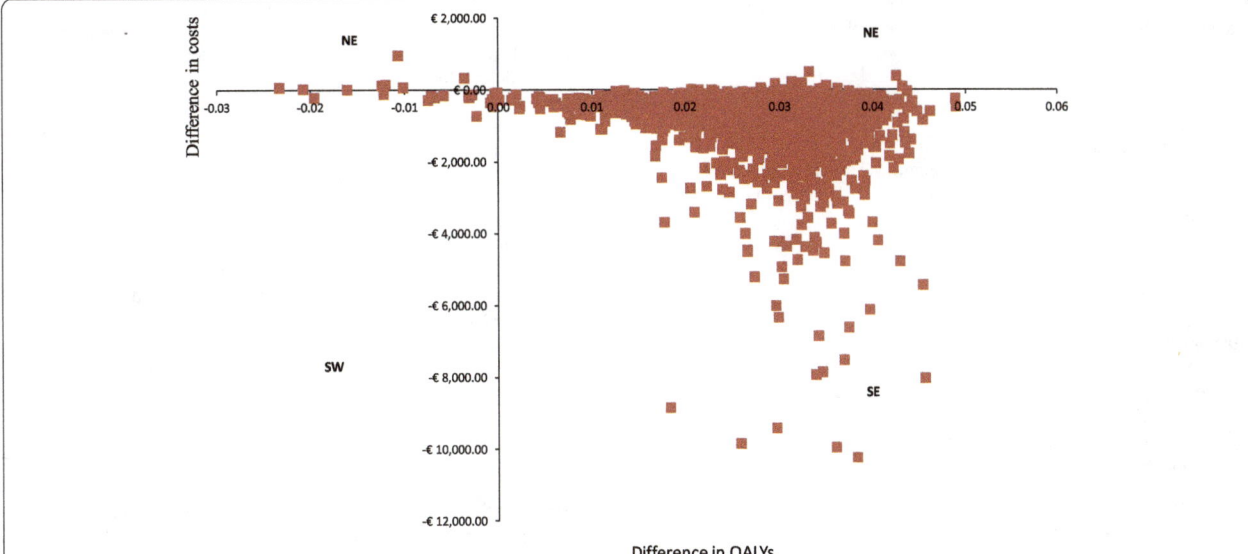

Fig. 3 Cost-effectiveness plane for sNPWT compared to standard care in patients following CABG surgery. The cost-effectiveness plane shows results of the probabilistic sensitivity analysis for the two interventions sNPWT and SC. Each point on the plot corresponds to one trial in the Monte-Carlo simulation (2000 simulations were conducted) comparing the incremental effectiveness and incremental costs of sNPWT compared to SC. Costs for sNPWT were consistently lower (read on the y-axis) and effectiveness highest (read on the x-axis) for the SSC prevention following CABG compared to SC. The figure therefore shows that sNPWT is cost-saving

Given the diversity of health systems across the world, the results of this analysis should be interpreted with caution. We acknowledge that the reimbursement systems, relative prices, and treatment practices, are important issues that vary from country to country hence country-specific assumptions may be required. However, we note that our cost-effectiveness results were tested in sensitivity analysis and the RCT measured SSI in a standard way using the ECDC matrix. A study by Hansen 2012, found that there was a high degree of concordance between European and US case definitions of healthcare-associated infections [25]. Therefore, the measurement of SSI in a standard way suggests that the results of the RCT which drive the cost-effectiveness are likely to be replicated in setting with similar baseline risks. Furthermore, our model is based on clinical data that comes from a single center RCT, multi center trials should be preferred as they yield data which is easily generalisable. We therefore encourage other scholars to update the economic model once additional evidence becomes available.

Conclusions

Our analysis found sNPWT to be less costly and more effective (dominant), resulting in an overall cost decrease of €586 per patient when used prophylactically in patients undergoing coronary artery by-pass surgery. These results remained stable in sensitivity analyses with bigger savings identified in sub-groups of patients with elevated risk of surgical site complications such as those patients with diabetes, obese and smokers. We however recommend that additional economic studies should be conducted as new evidence on the use of sNPWT in CABG patients becomes available to validate the results of this economic analysis.

Table 5 Sub-group analysis results for sNPWT compared to standard care in patients following CABG surgery

Sub-group	Cost saving with sNPWT	Additional QALYs due to sNPWT	Reduction in complications due to sNPWT
BMI ≥ 30	€ 1586	0.1147	0.1507
Diabetes	€ 1370	0.096	0.1262
Smoking	€ 1298	0.0898	0.118

Abbreviations: *sNPWT* single use negative pressure wound therapy, *BMI* body mass index, *QALYs* quality adjusted life years

Abbreviations
BMI: Body mass index; CABG: Coronary artery bypass grafting; ECDC: European Centre for Disease Prevention and Control; QALY: Quality adjusted life years; RCT: Randomised controlled trial; sNPWT: Single use negative pressure wound therapy dressings; SSC: Surgical site complications; SSI: Surgical site infections

Authors' contributions
LN conceived of the study, conducted the economic analysis and drafted the manuscript. PT conceived of the study, double checked the economic analysis and commented on the draft manuscript. MS advised on clinical aspects of the analysis and commented on the draft manuscript. FAF

advised on economic modelling aspects and commented on the draft manuscript. All authors read and approved the final manuscript.

Competing interests

LN and PT are employees of Smith & Nephew, Wound Management Hull, and may own shares of Smith & Nephew. MS and FAF have no competing financial interests.

Author details

[1]Smith & Nephew Advanced Wound Management, Global Market Access, 101 Hessle Road, Hull HU3 2BN, UK. [2]Vascular and Diabetic Centre Department of Heart Surgery, Asklepios Klinik St. Georg Cardiac, Lohmühlenstr 5, 20099 Hamburg, Germany. [3]Department of Health Professions, Manchester Metropolitan University, Manchester, UK.

References

1. European Centre for Disease Prevention and Control. Surveillance of surgical site infections in Europe 2010–2011. Stockholm: ECDC; 2013.
2. Gheorghe A, Moran G, Duffy H, Roberts T, Pinkney T, Calvert M, Health Utility Values Associated with Surgical Site Infection: A Systematic Review; DOI, https://doi.org/10.1016/j.jval.2015.08.004.
3. Reddy VS. Use of closed incision management with negative pressure therapy for complex cardiac patients. Cureus. 2016. https://doi.org/10.7759/cureus.506.
4. Shepard J, Ward W, Milstone A, Carlson T, Frederick J, Hadhazy E, Perl T. Financial impact of surgical site infections on hospitals: the hospital management perspective. JAMA Surg. 2013. https://doi.org/10.1001/jamasurg.2013.2246.
5. Dohmen PM, Gabbieri D, Weymann A, Linneweber J, Konertz W. Reduction in surgical site infection in patients treated with microbial sealant prior to coronary artery bypass graft surgery: a case control study. J Hosp Infect. 2009;72(2):119–26.
6. Graf K, Ott E, Vonberg RP, Kuehn C, Schilling T, Haverich A, Chaberny IF. Surgical site infections--economic consequences for the health care system. Langenbeck's Arch Surg. 2011. https://doi.org/10.1007/s00423-011-0772-0.
7. Lee BY, Wiringa AE, Bailey RR, Goyal V, Lewis GJ, Tsui BYK, et al. Screening cardiac surgery patients for MRSA: an economic computer model. Am J Manag Care. 2010;16:e163–73 PMID: 20645662.
8. Si D, Rajmokan M, Lakhan P, Marquess J, Coulter C, Paterson D. Surgical site infections following coronary artery bypass graft procedures: 10 years of surveillance data. BMC Infect Dis. 2014. https://doi.org/10.1186/1471-2334-14-318.
9. Grauhan O, Navasardyan A, Hofmann M, Müller P, Stein J, Hetzer R. Prevention of poststernotomy wound infections in obese patients by negative pressure wound therapy. J Thorac Cardiovasc Surg. 2013. https://doi.org/10.1016/j.jtcvs.2012.09.040.
10. Jenks PJ, Laurent M, McQuarry S, Watkins R. Clinical and economic burden of surgical site infection (SSI) and predicted financial consequences of elimination of SSI from an English hospital. J Hosp Infect. 2014;86(1):24–33.
11. Karlakki S, Whittall C, Kuiper JH, Hamad AK, et al. Incisional negative pressure wound therapy dressings (iNPWTd) in routine primary hip and knee replacements – a randomised controlled trial. Bone Joint Res. 2016;5:328–37.
12. Nherera LM, Trueman P, Karlakki SL. Cost-effectiveness analysis of single-use negative pressure wound therapy dressings (sNPWT) to reduce surgical site complications (SSC) in routine primary hip and knee replacements. Wound Repair Regen. 2017. https://doi.org/10.1111/wrr.12530.
13. Tuffaha HW, Gillespie BM, Chaboyer W, Gordon LG, Scuffham PA. Cost-utility analysis of negative pressure wound therapy in high-risk cesarean section wounds. J Surg Res. 2015;195(2):612–22.
14. Strugala V, Martin R. Meta-analysis of comparative trials evaluating a prophylactic single-use negative pressure wound therapy system for the prevention of surgical site complications. Surg Infect. 2017;18(7):810–9. https://doi.org/10.1089/sur.2017.156.
15. Hyldig N, Birke-Sorensen H, Kruse M, Vinter C, Joergensen JS, Sorensen JA, et al. Meta-analysis of negative-pressure wound therapy for closed surgical incisions. BJS. 2016. https://doi.org/10.1002/bjs.10084.
16. Cristofolini M, Worlitzsch D, Wienke A, Silber RE, Borneff-Lipp M. Surgical site infections after coronary artery bypass graft surgery: incidence, perioperative hospital stay, readmissions, and revision surgeries. Infection. 2012. https://doi.org/10.1007/s15010-012-0275-0.
17. Witt-Majchrzak A, Żelazny P, Snarska J. Preliminary outcome of treatment of postoperative primarily closed sternotomy wounds treated using negative pressure wound therapy. Pol Przegl Chir. 2015. https://doi.org/10.2478/pjs-2014-0082.
18. Germany Federal Statistical Office https://www.destatis.de/EN/FactsFigures/SocietyState/Population/Deaths/Deaths.html, (Accessed 15 Mar 2018).
19. Wu C, Camacho FT, Wechsler AS, Lahey S, Culliford AT, Jordan D, Hannan EL. A Risk Score for Predicting Long-Term Mortality Following Coronary Artery Bypass Graft Surgery. Circulation. 2012. https://doi.org/10.1161/CIRCULATIONAHA.111.055939.
20. The Aerzteblatt. https://www.aerzteblatt.de/archiv/43690/Krankenhaus-Management-Kompetenzzentren-sind-zukunftstraechtig, (Accessed 15 Mar 2018).
21. Zeidler J, Mittendorf T, Vahldiek G, von der Schulenburg JM. Comparative cost analysis of outpatient and inpatient rehabilitation for cardiac diseases. Herz. 2008. https://doi.org/10.1007/s00059-008-3126-0.
22. The Vdek association of health insurances. https://www.vdek.com/vertragspartner/heilmittel/rahmenvertrag/_jcr_content/par/download_19/file.res/Verg%C3%BCtungsvereinbarung_West_2016_UF_160321.pdf. (Accessed 15 Mar 2018).
23. Olsen MA, Lock-Burkley P, Hopkins D, Polish L, Sundt TM, Fraser VJ. The risk factors for deep and superficial chest surgical-site infections after coronary artery bypass graft surgery are different. J Thorac Cardiovasc Surg. 2002. https://doi.org/10.1067/mtc.2002.122306.
24. Posnett J, Franks PJ. The burden of chronic wounds in the UK. Nurs Times. 2008;104(3):44–5.
25. Hansen S, Sohr D, Geffers C, Astagneau P, Blacky A, Koller W, Gastmeier P. Concordance between European and US case definitions of healthcare-associated infections. Antimicrob Resist Infect Control. 2012. https://doi.org/10.1186/2047-2994-1-28.

Video assisted thoracic surgery vs. thoracotomy for locally advanced lung squamous cell carcinoma after neoadjuvant chemotherapy

Likui Fang, Luming Wang, Yiqing Wang, Wang Lv and Jian Hu*

Abstract

Background: Surgery is an important part of multidisciplinary treatment strategy for locally advanced lung squamous cell carcinoma (LSCC), but insufficient evidence supports the feasibility and safety of video assisted thoracic surgery (VATS) following neoadjuvant chemotherapy for locally advanced LSCC. This study aims to compare perioperative data and long-term survival of locally advanced LSCC patients between VATS and thoracotomy after neoadjuvant chemotherapy.

Methods: We retrospectively collected the clinical and pathological information of patients with locally advanced LSCC who underwent surgical resection after neoadjuvant chemotherapy from October 2013 to October 2017. All patients were divided into two groups (thoracotomy and VATS) and were compared the differences in perioperative, oncological and survival outcomes.

Results: A total of 81 patients were analyzed in this study (67 thoracotomy and 14 VATS). VATS provided less postoperative pain ($P = 0.005$) and produced less volume of chest drainage ($P = 0.019$) than thoracotomy, but the number of resected lymph nodes was less in VATS group ($P = 0.011$). However, there was no significant difference in the number of resected lymph node stations and the rate of nodal upstaging between two groups. The mean disease free survival (DFS) was 32.7 ± 2.7 months for the thoracotomy group and 31.8 ± 3.0 months for the VATS group ($P = 0.335$); the corresponding overall survival (OS) was 41.7 ± 2.2 months and 36.4 ± 4.1 months ($P = 0.925$).

Conclusion: In selected patients with locally advanced LSCC, VATS played a positive role in postoperative recovery and associated similar survival outcome compared with thoracotomy after neoadjuvant chemotherapy.

Keywords: Locally advanced lung squamous cell carcinoma, Neoadjuvant chemotherapy, Video assisted thoracic surgery, Thoracotomy

Introduction

Lung cancer is one of the most common cancers and the leading cause of cancer-related death in the world, and more than 80% of patients have a group of histological subtypes known as non-small cell lung cancer (NSCLC) [1]. Lung adenocarcinoma (LA) and lung squamous cell carcinoma (LSCC) are the most common subtypes of NSCLC [2]. Although operable early stage NSCLC has satisfactory prognosis with the improvement

of medical technology [3, 4], the 5-year survival rate of locally advanced NSCLC (LANSCLC) with surgery alone is only 20–35% [5]. So far, the treatment of LANSCLC has evolved from surgery alone to multidisciplinary pattern. It has been proven that neoadjuvant chemotherapy could significantly improve overall survival, time to distant recurrence, and recurrence-free survival [6], while preoperative radiotherapy do not add any survival benefit to neoadjuvant chemotherapy followed by surgery [7]. Neoadjuvant chemotherapy has been a valid treatment option for most of patients with LANSCLC. However, there also have been many controversial debates about

* Correspondence: dr_hujian@zju.edu.cn
Department of Thoracic Surgery, the First Affiliated Hospital, Zhejiang University School of Medicine, Hangzhou 310003, China

the operation based multidisciplinary treatment, one of which is the selection of surgical approaches after neoadjuvant chemotherapy, thoracotomy or video assisted thoracic surgery (VATS).

VATS is superior to open surgery for the resection of early stage NSCLC, because it can minimize complications, provide less pain and offer faster recovery with at least equivalent long-term survival rate [8, 9]. VATS was initially proposed only for operable early stage lung cancer, but in recent years it has been carried out by some experienced thoracic surgeons in LANSCLC with satisfactory outcome [10, 11]. However, there were only few studies reporting the outcome of VATS following neoadjuvant therapy [12, 13] and currently, no published study reported the comparison between VATS and thoracotomy following neoadjuvant chemotherapy in locally advanced LSCC staged by the eighth American Joint Committee on Cancer (AJCC 8) staging system.

In this study, we aimed to compare perioperative data and long-term survival of locally advanced LSCC patients between VATS and thoracotomy after neoadjuvant chemotherapy. The primary goal of this study was to explore the feasibility and safety of VATS following neoadjuvant chemotherapy for locally advanced LSCC in terms of intraoperative and postoperative outcomes.

Methods

Patients selection

The study protocol was approved by the Institutional Review Board of the First Affiliated Hospital of Zhejiang University, School of Medicine. The data in this study was collected retrospectively from hospital electronic medical records system, including demographic characteristics, preoperative investigations, intraoperative data and postoperative course between October 2013 and October 2017.

All patients included in the analysis were restaged by AJCC 8 staging system [14] and fitted the following criteria: (1) the disease was pathologically diagnosed as LSCC; (2) the patient did not have distant metastasis before neoadjuvant chemotherapy; (3) the surgery was preceded by neoadjuvant chemotherapy.

We excluded patients with a history of previous cancers, other concurrent malignant disease and patients who underwent pulmonary resection previously. Locally advanced squamous lung cancer was mainly defined as stageIII, while the patients with stage T3 was also regarded as locally advanced disease. Clinical lymph node (LN) status was assessed by CT scan, PET scan and/or endobronchial ultrasound. Tumor size was defined as the maximum diameter of the pathological specimens.

Patients were retrospectively classified into the thoracotomy group and VATS group on the basis of the surgical approach. Patients undergoing conversion in the VATS group were eliminated from the study group.

Treatment protocol and response assessment

Neoadjuvant chemotherapy consisted of platinum-based two-drug regimen with 2 cycles, while the cycle was adjusted with tumor response and adverse effects after systematic evaluation. Generally, the resection was performed within 6 weeks after neoadjuvant chemotherapy and adjuvant therapy was carried out depending on the recovery condition of patients. Tumor response was classified according to Response Evaluation Criteria in Solid Tumors version 1.1 (RECIST 1.1) criteria [15]. The patients who had received at least 1 cycle of chemotherapy were candidates for response assessment.

Surgical procedures

All patients underwent general anesthesia with single-lung ventilation and were placed in lateral decubitus position. Conventional posterolateral serratus divided thoracotomies were performed in the open procedures, and 3-ports approach was adopted in the thoracoscopic procedures. Generally, bronchi, pulmonary vasculature and parenchyma were resected by the corresponding endoscopic cut stapler. Prior closing, the cavity was rinsed by normal saline to detect potential air leak and one chest tube was placed in the appropriate position at the end of the procedure. The tube was removed when it was clearly confirmed no air leak and the volume of drainage was less than 200 mL/day. In contrast, when pneumonectomy was performed the tube was normally clipped after surgery and removed when there was no abnormal appearance in roentgenograms.

Follow-up

Follow-up data were collected by telephone calls and reviewing the records of reexamination in the outpatient clinic. The last follow-up time was February 2018. The outcomes of interest of the current study included disease-free survival (DFS) and overall survival (OS). DFS was calculated from the day of surgery to the date of cancer recurrence or death from any cause. Patients who did not have a recurrence or who did not die during the study period were censored at the date they were last confirmed to be alive with no evidence of disease. OS was calculated from the day of surgery to the time of death. Patients who did not die during the study period were censored at the date they were last confirmed to be alive.

Statistical analysis

The measurement data and numeration data were statistically analyzed with t test and χ^2 test respectively. DFS and OS were estimated using the Kaplan-Meier method.

All the above analysis was conducted by SPSS software (version 19.0, IBM SPSS Inc. United States). The statistical power analysis was further conducted by R (version 3.2.5; R Development Core Team) when the differences between the two groups were statistical significant. Statistical significance was set at P value < 0.05 (All P values presented were 2-sided).

Result

Patients' characteristics

From October 2013 to October 2017, a total of 83 patients fitted the criteria for inclusion in the study: 67 treated with thoracotomy and 16 treated with VATS. Two patients converted to thoracotomy because of severe adhesions were eliminated from the VATS group, so there were 67 patients in the thoracotomy group and 14 patients in the VATS group finally. The major demographic and clinical characteristics were listed in Table 1. There was no significant gender difference between thoracotomy group and VATS group, in which the male gender occupied 94.0 and 78.6%, respectively. The age was also similar between two groups. It was comparable in the two groups for the number of patients with other possible prognostic factors which might be predictive of survival, including body mass index (BMI) [16], weight loss (more than 5%) [17] and other nutritional status [18].

Disease characteristics

The disease characteristics of two groups were listed in Table 2 in detail. There was no significant difference between thoracotomy group and VATS group in the clinical stage before neoadjuvant chemotherapy with 54 (80.6%) and 13 (92.9%) patients in stage IIIA or IIIB, respectively. It was worth mentioning that 14 patients (13 in thoracotomy group and 1 in VATS group) with IIIA disease in seventh AJCC staging system were restaged as IIB disease in eighth AJCC staging system. More than half of the patients received the regimens consisted of gemcitabine and platinum with 2 cycles in both groups. T stage was similar in two groups either before neoadjuvant chemotherapy of after, as well as the number of T downstaging. Clinical complete response (cCR) was seen in 1 patient in both groups, retrospectively, while 43 (64.2%) patients in thoracotomy group and 11 (78.6%) patients in VATS group were evaluated as partial response (PR). Only 4 (6.0%) patients in thoracotomy group were classified in progressive disease (PD), with one patient having oligometastasis in 11th thoracic vertebra. However, the primary tumor of the patient with oligometastasis was detected with only few cancer cells under the microscope. The number of patients with downstaging after neoadjuvant chemotherapy which was a certain prognostic factor was comparable in two groups. There was also no statistical difference in pathologic stage and tumor size between two groups.

Table 1 The demographic and clinical characteristics in the thoracotomy and VATS group

Variables	Thoracotomy ($N = 67$)	VATS ($N = 14$)	P value
Male gender	63 (94.0%)	11 (78.6%)	0.177
Age (year)	60 (29–77)	61 (55–73)	0.182
Smoking	59 (88.1%)	11 (78.6%)	0.608
Drinking	29 (43.3%)	5 (35.7%)	0.602
BMI	23 (17–30)	23 (18–29)	1
Weight loss	15 (22.4%)	2 (14.3%)	0.752
Hypertension	12 (17.9%)	6 (42.9%)	0.091
Diabetes	5 (7.5%)	1 (7.1%)	1
COPD	1 (1.5%)	0 (0)	1
Lymphocyte (10^9/L)	1.5 (0.8–4.0)	1.6 (0.7–3.2)	0.954
Total protein (g/L)	68.8 (54.4–82.4)	67.3 (39.2–80.6)	0.077
Albumin (g/L)	41.6 (26.6–54.8)	39.2 (20.9–50.9)	0.128
Serum Creatinine (mmol/L)	69.0 (52.0–105.0)	68.5 (50.0–119.0)	0.507
Serum trioxypurine (mmol/L)	296.5 (192.0–455.0)	319.5 (157.0–462.0)	0.676
Triglyceride (mmol/L)	1.1 (0.4–4.1)	1.2 (0.7–3.0)	0.581
Cholesterol (mmol/L)	4.2 (2.7–6.1)	4.3 (2.7–8.0)	0.399

Values are N (percentage) or median (range)

BMI body mass index, *COPD* chronic obstructive pulmonary disease, *VATS* video assisted thoracic surgery

Table 2 The disease characteristics in the thoracotomy and VATS group

Variables	Thoracotomy (N = 67)	VATS (N = 14)	P value
T stage before neoadjuvant chemotherapy			0.135
1b	0 (0)	1 (7.1%)	
1c	1 (1.5%)	2 (14.3%)	
2a	25 (37.3%)	3 (21.4%)	
2b	7 (10.4%)	2 (14.3%)	
3	19 (28.4%)	3 (21.4%)	
4	15 (22.4%)	3 (21.4%)	
Clinical stage before neoadjuvant chemotherapy			0.508
IIB	13 (19.4%)	1 (7.1%)	
IIIA	32 (47.8%)	7 (50.0%)	
IIIB	22 (32.8%)	6 (42.9%)	
Neoadjuvant chemotherapy regimens			0.664
Docetaxel + platinum	16 (23.9%)	2 (14.3%)	
Paclitaxel + platinum	16 (23.9%)	3 (21.4%)	
Gemcitabine + platinum	35 (52.2%)	9 (64.3%)	
Cycles of neoadjuvant chemotherapy	2 (1–5)	2 (2–4)	0.930
T stage after neoadjuvant chemotherapy			0.058
0	1 (1.5%)	1 (7.1%)	
1b	1 (1.5%)	2 (14.3%)	
1c	0 (0)	1 (7.1%)	
2a	42 (62.7%)	8 (57.1%)	
2b	6 (9.0%)	0 (0)	
3	14 (20.9%)	1 (7.1%)	
4	3 (4.5%)	1 (7.1%)	
Clinical stage after neoadjuvant chemotherapy			0.308
0	1 (1.5%)	1 (7.1%)	
IB	15 (22.4%)	4 (28.6%)	
IIA	1 (1.5%)	0 (0)	
IIB	12 (17.9%)	0 (0)	
IIIA	25 (37.3%)	7 (50.0%)	
IIIB	12 (17.9%)	2 (14.3%)	
VI	1 (1.5%)	0 (0)	
Response assessment			0.261
cCR	1 (1.5%)	1 (7.1%)	
PR	43 (64.2%)	11 (78.6%)	
SD	19 (28.4%)	2 (14.3%)	
PD	4 (6.0%)	0 (0)	
T downstaging	28 (41.8%)	9 (64.3%)	0.124
TNM downstaging	29 (43.3%)	8 (57.1%)	0.344
Pathologic stage			0.221
IA	1 (1.5%)	3 (21.4%)	
IB	22 (32.8%)	3 (21.4%)	
IIA	2 (3.0%)	0 (0)	
IIB	18 (26.9%)	3 (21.4%)	

Table 2 The disease characteristics in the thoracotomy and VATS group *(Continued)*

Variables	Thoracotomy (*N* = 67)	VATS (*N* = 14)	*P* value
IIIA	18 (26.9%)	4 (28.6%)	
IIIB	5 (7.5%)	1 (7.1%)	
VI	1 (1.5%)	0 (0)	
Tumor size (cm)[a]	3.1 (0.8–8.0)	2.5 (1.0–7.0)	0.335

Values are N (percentage) or median (range)

cCR clinical complete response, *PR* partial response, *SD* stable disease, *PD* progressive disease

[a]Only few cancer cells in 4 patients were observed microscopically (3 patients in thoracotomy group and 1 in VATS group), so the tumor size of the 4 cases was unable to measure

Perioperative data

The detailed information of surgical outcome was presented in Table 3. Surgical procedure was comparable in both groups, although there was no double sleeve lobectomy and pneumonectomy in VATS group. In contrast, the number of resected lymph nodes in thoracotomy group was more than that in VATS group (*P* = 0.011, power = 80.4%), but there was no significant difference in the number of resected lymph node stations and the case of nodal upstaging. The rate of negative surgical margin in VATS group reached up to 92.9% which was seemed to be higher than that in thoracotomy group but the difference was not of statistical significance. The operation time and blood loss were also similar in two groups, but the volume of chest drainage in VATS group was less than that in thoracotomy group (*P* = 0.019, power = 80.1%), although the duration of chest drainage was comparable. In addition, the VATS group had a clear advantage over the thoracotomy group in terms of postoperative pain (*P* = 0.005, power = 62.2%) which was recorded by numerical rating scale (NRS) [19]. Perioperative complications ranked by Clavien-Dindo classification [20] were comparable in thoracotomy and VATS groups with 9 (13.4%), 9 (13.4%), 2 (3.0%) and 1 (7.1%), 2 (14.3%), 0 (0) in GradeI, GradeII, GradeIII, respectively. The length of postoperative hospital stay was also comparable in two groups. The delay and protocol of adjuvant therapy after surgery in thoracotomy group were similar to those in VATS group as well.

Survival outcome

Follow-up information was successfully collected from 73 of 81 patients with median follow-up time of 15 months (range: 3 to 48 months). Tumor recurrence and death occurred in 18 cases (9 deaths, 9 alive with disease). Four patients evaluated as PD after neoadjuvant chemotherapy were all alive during the follow-up period. The patient who had oligometastasis in 11th thoracic vertebra received concurrent chemoradiotherapy and had been living for more than 3 months after surgery with satisfactory life quality. Other patients had been living for 9, 13 and 16 months after surgery, respectively, with one patient alive with disease. The mean DFS and

OS were 32.7 ± 2.7 months, 41.7 ± 2.2 months for the thoracotomy group and 31.8 ± 3.0 months, 36.4 ± 4.1 months for the VATS group, respectively. The differences between two groups were not statistically significant (Figs. 1 and 2).

Discussion

In spite of the increased prevalence of early stage NSCLC with satisfactory survival outcome, the treatment of LANSCLC remains challenging. Early stage NSCLC patients are commonly treated with radical resection, but unfortunately most patients with LANSCLC do not benefit clearly by surgery alone or even by chemoradiotherapy [21]. In the result, neoadjuvant therapy has been proposed in order to better achieve local and distant disease control in LANSCLC. Although neoadjuvant chemoradiotherapy followed by surgery had been proven to be a feasible and safe treatment strategy [22, 23], several subsequent studies reported that preoperative radiotherapy significantly increased the occurrence of bronchopleural fistula after surgery [24] and did not add any survival benefit to neoadjuvant chemotherapy followed by surgery [7, 25]. Of course, neoadjuvant chemotherapy had some controversial problems, one of which was the challenges in surgery, including perioperative complications, interval time and the surgical approach.

In spite of lacking multicenter prospective researches, a large number of retrospective studies proved that neoadjuvant chemotherapy did not add any extra risk to the occurrence of perioperative complications and mortality [7, 26, 27] even though mediastinal structures become differently affected after neoadjuvant chemotherapy. In addition, the optimal interval time from the end of neoadjuvant chemotherapy to surgery was proven to be not more than 6 weeks [28]. However, there was little evidence suggesting the preferable surgical approach after neoadjuvant chemotherapy in LANSCLC, especially in local advanced LSCC, thoracotomy or VATS. Historically, VATS was initially recommended only for early stage disease, but with the technological improvement and growing experience, a few experts started to use the VATS platform to carry out pulmonary resection in

Table 3 Perioperative data in the thoracotomy and VATS group

Variables	Thoracotomy (N = 69)	VATS (N = 14)	P value	Cohen's d value	Statistical power
Surgical procedure			0.078		
Sublobar resection	1 (1.5%)	2 (14.3%)			
Lobectomy	39 (58.2%)	8 (57.1%)			
Bilobectomy	6 (9.0%)	3 (21.4%)			
Sleeve lobectomy	9 (13.4%)	1 (7.1%)			
Double sleeve lobectomy	2 (3.0%)	0 (0)			
Pneumonectomy	10 (14.9%)	0 (0)			
Surgical margin			0.760		
R0	59 (88.1%)	13 (92.9%)			
R1	7 (10.4%)	1 (7.1%)			
R2	1 (1.5%)	0 (0)			
Number of resected LNs	20 (2–57)	16 (1–28)	0.011	0.838	80.4%
Number of resected LN stations	7 (2–12)	7 (1–10)	0.856		
Nodal upstaging	13 (19.4%)	4 (28.6%)	0.685		
Operation time (minutes)	146 (87–410)	145 (73–364)	0.411		
Blood loss (ml)	100 (20–400)	83 (10–500)	0.819		
Numerical pain rating scale	2 (1–7)	2 (1–3)	0.005	0.676	62.2%
Chest drainage (ml)	1035 (150–5850)	550 (30–2100)	0.019	0.835	80.1%
Duration of chest drainage (days)	5 (2–20)	4 (2–15)	0.285		
Complications	20 (29.9%)	3 (21.4%)	0.729		
GradeI	9 (13.4%)	1 (7.1%)			
GradeII	9 (13.4%)	2 (14.3%)			
GradeIII	2 (3.0%)	0 (0)			
Postoperative hospital stay (days)	7 (4–21)	6 (4–16)	0.066		
Mortality within 30 days	0 (0)	0 (0)	/		
Delay of adjuvant therapy (days)	40 (21–127)	36 (23–57)	0.353		
Protocol of Adjuvant therapy			0.275		
Chemotherapy	36 (53.7%)	10 (71.4%)			
Radiotherapy	6 (9.0%)	0 (0)			
Chemoradiotherapy	16 (23.9%)	4 (28.6%)			
Unknown	9 (13.4%)	0 (0)			

Values are N (percentage) or median (range)
LN lymph node

LANSCLC. Jun Huang et al. [13] publishing a single institution retrospective series of 43 cases reported that VATS following neoadjuvant therapy was safe and feasible for the treatment of LANSCLC with low incidence of postoperative complications and mortality. Unfortunately, this study did not compare the surgical and survival outcomes of VATS with those of thoracotomy. Another study reported by Bernard J. Park et al. [12] compared minimally invasive lobectomy (VATS and robotic) with open lobectomy and concluded that minimally invasive surgery possessed good feasibility, good safety and an acceptable survival time in appropriately selected patients with LANSCLC after neoadjuvant

chemotherapy. However, this study mainly focused on lung adenocarcinoma and lobectomy. Meanwhile, the age between two groups had statistical difference, which might cause potential bias in the conclusion.

In this study, we explored whether VATS was suitable to be applied in locally advanced LSCC staged by AJCC 8 staging system or not. We observed similar operative time and blood loss between VATS and thoracotomy, but VATS had advantages in postoperative pain and chest drainage. Interestingly, duration of chest drainage was similar in two groups, but the length of postoperative hospital stay was seemed to be shorter in VATS group although the difference was not statistically

Video assisted thoracic surgery vs. thoracotomy for locally advanced lung squamous cell carcinoma...

173

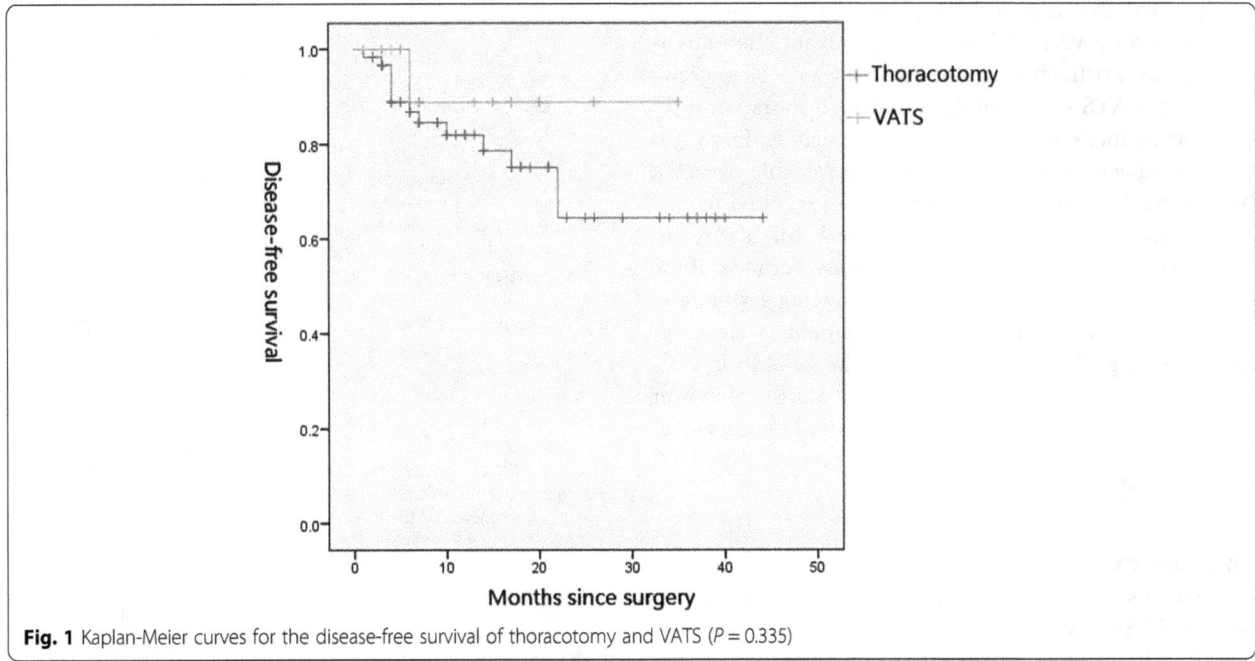

Fig. 1 Kaplan-Meier curves for the disease-free survival of thoracotomy and VATS (*P* = 0.335)

significant. The rate and the severity of complications were also comparable. These results suggested that VATS played a positive role in enhanced recovery after surgery (ERAS) in locally advanced LSCC with equivalent survival to thoracotomy.

Systematic lymph node resection is an important part of surgical treatment for LANSCLC. It is a controversial problem about the quality of nodal assessment provided by VATS when compared to thoracotomy and its impact on long-term survival. Some publications indicated more lymph nodes were resected and a higher nodal upstaging rate was found in open surgery [29], while other studies suggested no correlation between the surgical approach and the number of lymph nodes resected [30]. In this study, we thoroughly analyzed the quality of lymph node resection between VATS and thoracotomy after neoadjuvant chemotherapy. Although the number of resected lymph node in VATS group was less than that in thoracotomy group, the number of resected stations and the rate of nodal upstaging were both similar in two groups.

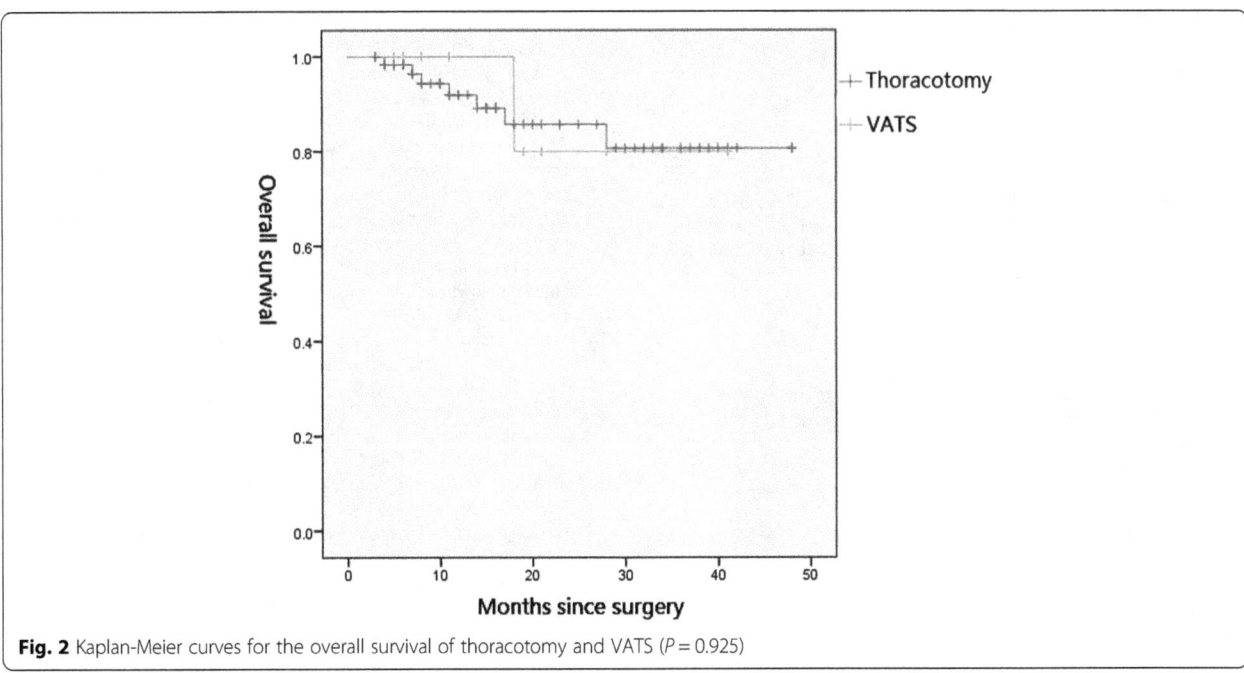

Fig. 2 Kaplan-Meier curves for the overall survival of thoracotomy and VATS (*P* = 0.925)

It suggested that a radical lymph node dissection could be achieved by VATS following neoadjuvant chemotherapy. It was worthwhile to note that the rate of negative margin of VATS was equivalent to that of thoracotomy.

However, there are some limits in this study. First, it is the retrospective study that has unavoidable selected bias, so further prospective evidence is warranted to verify the validity of our findings. Second, this study included some patients restaged IIB disease because of the difference between the seventh AJCC staging system and the eighth in the T stage, but most patients were diagnosed as stage IIIA or IIIB. Lastly, the sample is relatively small in this study, although the statistical power analysis was further conducted when the differences between the two groups were statistically significant.

Conclusions

This study suggested that in selected patients with locally advanced LSCC VATS following neoadjuvant chemotherapy played a positive role in ERAS and associated similar oncological and survival outcome with thoracotomy.

Abbreviations

LSCC: Lung squamous cell carcinoma; LA: Lung adenocarcinoma; NSCLC: Non-small cell lung cancer; LANSCLC: Locally advanced non-small cell lung cancer; VATS: Video assisted thoracic surgery; DFS: Disease free survival; OS: Overall survival; AJCC 8: The eighth American Joint Committee on Cancer; LN: Lymph node; BMI: Body mass index; cCR: Clinical complete response; PR: Partial response; SD: Stable disease; PD: Progressive disease; ERAS: Enhanced recovery after surgery; COPD: Chronic obstructive pulmonary disease

Acknowledgements

Not applicable.

Funding

This study was funded by Major science and technology projects of Zhejiang province (2014C03032), Key research project of traditional Chinese medicine science and technology plan in Zhejiang Province (2015ZZ007) and National Key R&D Program of China (2017YFC0113500). The funders had no role in study design, data collection and analysis, decision to publish, or preparation of the manuscript.

Authors' contributions

JH and LF contributed to the conception and design of the work. LF contributed to conception, design, data analysis and editing the manuscript. LF, LW and YW contributed to data acquisition, statistical analysis and interpretation of the data. WL contributed to the revision of the manuscript. All authors have approved the final draft of the manuscript and there are no conflicts of interest.

Competing interests

The authors declare that they have no competing interests.

References

1. Torre LA, Bray F, Siegel RL, Ferlay J, Lortet-Tieulent J, Jemal A. Global cancer statistics, 2012[J]. CA Cancer J Clin. 2015;65(2):87–108.
2. Molina JR, Yang P, Cassivi SD, Schild SE, Adjei AA. Non-small cell lung cancer: epidemiology, risk factors, treatment, and survivorship [J]. Mayo Clin Proc. 2008;83(5):584–94.
3. Darling GE, Allen MS, Decker PA, Ballman K, Malthaner RA, Inculet RI, Jones DR, McKenna RJ, Landreneau RJ, Rusch VW, Putnam JB Jr. Randomized trial of mediastinal lymph node sampling versus complete lymphadenectomy during pulmonary resection in the patient with N0 or N1 (less than hilar) non-small cell carcinoma: results of the American College of Surgery Oncology Group Z0030 Trial [J]. J Thorac Cardiovasc Surg. 2011;141(3):662–70.
4. van den Berg LL, Klinkenberg TJ, Groen HJ, Widder J. Patterns of recurrence and survival after surgery or stereotactic radiotherapy for early stage NSCLC [J]. J Thorac Oncol. 2015;10(5):826–31.
5. Berghmans T, Paesmans M, Sculier JP. Prognostic factors in stage III non-small cell lung cancer: a review of conventional, metabolic and new biological variables [J]. Ther Adv Med Oncol. 2011;3(3):127–38.
6. Group NM-aC. Preoperative chemotherapy for non-small-cell lung cancer: a systematic review and meta-analysis of individual participant data [J]. Lancet. 2014;383(9928):1561–71.
7. Pless M, Stupp R, Ris H-B, Stahel RA, Weder W, Thierstein S, Gerard M-A, Xyrafas A, Früh M, Cathomas R, Zippelius A, Roth A, Bijelovic M, Ochsenbein A, Meier UR, Mamot C, Rauch D, Gautschi O, Betticher DC, Mirimanoff R-O, Peters S. Induction chemoradiation in stage IIIA/N2 non-small-cell lung cancer: a phase 3 randomised trial [J]. Lancet. 2015;386(9998):1049–56.
8. Hanna WC, de Valence M, Atenafu EG, Cypel M, Waddell TK, Yasufuku K, Pierre A, De Perrot M, Keshavjee S, Darling GE. Is video-assisted lobectomy for non-small-cell lung cancer oncologically equivalent to open lobectomy?[J]. Eur J Cardiothorac Surg. 2013;43(6):1121–5.
9. Klapper J, D'Amico TA. VATS versus open surgery for lung cancer resection: moving toward a minimally invasive approach [J]. J Natl Compr Cancer Netw. 2015;13(2):162–4.
10. Zhou S, Pei G, Han Y, Yu D, Song X, Li Y, Xiao N, Liu S, Liu Z, Xu S. Sleeve lobectomy by video-assisted thoracic surgery versus thoracotomy for non-small cell lung cancer [J]. J Cardiothorac Surg. 2015;10:116.
11. Gonzalez-Rivas D, Yang Y, Stupnik T, Sekhniaidze D, Fernandez R, Velasco C, Zhu Y, Jiang G. Uniportal video-assisted thoracoscopic bronchovascular, tracheal and carinal sleeve resectionsdagger [J]. Eur J Cardiothorac Surg. 2016;49(Suppl 1):i6–16.
12. Park BJ, Yang HX, Woo KM, Sima CS. Minimally invasive (robotic assisted thoracic surgery and video-assisted thoracic surgery) lobectomy for the treatment of locally advanced non-small cell lung cancer [J]. J Thorac Dis. 2016;8(Suppl 4):S406–13.
13. Huang J, Xu X, Chen H, Yin W, Shao W, Xiong X, He J. Feasibility of complete video-assisted thoracoscopic surgery following neoadjuvant therapy for locally advanced non-small cell lung cancer [J]. J Thorac Dis. 2013;5(Suppl 3):S267–73.
14. Rami-Porta R, Asamura H, Travis WD, Rusch VW. Lung cancer - major changes in the American joint committee on Cancer eighth edition cancer staging manual [J]. CA Cancer J Clin. 2017;67(2):138–55.
15. Eisenhauer EA, Therasse P, Bogaerts J, Schwartz LH, Sargent D, Ford R, Dancey J, Arbuck S, Gwyther S, Mooney M, Rubinstein L, Shankar L, Dodd L, Kaplan R, Lacombe D, Verweij J. New response evaluation criteria in solid tumours: revised RECIST guideline (version 1.1) [J]. Eur J Cancer. 2009;45(2):228–47.
16. Yang Y, Dong J, Sun K, Zhao L, Zhao F, Wang L, Jiao Y. Obesity and incidence of lung cancer: a meta-analysis [J]. Int J Cancer. 2013;132(5): 1162–9.
17. Finkelstein DM, Ettinger DS, Ruckdeschel JC. Long-term survivors in metastatic non-small-cell lung cancer: an eastern cooperative oncology group study [J]. J Clin Oncol. 1986;4(5):702–9.
18. Akamine T, Toyokawa G, Matsubara T, Kozuma Y, Haratake N, Takamori S, Katsura M, Takada K, Shoji F, Okamoto T, Maehara Y. Significance of the preoperative CONUT score in predicting postoperative disease-free and overall survival in patients with lung adenocarcinoma with obstructive lung disease [J]. Anticancer Res. 2017;37(5):2735–42.
19. Hartrick CT, Kovan JP, Shapiro S. The numeric rating scale for clinical pain measurement: a ratio measure?[J]. Pain Pract. 2003;3(4):310–6.

20. Dindo D, Demartines N, Clavien PA. Classification of surgical complications: a new proposal with evaluation in a cohort of 6336 patients and results of a survey [J]. Ann Surg. 2004;240(2):205–13.

21. Koletsis EN, Prokakis C, Apostolakis E, Chatzimichalis A, Dougenis D. Surgery after induction chemoradiotherapy for non small cell lung cancer: when and why [J]. J buon. 2007;12(4):453–61.

22. Stupp R, Mayer M, Kann R, Weder W, Zouhair A, Betticher DC, Roth AD, Stahel RA, Majno SB, Peters S, Jost L, Furrer M, Thierstein S, Schmid RA, Hsu-Schmitz SF, Mirimanoff RO, Ris HB, Pless M. Neoadjuvant chemotherapy and radiotherapy followed by surgery in selected patients with stage IIIB non-small-cell lung cancer: a multicentre phase II trial [J]. Lancet Oncol. 2009; 10(8):785–93.

23. Kusumoto S, Hirose T, Fukayama M, Kataoka D, Hamada K, Sugiyama T, Shirai T, Yamaoka T, Okuda K, Ohnishi T, Ohmori T, Kadokura M, Adachi M. Induction chemoradiotherapy followed by surgery for locally advanced non-small cell lung cancer [J]. Oncol Rep. 2009;22(5):1157–62.

24. Li S, Fan J, Liu J, Zhou J, Ren Y, Shen C, Che G. Neoadjuvant therapy and risk of bronchopleural fistula after lung cancer surgery: a systematic meta-analysis of 14 912 patients [J]. Jpn J Clin Oncol. 2016;46(6):534–46.

25. Sher DJ, Fidler MJ, Liptay MJ, Koshy M. Comparative effectiveness of neoadjuvant chemoradiotherapy versus chemotherapy alone followed by surgery for patients with stage IIIA non-small cell lung cancer [J]. Lung Cancer. 2015;88(3):267–74.

26. Brouchet L, Bauvin E, Marcheix B, Bigay-Game L, Renaud C, Berjaud J, Falcoze PE, Venissac N, Raz D, Jablons D, Mazieres J, Dahan M. Impact of induction treatment on postoperative complications in the treatment of non-small cell lung cancer [J]. J Thorac Oncol. 2007;2(7):626–31.

27. Glover J, Velez-Cubian FO, Toosi K, Ng E, Moodie CC, Garrett JR, Fontaine JP, Toloza EM. Perioperative outcomes and lymph node assessment after induction therapy in patients with clinical N1 or N2 non-small cell lung cancer [J]. J Thorac Dis. 2016;8(8):2165–74.

28. Gao SJ, Corso CD, Wang EH, Blasberg JD, Detterbeck FC, Boffa DJ, Decker RH, Kim AW. Timing of surgery after neoadjuvant Chemoradiation in locally advanced non-small cell lung Cancer [J]. J Thorac Oncol. 2017;12(2):314–22.

29. Merritt RE, Hoang CD, Shrager JB. Lymph node evaluation achieved by open lobectomy compared with thoracoscopic lobectomy for N0 lung cancer [J]. Ann Thorac Surg. 2013;96(4):1171–7.

30. Zhong C, Yao F, Zhao H. Clinical outcomes of thoracoscopic lobectomy for patients with clinical N0 and pathologic N2 non-small cell lung cancer [J]. Ann Thorac Surg. 2013;95(3):987–92.

26

The midterm results of coronary endarterectomy in patients with diffuse coronary artery disease

Zhibing Qiu[1], L. Auchoybur Merveesh[1], Yueyue Xu[1], Yinshuo Jiang[1], Liming Wang[1], Ming Xu[1], Fei Xiang[1] and Xin Chen[1,2]*

Abstract

Background: Diffuse coronary artery disease is a challenge for both percutaneous coronary intervention (PCI) and coronary artery bypass grafting (CABG). Coronary artery endarterectomy (CE) coupled with CABG is an alternative method to achieve complete revascularization. The mid- and long-term results of CE are largely questionable. The aim is to evaluate the early and mid-term graft patency of concomitant coronary artery endarterectomy and CABG.

Methods: A total of 304 patients who had undergone concomitant CE and CABG for diffuse coronary artery disease were identified from our database. A total of 238 patients (1) with complete operative records, (2) with good graft flow during surgery, (3) who were discharged, (4) with a one-year/ three-year follow-up were included in our study. The follow-up information was obtained directly from our out-patient department and by telephone contact. The categorical and continuous values were analyzed by Chi Square test and student's test respectively.

Results: CE was performed on 238 patients who represented a total of 269 target coronary vessels. The mean age of the patients was 67.8 ± 6.8 years old; male to female patient ratio was 170:68. The mean intensive care unit stay was 1.7 ± 8 days, and mean post-operative length of hospital stay was 11 ± 3 days. The average follow up time was 41.8 ± 21.4 months. At follow-up, the overall graft patency was 78.4% at one year and 69.8% at three years. The left coronary graft patency rate was significantly higher than the right coronary graft patency rate (87.4% vs 73.1% at one-year and 78.2% vs 64.8% at three years). There was no significant difference in graft patency rates between the on-pump CE + CABG vs off-pump CE + CABG groups at one year (80.0% vs 76.9%) and at three years (92.3% vs 91.7%). At the one-year follow up, 92.3% of grafts showed grade A patency in the on-pump group versus 91.7% in the off-pump group; 7.7% of grafts showed grade B patency in the on-pump group versus 8.3% in the off-pump group. At the three-year follow up, 80.6% of grafts showed grade A patency in the on-pump group versus 77.4% in the off-pump group; 19.4% of grafts showed grade B patency in the on-pump group versus 22.6% in the off -pump group. The Predictors of better graft patency are use of LIMA graft, CE on LAD, and intra-operative graft flow meter and PI.

Conclusions: In patients with diffuse coronary disease, CE is a safe and feasible technique for a select group of patients with excellent mid-term survival rates and graft patency rates. CE produces better overall results when performed on the LAD, and grafted over with the LIMA. Similar outcomes are obtained with both on-pump and off-pump surgery. For a select group of patients, coronary endarterectomy (CE) offers an alternative choice of coronary artery reconstruction and complete coronary revascularization.

Keywords: Coronary endarterectomy, Coronary artery bypass grafting, Graft patency, Follow-up results

* Correspondence: stevecx@njmu.edu.cn
[1]Department of Thoracic and Cardiovascular Surgery. Nanjing First Hospital, Nanjing Medical University, Changle Rd 68, Nanjing 210006, Jiangsu, China
[2]Department of Cardiothoracic and vascular Surgery, Nanjing First Hospital, Nanjing Medical University, 68 Changle Rd, Nanjing 210006, China

Background

Revascularization of diffuse coronary artery disease is still challenging for both percutaneous coronary intervention (PCI) and coronary artery bypass grafting (CABG). These techniques often prove to be inadequate when dealing with severe diffuse coronary atherosclerosis. An alternative to achieve complete revascularization is coronary endarterectomy (CE) which was introduced in the 1950s with the first procedures performed without cardiopulmonary bypass [1]. Initially, CE followed by CABG lost popularity due to higher associated rates of perioperative morbidity and mortality as compared to CABG alone [2]. Moreover, the complications are even more fatal when CE is performed on arteries that are crucial to achieve optimal effect, such as the left anterior descending (LAD) artery, where failure to obtain optimal blood flow results in catastrophic clinical outcomes. It is debatable, however, that the difference in favorable outcomes between CE + CABG and CABG alone is due to lesion complexity. Fukui T et al., postulate that the higher risks associated with CE are due to the profile of patients with diffuse coronary vessel lesions which makes grafting challenging due to the unavailability of a soft region [3]. Data from the last 15 years report better survival rates after CE [4–6]. Many surgeons are still reluctant to perform CE due to the absence of guidelines and varying outcomes from across centers [7, 8]. The aim of this retrospective study is to evaluate the mid-term results of coronary endarterectomy followed by coronary artery bypass grafting (CE + CABG).

Methods

Study design

A retrospective analysis was performed on 238 consecutive patients who underwent CE + CABG at our center. This study was approved by the institutional review board of Nanjing First Hospital, Nanjing Medical University in compliance with health insurance portability and accountability act regulations and the declaration of Helsinki.

Patient population

The data of 304 patients who underwent CE and CABG at our center under the same surgeon from January 2010 to January 2017 was reviewed. Of these, 78%(238 patients) who (1)had complete operative records, (2)good graft flow during surgery, (3) were successfully discharged, and (4) were followed up at the one-year mark were included in this study. Our study was commissioned and approved by the ethical commission of Nanjing first hospital. The patients were informed of our treatment and follow-up protocol, and written consent was obtained from all of them. The decision to perform endarterectomy was based on the preoperative angiograms and intra-operative findings. Most of the CE were scheduled before the operation, but the final decision as to use which strategy of revascularization and technique of CE was made during the operation as per the surgeon's preference.

Surgical procedure

All patients underwent routine median sternotomy. On pump CABG surgery was performed on 146 patients (61.3%), while the remaining underwent off-pump CABG surgery with 92 patients(38.7%). The decision to carry-out CE was made pre-operatively from the coronary artery angiographic results and intra-operatively according to the length of stenosed segment and availability of graftable regions on the calcified coronaries. CE was performed if the target coronary artery had diffuse disease with severe calcifications, and occluded or semi-occluded lumen distal to the proximal stenosed segment. A 10-20 mm longitudinal incision was made near the proximal stenosed end. Using coronary forceps, the calcified intima was gently pulled out while the coronary adventitia was simultaneously pushed in the opposite direction (closed endarterectomy). The procedure was repeated until all calcified segments were removed. Alternatively, we also used longer arteriotomies for direct vision removal of the calcified segment (open endarterectomy). The coronaries were flushed to remove any debris. Subsequently, CABG was performed. We used 3 methods of anastomosis, namely, the (1)on-lay LIMA graft to the LAD, (2) saphenous vein patch + LIMA graft to the LAD, and (3) on-lay saphenous vein graft to other territories. Before chest closure, the graft flow rate and PI value were measured and recorded using Medi-Stim Butterfly flowmeter (Medi-Stim As, Oslo, Norway).

Study endpoints and follow-up

The primary endpoint of this study is post-procedural graft patency at one-year and three-year follow up respectively. Graft patency were classified as 1) Grade A: excellent graft patency, < 50% stenosis, 2) Grade B: graft stenosis> 50%, and 3) Grade O: total graft occlusion. The patients underwent either a coronary angiography (CAG) or a computer tomography angiogram (CTA) to assess the degree of in-graft stenosis. The secondary end-point was the incidence of major adverse cardiac and cerebrovascular events (MACCE), defined as all-cause death, non-fatal myocardial infarction and cerebrovascular event during the 3-year clinical follow-up. Follow-up data was obtained from the patients by telephone contact after surgery and/or follow-up at the out-patient department.

Statistical analysis

Continuous data were expressed as mean ± standard deviation or median with the interquartile range and categorical data as percentages. Cumulative survival was evaluated with the Kaplan–Meier method. All reported P values are two-sided, and P values of < 0.05 were considered to indicate statistical significance. All statistical analyses were performed with SPSS 22.0 (SPSS, Inc., Chicago, IL, USA). All statistical analyses were performed with the assistance of a departmental statistician. Categorical variables were compared using either Pearson's chi-square or Fisher's exact tests and are expressed as a percentage of the group of origin.

Multiple variable models were constructed to determine independent factors influencing the following outcomes: advanced age, diabetes mellitus, dyslipidaemia, off-pump surgery, LIMA graft, CE on LAD and Intraoperative graft flow-meter and PI.

Results

A total of 238 patients underwent CE + CABG during the study period. The mean age of the patients was 65 ± 8 years in the on-pump group and 63 ± 9 years in the off-pump group; the male to female ratio was 201:37.

59.8% of patients undergoing off-pump surgery had a high lipid profile (vs 43.8% on-pump), 14.1% had suffered from previous cerebrovascular accident (vs 2.1% on-pump), 23.9% suffered from concomitant COPD (vs 4.1% on-pump), 48.9% had a calcified ascending aorta (vs 2.7% on-pump), 96.7% had RCA critical stenosis > 90% (vs 55.5% on-pump). We preferred off-pump CE + CABG in patients with known hyperlipidemia, previous cerebrovascular accidents, COPD, calcified ascending aorta, and RCA critical stenosis> 90. The complete pre-operative patient characteristics are summarized in Table 1. Our patient cohort represented 269 target coronary lesions, of which 108 (40.1%) were located on the left anterior descending (LAD) artery and sub-branches, 140 (52%) were located on the right coronary artery (RCA) and sub-branches, and 21 (8.8%) were located on the left circumflex artery and/or obtuse marginal artery (LCX/OM). The mean number of bypasses performed was 4.0 ± 0.9 (on-pump) vs 3.8 ± 0.7 (off-pump), 8.9% of on-pump patients required intra-aortic balloon pump (vs 1.1% in the off-pump group). The left internal mammary artery was used in all of the patients, saphenous vein grafts were used in more than 90% of the patients, and the radial artery was used in one-fifth of the patients

Table 1 Preoperative Patient Characteristics in CE

Variable	Group on-pump ($n = 146$)	Group off-pump ($n = 92$)	P Value
Clinical demographics			
Age (y)	65 ± 8	63 ± 9	0.0749
Female sex	25 (17.1%)	12(13.0%)	0.398
Coronary risk factors			
Hypertension	95(65.1%)	59(64.1%)	0.883
Diabetes	122(83.6%)	76(82.6%)	0.080
Hyperlipidemia	64(43.8%)	55(59.8%)	**0.017**
Smoking	67(45.9%)	41(44.6%)	0.842
Peripheral vascular disease	28(19.2%)	15(16.6%)	0.575
Previous renal impairment	8(5.5%)	4(4.3%)	0.698
Cerebrovascular accident	3(2.1%)	13(14.1%)	**0.000**
COPD	6(4.1%)	22(23.9%)	**0.000**
Calcified ascending aorta	4(2.7%)	45(48.9%)	**0.000**
Cardiac profile			
Previous myocardial infarction	93(63.7%)	55(62.2%)	0.544
Unstable angina	106(72.6%)	68(73.9%)	0.824
previous PCI	23(15.8%)	15(16.3%)	0.910
Mean ejection fraction	0.58 ± 0.12	0.56 ± 0.11	0.1974
Poor ejection fraction(<0.35)	15(10.3%)	9(9.8%)	0.902
Left main disease	29(19.8%)	17(18.5%)	0.792
RCA Critical stenosis > 90%	81(55.5%)	89(96.7%)	**0.000**
Number of diseased vessels	3.5 ± 0.5	3.4 ± 0.6	0.1689

COPD chronic obstructive pulmonary disease, *PCI* percutaneous coronary intervention, *RCA* right coronary artery

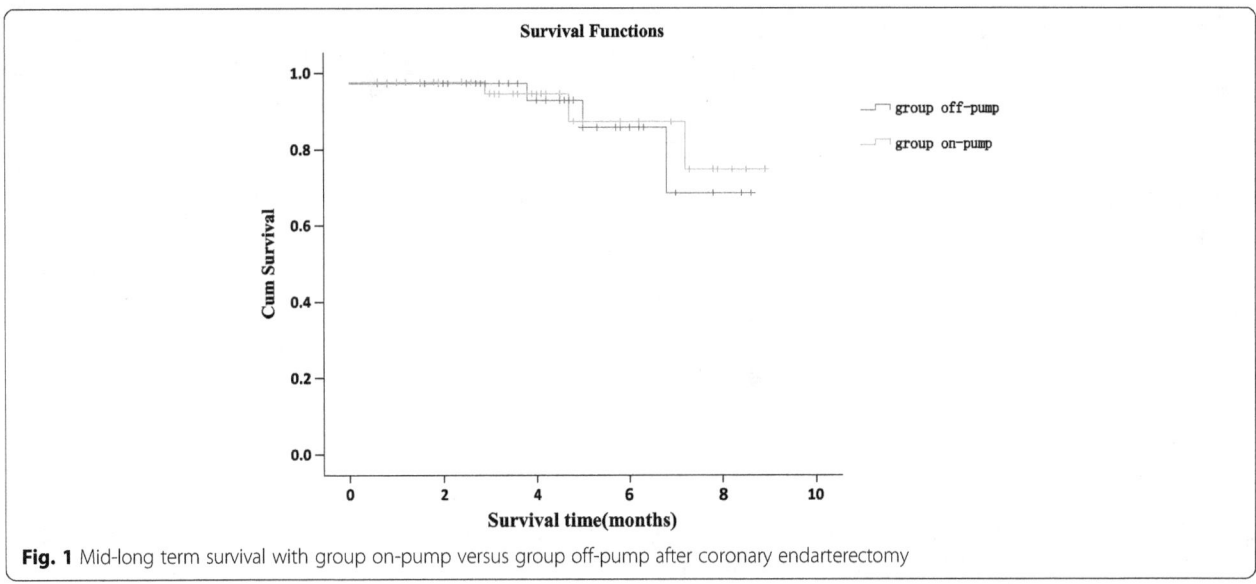

Fig. 1 Mid-long term survival with group on-pump versus group off-pump after coronary endarterectomy

(see Table 2: operative characteristics). The mean graft flow rates measured intra-operatively after endarterectomy and bypass grafting was 36 ± 8 ml/min with a mean PI value of 3.1 ± 0.8.

The mean intensive care unit stay was 2.5 ± 0.5 days for the patients who underwent on-pump surgery and 2.6 ± 0.7 days for the patients who underwent off-pump surgery. There was no significant difference in preoperative death and MACCE rates between the two groups. The occurrence of ventricular arrhythmia was significantly greater in the off-pump group (14.1% vs 4.8% in the on-pump group) (Table 3: perioperative mortality and morbidity). The average follow up time was 41.8 ± 21.4 months. Follow-up on the patients postoperatively showed a significant reduction in angina and dyspnea across the entire cohort as compared to the pre-operative period ($P < 0.001$). Six patients died during the 3-year follow-up period, two of whom died of neoplasms, three of cerebrovascular events and one died of

unknown reasons and was considered MACCE-related for statistical purposes.

At the one-year follow-up, data of 208 (232 endarterectomized target vessels; 88.5% of the original cohort) patients were obtained. The overall graft patency was 78.4% at 1 year and 69.8% at 3 years. The left coronary graft patency rate was significantly higher than the right coronary graft patency rate (87.4% vs 73.1% at one-year, $p = 0.011$ and 78.2% vs 64.8% at 3 years, $p = 0.032$) (Table 4: follow up graft patency analysis of coronary endarterectomy). There was no significant difference in graft patency rates between the on-pump CE + CABG vs off-pump CE + CABG groups at 1 year (80.0% vs 76.9%; $p = 0.599$) and at 3 years (92.3% vs 91.7%; $p = 0.884$). At the one-year follow up, 92.3% of grafts showed grade A patency in the on-pump group versus 91.7% in the off-pump group (p = 0.884); 7.7% of grafts showed grade B patency in the on-pump group versus 8.3% in the off-pump group ($p = 0.988$). At the three-year follow up,

Table 2 Operative Characteristics

Variable	Group on-pump ($n = 146$)	Group off-pump ($n = 92$)	P Value
Length of the ateriotomy	14.5 ± 2.5	14.1 ± 2.8	0.2525
Operative time (min)	253 ± 42	260 ± 48	0.2375
The number of distal anastomoses	4.0 ± 0.9	3.8 ± 0.7	0.0711
Associatied procedure	38(26.0%)	26(28.3%)	0.705
Intra-aortic balloon pump	13(8.9%)	1(1.1%)	**0.013**
Conduit to anastomosis vessel			
LIMA	146(100%)	92(100%)	1.000
Radial artery	29(19.9%)	19(20.7%)	0.883
Saphenous vein	138(94.5%)	88(95.7%)	0.698

LIMA Left internal mammary artery

Table 3 Perioperative Mortality and Morbidity

Variable	Group on-pump (n = 146)	Group off-pump (n = 92)	P Value
Death (30-day)	2(1.4%)	1(1.1%)	1.000
Perioperative myocardial infarction	6(4.1%)	3(5.4%)	1.000
Ventricular arrhythmia	7(4.8%)	13(14.1%)	**0.011**
Re-exploration for bleeding	2(1.4%)	1(1.1%)	1.000
Cerebral vascular accident	1(0.7%)	1(1.1%)	1.000
Acute renal failure	7(4.8%)	5(5.4%)	1.000
Intensive care unit stay(days)	2.5 ± 0.5	2.6 ± 0.7	0.2005
Infection	4(2.7%)	2(2.2%)	1.000

80.6% of grafts showed grade A patency in the on-pump group versus 77.4% in the off-pump group (p = 0.636); 19.4% of grafts showed grade B patency in the on-pump group versus 22.6% in the off -pump group (p = 0.636); (see: Table 5. Follow-up graft patency analysis between group on-pump and off-pump CE).

Moreover, the predictors of better graft patency are use of LIMA graft (P = 0.021), CE on LAD (P = 0.013), and intra-operative graft flow meter and PI (P = 0.002)(Table 6). Kaplan-Meier survival estimates in the on-pump CE + CABG group at one, 3 and 5 years were 0.96, 0.89 and 0.73 respectively and 0.95, 0.88 and 0.71 respectively in the off-pump CE + CABG group (Fig. 1: Mid-long term survival with group on-pump versus group off-pump after coronary endarterectomy).

Discussion

Before the widespread use of CABG to treat coronary artery disease, CE was the mainstay treatment for improving blood flow to severely stenosed coronary arteries. Although the technique was introduced more than five decades ago, it rapidly fell out of usage [1]. Acute post-operative MI, a key complication following CE, might be associated to endothelial damage during the procedure and subsequent thrombosis. Intact coronary endothelium produces vasoactive factors to neutralize leukocyte adhesion and platelet aggregation, consequently reducing inflammation and thrombosis in blood vessels [9]. Furthermore, MI caused by residual lesion-induced occlusion also contribute to the post-operative morbidity and mortality of CE [10, 11].

The aim of endarterectomy is to extract the calcified intima distal to the incision and ensure adequate revascularization. Distal intimal extraction is considered adequate if obvious bleeding of the distal vascular segment and a patent vessel with normal distal intima (with thin and soft tissues) on the top is observed after endarterectomy. There are two methods of performing endarterectomy, namely the 'open' and 'closed' techniques [12, 13]. The decision to use either 'open' or 'closed' CE was by the operating surgeon using the following criteria: 1) type of occlusion (complete total occlusion, or > 50% occlusion, or > 75% occlusion), 2) length of stenosed segment, 3) location of the lesion (medial or distal), and 4)number of bypasses to be performed. In hospital-mortality, defined as death due to any cause within 30 days of the operation, was 1.3% for both groups. 3.8% of the patients developed myocardial infarction during the peri-operative period, and 8.4% developed ventricular arrhythmias. During the three-year follow-up period, six deaths occurred, of which four were considered to be MACCE-related (1.7%). A 2015 meta-analysis performed by Kirill LK et al. show a 2.07% mortality at 30 days, 6.0% at 1 year, and 12.10% at 3 years post CABG surgery. Although the authors predominantly investigate outcomes in an elderly patient cohort (> 50% of patients were > 70 years old), we consider 1.3% mortality rate at 30-days, and a 3-year MACCE rate of 1.7% to be acceptable for concomitant CE and CABG. At the very least, it indicates that CE doesn't significantly increase the risk margin of the procedure [14].

As mentioned above, the patient cohort undergoing CE have a higher risk profile and the surgery itself is technically more challenging. For on-pump CE + CABG, this invariably translates to longer aortic cross-clamp, CPB times; and a greater incidence of intra-operative intra-aortic balloon pump implantation as compared to off-pump CABG (8.9% vs 1.1% respectively). We also performed off-pump CE + CABG on 38.7% of our

Table 4 Follow-up graft patency analysis of coronary endarterectomy

Follow-up time/patency rate	Total patency rate	Left coronary graft patency rate	Right coronary graft patency rate	P value
One year	78.4%(182/232)	87.4%(76/87)	73.1%(106/145)	0.011
Three year	69.8%(162/232)	78.2%(68/87)	64.8%(94/145)	0.032

Table 5 Follow-up graft patency analysis between group on-pump and off-pump CE

Variable	Group on-pump (n = 130)	Group off-pump (n = 78)	P Value
Early patency rate(1 year)	80.0%(104/130)	76.9%(60/78)	0.599
Grade A	92.3%(96/104)	91.7%(55/60)	0.884
Grade B	7.7%(8/104)	8.3%(5/60)	0.988
Midterm patency rate(3 year)	71.5%(93/130)	67.9%(53/78)	0.584
Grade A	80.6%(75/93)	77.4%(41/53)	0.636
Grade B	19.4%(18/93)	22.6%(12/53)	0.636

Grade A stands for excellent graft patency, Grade B for graft stenosis of greater than 50%, and Grade O for occlusion

cohort. In our study, we found that patients with a certain profile are more likely to be referred for off-pump surgery instead of on-pump surgery. Some patient characteristics include younger age, previous cerebrovascular accident, COPD, and calcified ascending aorta. One drawback of off-pump surgery is that it significantly increases the rate of peri-operative ventricular arrhythmias. There was no significant difference in early and late patency rates between the on-pump and off-pump CE + CABG groups. Off-pump CABG has beneficial effects on the recovery of the patient in the early post-operative period, as it decreases the operative time, and lowers the rate of MI, reduces the duration of inotropic support and ICU stay, and decreases the rate of peri-operative bleeding [15]. Our analysis on the on-pump and off-pump groups, show no significant difference in one-year and three-year graft patency rates; The results are similar to the study performed by Li S et al., where they also found no significant difference in survival at one-year between on-pump CABG and off-pump CABG [16]. Kaplan-Meier survival estimates at one-, three-, and five-years do not show a significant difference between the on-pump and off-pump CABG groups. It appears that the choice of either off-pump or on-pump in the setting of CE + CABG does not have deleterious effects on the early and mid-term outcomes of the procedure. In our study cohort, the mean discharge time after transfer to the ICU was (11 ± 3) days vs the 9.01 days and 7.7 days, reported by LaPar et

al. for patients undergoing CE + CABG and CABG respectively; Nevertheless, we report lower mortality rates (1.42% vs 4.0%) despite our longer follow-up time (41.8 ± 21.4 months vs 27.7 ± 17.7 months) [17].

Complete revascularization is accompanied by added benefits such as ischemia reduction, improvement of LV function, reduction of arrhythmias, and preserved ejection fraction [17]. Moreover, the composite endpoint of death/MI/stroke is significantly more likely with higher degrees of incomplete revascularization [18]. The 2011 ACC/AHA guideline for coronary artery bypass graft surgery and the 2014 ESC/EACTS guideline on myocardial revascularization have no reference to the clinical recommendation of CE due to the absence of randomized controlled trials [19–21]. Despite a lack of guidelines for the feasibility of complete or incomplete revascularization in the case of concomitant CE + CABG, we decided that a strategy of complete revascularization would better fit the high risk profile of our patient cohort. We obtained satisfactory results while keeping a high number of distal anastomoses (4.0 ± 0.9 vs 3.8 ± 0.7 for on-pump vs off-pump group respectively), thus ensuring a graft vessel to each perfusion territory of myocardium.

Another significant result from our study, is the higher patency of the left coronary graft at both one and 3 years, as compared to the right coronary graft (87.4% vs 73.1%, $p = 0.011$ at one year; 78.2% vs 64.8%, $p = 0.032$ at 3 years respectively). Since all endarterectomies and bypasses were performed by the same surgeon (CX) to assure consistency of technique, this suggests that the use of LIMA graft is an independent factor accounting for the superior patency rates [22]. The endothelium of internal mammary arteries produce vasodilators, are better protected from atherosclerosis, and due to postsurgical blood flow remodeling of the graft vessel, are better conduits for bypass as compared to the saphenous vein. The LIMA graft is also a predictor for better graft patency during follow-up ($P = 0.021$) [23, 24]. Other predictors of graft patency at follow up are presence of using LIMA graft, performing coronary endarterectomy on the LAD, and good intra-operative flow and PI values. The presence of the above mentioned factors, are

Table 6 Predictors of better graft patency during follow-up

Characteristics	Odds ratio	95% CI	P-value
Advanced age	5.7	0.71–49.3	0.102
Diabetes mellitus	0.91	0.85–0.997	0.12
Dyslipidaemia	0.9	0.86–1.059	0.82
Off-pump surgery	1.125	0.98–1.356	0.056
LIMA graft	1.15	1.31–105.3	**0.021**
CE on LAD	23.8	1.29–46.9	**0.013**
Intraoperative graft flow-meter and PI	1.29	1.09–1.53	**0.002**

LIMA left internal mammary artery, CE coronary endarterectomy, LAD left anterior descending, PI pulsation index highly indicative of successful CE which translates into good graft patency, and hence, can be used to score a CE procedure.

Limitations

The main limitation of this study is its retrospective nature. This is also a single-institution study, which limits its generalizability. Whether a larger series of patients with more power would have shown more benefits is unknown.

Conclusions

In patients with diffuse coronary disease, CE is a safe and feasible technique for a select group of patients with excellent mid-term survival rates and graft patency rates. CE produces better overall results when performed on the LAD, and grafted over with the LIMA. Similar outcomes are obtained with both on-pump and off-pump surgery. For a select group of patients, coronary endarterectomy (CE) offers an alternative choice of coronary artery reconstruction and complete coronary revascularization.

Abbreviations

CABG: Coronary artery bypass grafting; CE: Coronary endarterectomy; CPB: Cardiopulmonary bypass; CTA: Computer tomography angiogram; EF: Ejection fraction; LIMA: Left internal mammary artey; NYHA: New York Heart Association; PI: Pulsation index

Acknowledgments

We thank all the participants of our hospital for their tireless efforts to ensure the timeliness, completeness, and accuracy of the registry data.

Funding

This study was supported by grants from Jiangsu Top Expert Program in Six Professions(2014 WSW 052);Jiangsu Provincial Special Program of Medical Science (BE2015612).

Congresses

The abstract of the article has already been presented at international Coronary Congress, in NewYork, USA, 18–20 August 2017.

Authors' contributions

QZB and CX had helped with design of the study, data interpretation and in writing of the paper. QZB and Auchoybur Merveesh. L contributed to the work equally and should be regarded as co-first authors. XYY has made the statistical analysis and took part in the writing process. QZB and Auchoybur Merveesh. L also took part in the correction of the manuscript according to the reviewers' suggestions. JYS and WLM had helped in gathering patient information and performed graphic measurements. XF and XM performed graphics and tables and added comments to the paper. All authors read and approved the final manuscript.

Competing interests

The authors declare that they have no competing interests.

References

1. Bailey CP, May A, Lemmon WM. Survival after coronary endarterectomy in man. J Am Med Assoc. 1957;164:641–6.
2. Abrahamov D, Tamaris M, Guru V, Fremes S, Christakis G, Bhatnagar G, Sever J, Goldman B. Clinical results of endarterectomy of the right and left anterior descending arteries. J Card Surg. 1999;14:16–25.
3. Fukui T, Takanashi S, Hosoda Y. Long term segmental reconstruction of diffusely diseased left anterior descending coronary artery with left internal thoracic artery with or without endarterectomy. Ann Thorac Surg. 2005;80: 2098–105.
4. Byrne JG, Karavas AN, Gudbjartson T, Leacche M, Rawn JD, Couper GS, Rizzo RJ, Cohn LH, Aranki SF. Left anterior descending coronary endarterectomy: early and late results in 196 consecutive patients. Ann Thorac Surg. 2004;78: 867–73.
5. Marinelli G, Chiappini B, Di Eusanio M, Di Bartolomeo R, Caldarera I, Marrozzini C, Marzocchi A, Pierangeli A. Bypass grafting with coronary endarterectomy: immediate and long-term results. J Thorac Cardiovasc Surg. 2002;124:553–60.
6. Sirivella S, Gielchinsky I, Parsonnet V. Results of coronary artery endarterectomy and coronary artery bypass grafting for diffuse coronary artery disease. Ann Thorac Surg. 2005;80:1738–44.
7. Livesay JJ, Cooley DA, Hallman GL, Reul GJ, Ott DA, Duncan JM, Frazier OH. Early and late results of coronary endarterectomy. Analysis of 3,369 patients. J Thorac Cardiovasc Surg. 1986;92:649–60.
8. Minale C, Nikol S, Zander M, Uebis R, Effert S, Messmer BJ. Controversial aspects of coronary endarterectomy. Ann Thorac Surg. 1989;48:235–41.
9. Bonetti PO, Lerman LO, Lerman A. Endothelial dysfunction: a marker of atherosclerotic risk. Arterioscler Thromb Vasc Biol. 2003;23:168–75.
10. Lawrie GM, Morris GC Jr, Silvers A, Wagner WF, Baron AE, Beltangady SS, Glaeser DH, Chapman DW. The influence of residual disease after coronary bypass on the 5-year survival rate of 1274 men with coronary artery disease. Circulation. 1982;66:717–23.
11. Widimsky P, Straka Z, Stros P, Jirasek K, Dvorak J, Votava J, Lisa L, Budesinsky T, Kolesar M, Vanek T, Brucek P. One year coronary bypass graft patency. Circulation. 2004;110:3418–23.
12. Keogh BE, Bidstrup BP, Taylor KM, Sapsford RN. Angioscopic evaluation of intravascular morphology after coronary endarterectomy. Ann Thorac Surg. 1991;52:766–71.
13. Tiruvoipati R, Loubani M, Peek G. Coronary endarterectomy in the current era. Cyrr Opin Cardiol. 2005;20:517–20.
14. Kozlov KL, Bogachev AA. Coronary revascularization in the elderly. J Geriatr Cardiol. 2015;12(5):555–68.
15. Hussain G, Azam H, Baig MA, Ahmad M. Early outcomes of on-pump versus off-pump coronary artery bypass grafting. Pak J Med Sci. 2016;32:917–21.
16. LI S, Gong W, QI Q, Yuan Z, Chen A, Liu J, Cai J, Zhou M, Wang Z, Ye X, Zhao Q. Outcomes of off-pump versus on-pump coronary artery bypass graft surgery in patients with severely dilated left ventricle. Ann Transl Med. 2016;4:340.
17. LaPar DJ, Anvari F, Irvine JN, Kern JA, Swenson BR, Kron IL, Ailawadi G. The impact of coronary artery endarterectomy on the outcomes during coronary artery bypass grafting. J Card Surg. 2011;26:247–53.
18. Sandoval Y, Brilakis ES, Canoniero M, Yannopoulos D, Garcia S. Complete versus incomplete coronary revascularization of patients with multivessel coronary artery disease. Curr Treat Options Cardio Med. 2015;17:8.
19. Schwartz L, Bertolet M, Feit F, Fuentes F, Sako EY, Toosi MS, Davidson CJ, Ikeno F, King SB. 20. Impact of completeness of revascularization on long-term cardiovascular outcomes in patients with type 2 diabetes mellitus. Circ Cardiovasc Interv. 2012;5:166–73.
20. Hillis LD, Smith PK, Anderson JL, Bittl JA, Bridges CR, Byrne JG, et al. 2011 ACCF/ AHA guideline for coronary artery bypass graft surgery: a report of

    the American College of Cardiology Foundation/ American Heart Association task force on Practive guidelines. Circulation. 2011;124:e652–735.
21. Kolh P, Windecker S, Alfonso F, Collet JP, Cremer J, Falk V, et al. ESC/EACTS Guidelines on myocardial revascularization: The Task Force on Myocardial Revascularization of the European Society of Cardiology (ESC) and the

European Association for Cardio-thoracic Surgery (EACTS), developed with the special contribution of the European Association Of Percutaneous Cardiovascular Interventions (EAPCI). Eur J Cardiothorac Surg. 2014;46:517–92.

22. Qiu Z, Chen X, Jiang Y, Wang L, Xu M, Huang F, Shi H, Zhang C. Comparison of off-pump and on-pump coronary endarterectomy for patients with diffusely diseased coronary arteries: early and midterm outcome. J Cardiothorac Surg. 2014;9:186–94.

23. Garcia S, Sandoval Y, Roukoz H, Adabag S, Canoniero M, Yannopoulos D, Emmanouil SB. Outcomes after complete versus incomplete revascularization of patients with multivessel coronary artery disease. JACC. 2013;62:1421–31.

24. Taqusari O, Kobayashi J, Bando K, Niwaya K, Nakajima H, Ishida M, Nakatani T, Yagihara T, Kitamura S. Early adaptation of the left internal thoracic artery as a blood source of y-composite radial artery grafts in off-pump coronary artery bypass grafting. Heart Surgery Forum. 2003;6:E93–8.

27

Postpneumonectomy transthoracic Esophagectomy – a case report: using anatomic change to create Extrathoracic Esophagogastric anastomosis

Qiuyuan Li[1,2], Jing Guo[1], Chenwei Li[1] and Xinjian Li[1*] ⓘ

Abstract

Background: Resection of primary esophageal cancer following previous pneumonectomy is a challenging procedure and was scarcely reported.

Case presentation: Here we report a case in which reduced thoracic space was used in left transthoracic esophagectomy to counter the difficulties caused by previous left pneumonectomy.

Conclusion: Retrograde dissection and infra-diaphragmatic esophagogastric anastomosis are examples of using postpneumonectomy changes to facilitate subsequent transthoracic esophagectomy for cancers of the lower esophagus.

Keywords: Pneumonectomy, Transthoracic esophagectomy, Esophageal cancer, Dissection, Esophagogastric anastomosis

Background

The occurrence of primary esophageal cancer after preceding pneumonectomy for primary lung cancer is rare. For patients with previous pneumonectomy, transthoracic esophagectomy is always technically challenging given the postpneumonectomy anatomic deviations and a solitary lung as the remaining pulmonary reserve [1, 2]. We herein report a case of an adult patient who had a history of left pneumonectomy for lung cancer 12 years ago, and further received left transthoracic esophagectomy for a newly diagnosed esophageal cancer.

Case presentation

A 72-year-old man came to our department with progressive dysphagia for nearly 2 months. At presentation, he could only take down fluid. The patient used tobacco and alcohol before he underwent left pneumonectomy for a pT2N0M0 primary squamous cell lung cancer 12 years ago, which was followed by 4 cycles of gemcitabine/

carboplatin doublet chemotherapy. At postoperative follow-ups, he had been shown to be recurrence free.

Barium swallow and esophagogastroduodenoscopy were ordered and a distal esophageal mass was identified which was 36 cm from the incisors with extension to the cardia. Biopsy confirmed poorly differentiated adenocarcinoma. Computed tomography (CT) of the chest and abdomen demonstrated marked anatomic changes as a result of previous pneumonectomy, i.e. hyperexpansion of the right lung, mediastinal shift to the left hemithorax, elevation of the left hemidiaphragm and reduced left intrathoracic space with heterogeneous opacification (Fig. 1). No metastasis or lymphadenopathy was found after thorough examination including brain magnetic resonance imaging (MRI) and bone scan. Pulmonary function test showed a forced expiratory volume in one second (FEV1) of 0.98 L (46.6% of predicted) and a forced vital capacity (FVC) of 1.12 L (40.8% of predicted). No neoadjuvant treatment was given to the patient.

Based on the patient's will and examination results, a left transthoracic esophagectomy with the ad hoc design of retrograde esophageal dissection and superior diaphragmatic reconstruction was pursuit for curative intent. This procedure was initiated with a regular posterolateral thoracotomy.

---

* Correspondence: dxjs1961@sina.com
[1]Department of Thoracic Surgery, Ningbo First Hospital, Ningbo 315010, China
Full list of author information is available at the end of the article

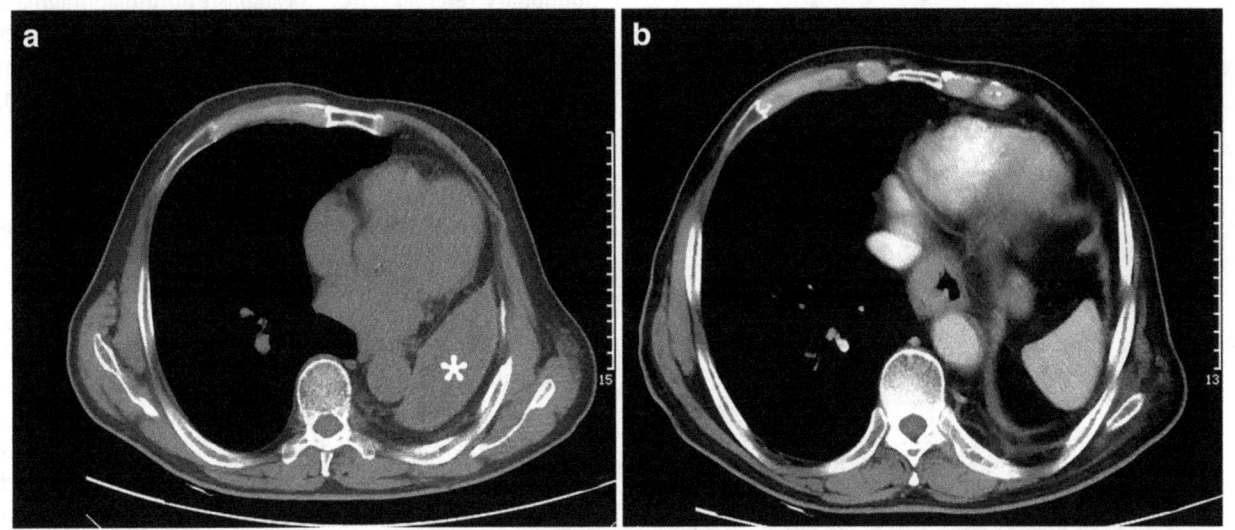

Fig. 1 Preoperative computed tomography imaging of the patient showed typical postpneumonectomy changes, characterized by **a** hyperexpansion of the residual lung, mediastinal shift to the opacified postpneumonectomy space (asterisk) as well as **b** elevation of the hemidiaphragm superior to the level of the esophageal mass

Thoracic probing identified the imaging-proven anomalies that highly obscured normal anatomy. As such, retrograde dissection starting from the abdomen was justified.

This was achieved by the standard abdominal component of a typical left transthoracic esophagectomy (Fig. 2), which included exploration of the upper abdomen, gastric mobilization with vascular pedicles and lymph node dissection.

Retrograde dissection of the esophagus was facilitated by the elevated diaphragm, which stretched and widened the esophageal hiatus. It was carried cephalad until 5 cm proximal to the esophageal mass, at which point the esophagus was transected. After the frozen section confirmed negative margin, the gastric conduit was prepared, and an end-to-end esophagogastric anastomosis was performed with an intraluminal circular stapler (Frankeman International Ltd., Suzhou, China), reinforced by several 4–0 absorbable sutures. An abdominal drainage tube was placed, and the diaphragmatic was reanastomosed superior to the esophagogastric anastomosis for an intentional precaution of postoperative anastomotic complications (Fig. 3). In the end, one chest tube was inserted, and decompression and nasojejunal feeding were initiated right after surgery.

In the postoperative course, ambulation was initiated on postoperative day (POD) 4. Oral feeding was restored on POD 7. Thoracic and abdominal drainage were terminated on POD 11 and POD 12 respectively after confirmation of anastomotic integrity. The patient was discharged on POD 14 with a normal chest CT. Postoperative pathology revealed a stage IIA primary adenosquamous esophageal carcinoma adventitia involvement (pT3N0M0).

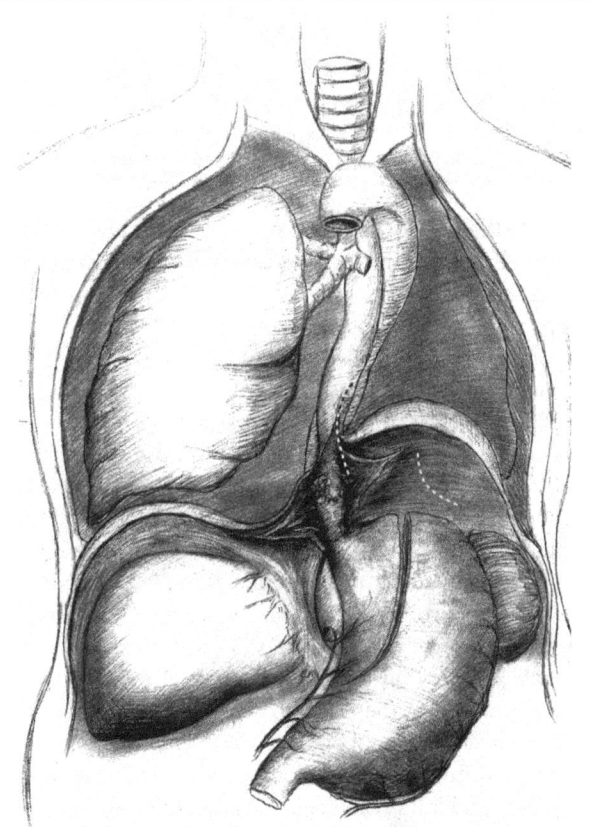

Fig. 2 The retrograde dissection was initiated at the hiatus and carried cephalad after the abdominal operation was completed. The dashed lines denote the incision line of the diaphragm and the mediastinal pleura

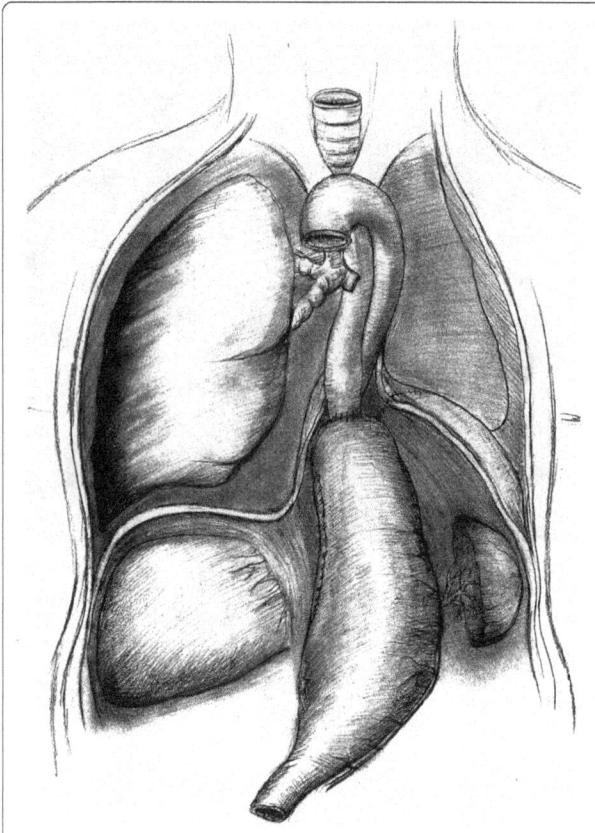

Fig. 3 Reconstruction of the gastrointestinal tract with the diaphragm being anastomosed superior to its original position so that the esophagogastric anastomosis was left in the abdomen

The patient was followed up for 12 m, and was re-admitted once for incision wound infection on POD 30, which required open drainage but no antibiotic use. No relapse was found.

Discussion and conclusions

Esophagectomy in the setting of prior pneumonectomy is challenging and only few cases have been reported to date [1–5]. A dilemma remains regarding the approaching side, as pneumonectomy has left substantial deformity in the ipsilateral thoracic space, whereas operating on the healthy side puts the residual lung at stake. Several techniques including endobronchial blockers [4] and extracorporeal membrane oxygenation (ECMO) [5] have been introduced to enable surgery on the side contralateral to pneumonectomy. However, in the current case, we opted to enter the pneumonectized hemithorax and performed transthoracic esophagectomy with adaptations of retrograde esophageal dissection and infra-diaphragmatic anastomosis.

The objectives of this method were three-fold: first, to aid the dissection in the unfamiliar postpneumonectomy area under the guidance of improved vision from the abdominal side; second, to keep the contralateral hemithorax intact so as to minimize impact on the residual pulmonary reserve; third, to establish infra-diaphragmatic anastomosis to allow for improved management improved management for potential anastomotic leak. These are important as they circumvent the technical hurdles arising from the previous pneumonectomy while maintaining safety at a reasonable level. Also, this procedure distinguished itself by taking advantage of the existing anatomic abnormalities without additional use of dedicated devices, thus making it more affordable and less technology demanding.

As an alternative, transhiatal esophagectomy could be an approach that avoid thoracic entry. However, this approach was also compromised by postpneumonectomy changes, and risk was further added by previous mediastinal lymph node dissection. Albeit our treatment proved to be useful in this patient, the surgical approach should be optimized on an individual basis, and the procedure presented here is only applicable for tumor of the lower esophagus. The lesson we took from this case is that a mindset of out-of-the-box thinking should always be ready for various real-life clinical scenarios.

In summary, transthoracic esophagectomy post ipsilateral pneumonectomy is feasible, and safe dissection and extra-thoracic esophagogastric anastomosis can be achieved by even harnessing postpneumonectomy changes. An example is retrograde dissection plus infra-diaphragmatic esophago-gastric anastomosis, which facilitates transthoracic esophagectomy for cancers of the lower esophagus.

Abbreviations
CT: Computed tomography; MRI: Magnetic resonance imaging; FEV1: Forced expiratory volume in one second; FVC: Forced vital capacity; POD: Postoperative day; ECMO: Extracorporeal membrane oxygenation

Authors' contributions
QL Conception, manuscript writing, JG Conception, data collection, manuscript writing, CL Data collection, resource, XL Conception, data collection, resource, manuscript writing. All authors read and approved the final manuscript.

Consent for publication
Written informed consent was obtained from the patient for the publication of this report and any accompanying images.

Competing interests
The authors declare that they have no competing interests.

Author details
[1]Department of Thoracic Surgery, Ningbo First Hospital, Ningbo 315010, China. [2]Department of Thoracic Surgery, Shanghai Pulmonary Hospital Tongji University, Shanghai, China.

References

1. Petri R, Brizzolari M, Sorrentino M, Bassi F, Muzzi R, Zuccolo M. Minimally invasive esophagectomy in a previously pneumonectomized patient. J Laparoendosc Adv Surg Tech A. 2012;22(7):695–700.
2. Reardon MJ, Estrera AL, Conklin LD, Reardon PR, Brunicardi FC, Beall AC. Esophagectomy after pneumonectomy: a surgical challenge. Ann Thorac Surg. 2000;69(1):286–8.
3. Velotta JB, Vasquez CR, Sugarbaker DJ. Transhiatal esophagectomy after previous right pneumonectomy. J Thorac Cardiovasc Surg. 2014;148(2):e150–2.
4. Wang H, Liu J, Jiang C, Liu M, Jiang G. Transthoracic esophagectomy using endobronchial blocker after previous pneumonectomy. Ann Thorac Surg. 2014;97(2):723–5.
5. Xu HC, Ye P, Bao FC, Pan H, Yang YH, Wang LM, Wang ZT, Li ZB, He ZH, Han WL, et al. ECMO-assisted esophagectomy after left pneumonectomy. Int J Artif Organs. 2013;36(4):259–62.

28

Feasibility, safety, and short-term outcome of totally thoracoscopic mitral valve procedure

Qin Jiang[1*†], Tao Yu[1], Keli Huang[1†], Lihua Liu[1†], Xiaoshen Zhang[2†] and Shengshou Hu[3]

Abstract

Background: The totally thoracoscopic procedure for mitral valve (MV) disease is a minimally invasive method. We investigated the procedure's feasibility, safety and effectiveness when it was performed by an experienced operator.

Methods: We retrospectively analysed 53 consecutive patients with MV disease treated between December 2014 and April 2017 by minimally invasive procedures. The procedures were performed on femoral artery-vein bypass through three 2–4 cm incisions, with one additional penetrating point on the right chest wall under totally thoracoscopic visual guidance and surveillance of transoesophageal echocardiography.

Results: Two patients who underwent intraoperative conversion to sternotomy were excluded due to indivisible pleural cavity adhesion. Of the others (38 female patients, average age, 49 ± 14 years, left ventricular ejection fraction, $59 \pm 7\%$), 34 received MV replacement for rheumatic mitral lesions, which was redone for one patient after the discovery of serious paravalvular leakage, 17 received MV repair for mitral regurgitation (with 4 secondary to atrial septum defect, 2 diagnosed with left atrial myxoma, and 2 redone for mitral valve replacement due to repair failure), 28 received additional tricuspid valvuloplasty, and one patient received a Warden procedure. The cardiopulmonary bypass and aortic cross clamp times were 144 ± 39 min and 80 ± 22 min, respectively. Postoperational chest tube drainage in the first 48 h was 346 ± 316 ml. The ventilation time and intensive care unit stay length were 11 ± 11 h and 23 ± 2 h, respectively. One patient died of disseminated intravascular coagulation and prosthesis thrombosis with fear of anticoagulation-related bleeding.

Conclusions: The totally thoracoscopic procedure on mitral valves by an experienced surgeon is technically feasible, safe, effective and worthy of widespread adoption in clinical practice.

Keywords: Minimally invasive surgical procedures, Thoracoscopy, Mitral valve, Cardiac surgical procedures

Introduction

Accumulating knowledge of the structure, function, and pathology of the mitral valve (MV) has led to favourable surgical results in MV procedures. Advances in imaging and surgical instruments have allowed surgeons to perform less invasive sternum-sparing MV surgery [1]. Several kinds of minimally invasive access for MV procedures in adult patients have been popularly introduced into clinical practice. Lower hemisternotomy was used as a popular form of a minimally invasive MV procedure [2]. Right anterolateral minithoracotomy for MV surgery was a safe approach with very low operative mortality comparable to standard median sternotomy [3, 4]. MV surgery through a right minithoracotomy did not result in increased morbidity, mortality or procedural duration; therefore, long-term survival outcomes were satisfactory [5, 6].

Endeavours to reduce surgical trauma, hasten patient recovery, improve cosmetics, and increase patient satisfaction continued to further promote minimally invasive procedures. Additional minimally invasive surgical approaches, such as total video-assisted thoracoscopy or robotic assistance, have also been applied to repair

* Correspondence: jq349@163.com
†Qin Jiang, Keli Huang, Lihua Liu and Xiaosheng Zhang contributed equally to this work.
[1]Department of Cardiac Surgery, Sichuan Provincial People's Hospital, Affiliated Hospital of University of Electronic Science and Technology, No.32, West Second Section First Ring Road, Chengdu, China
Full list of author information is available at the end of the article

congenital heart defects to minimize surgical trauma and improve cosmetic results [7–9]. Apart from comparable merits in cosmetics to robotic surgery, an approach using totally thoracoscopy assistance to repair MV without complicated hardware equipment has a remarkable advantage [10].

However, the application of totally video-assisted thoracoscopic procedures on MV has been very limited in clinical practice. It was demonstrated that adverse events, including intraoperative conversion to sternotomy, re-exploration for bleeding, and valve-related reoperation within the same hospital stay, occurred with a predicted 25% rate at the beginning; this trend remained sluggish with declines in conjunction with increased operation training [11]. In this study, we reported the two-year experience of our department regarding the totally endoscopic procedure on MV performed by a single experienced surgeon (Z.XS.).

Materials and methods

Patients

This was a single-centre, retrospective, observational study of prospectively collected data from consecutively recruited patients. This study was approved by the Institutional Review Board of Sichuan Provincial People's Hospital. Written informed consent was preoperatively obtained from each participant and/or their parents or guardians, and the patients were fully informed about the technique and were able to choose a standard median sternotomy according to their preference. We initiated the protocol at the end of 2014, and since that time, totally endoscopic procedure on MV has become the preferred approach for selected patients with MV disease, no matter whether the disease was isolated or combined with tricuspid valve (TV) disease and atrial septal defect (ASD). The selection criteria were as follows: (1) no combination with serious aortic or coronary artery disease; (2) available to the operator; (3) no previous history of a right thoracotomy with expected pleural cavity adhesion; and (4) no expected difficulty in femoral vessels cannulation or vena cava occlusion; and (5) a weight above 40 kg.

Position

After the induction of general anaesthesia, a 35F left-sided double-lumen endotracheal tube was placed to allow for single-lung ventilation. Adult electrodes were attached to the anterior and posterior chest walls as indicated in the instructions (Zoll Medical Corporation, MA, USA). The patients were positioned in the supine position with the right hemithorax elevated to 20°. After systemic heparinization, the femoral vessels were cannulated using a Seldinger technique. The setup of a bypass circuit was initiated by positioning a 16-24F catheter in

the abdominal aorta through the right femoral artery. A 28F venous cannula was precisely introduced and positioned into the inferior vena cava (IVC) at the junction with the right atrium (RA) under the surveillance of transoesophageal echocardiography (TEE), and a 16F catheter was percutaneously punctured into right jugular vein (RJV) or inserted into superior vena cava (SVC) through a stab incision in the centre of the purse string suture after pericardiotomy. The arterial and venous cannulas were purchased from Edward Lifesciences corporation (Irvine, California, USA) or Kangxin medical instrument corporation (Changzhou, Jiangsu, China).

Ports

Three small incisions and soft tissue retractors were established on the right side of the chest. Port 1 (2–3 cm) was located in the third intercostal space on the right anterior axillary line. This port was the entryway of surgical instruments, such as tissue forceps or suture needles. The drainage for the SVC and right superior pulmonary vein was also passed through the port, in addition to the cardioplegia irrigation tube and aortic clamp forcep. Port 2 (2–4 cm) was located in the fourth intercostal space on a midclavicular line as an entryway for instruments, such as scissors and prosthesis, or tissue removal. Port 3 (2–3 cm) was located in the fifth intercostal space on the right anterior axillary line. This port was for the placement of an thoracoscopy and a subsequent chest drainage tube. A left atrium (LA) blade retractor was introduced into the right chest cavity through a 2-mm shaft penetrating parasternally in the fourth intercostal space and was held on the operating table on the upper end (Fig. 1). A specific thoracoscopy 6800 (Karl Storz Endoskope, Tuttlingen, Germany) was conventionally used.

Procedures

Once the previous 3 ports were secured, a pericardiotomy was performed, and 3 to 4 sutures were placed to suspend the pericardium. Caval snares were placed in the SVC and IVC to install total cardiopulmonary bypass (CPB). After CPB initiation and cooling to 32 °C, a transthoracic Chitwood clamp (Scanlan International, MN, USA) was positioned on the ascending aorta. A 7-F long cardioplegia cannula needle (CalMed Technologies, CA) was inserted through port 1 into the aortic root for the delivery of cold blood cardioplegic solution to achieve cardiac arrest [12]. After snaring of the superior and inferior vena cavae, LA traditional access of incision to MV parallel to the interatrial sulcus was opened. The anterior wall of the LA was raised up by means of a specific LA blade retractor as shown in Fig. 2 [13]. The diseased MV was resected and then replaced with a prosthesis valve on the condition of rheumatic mitral

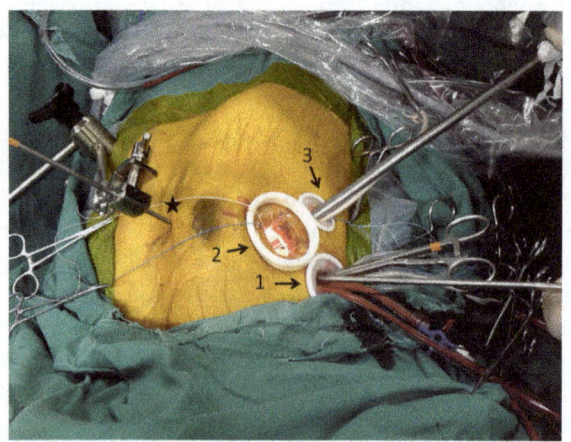

Fig. 1 The operative layout for the totally thoracoscopic mitral valve procedure. Drainage of the superior vena cava and right superior pulmonary vein, and cardioplegia perfusion cannula was passed through port 1 directly. Port 2 was located in the fourth intercostal space on a midclavicular line for the entry of instruments, such as scissors and prosthesis, or tissue removal. Port 3 was located in the fifth intercostal space on the right anterior axillary line (arrows). The left atrium was raised by a blade retractor and introduced through a 2-mm shaft penetrating parasternally in the fourth intercostal space and was held on the operating table (asterisk)

stenosis or repaired if mitral regurgitation occurred at the discretion of the operator. Artificial chordae tendineae (Gore-Tex) were used if MV prolapsed or chordae ruptured. The repair was completed by the insertion of an annuloplasty ring as shown in Fig. 3. All annular stitches were exteriorized through the working port and fixed in suture guides. The knots with interrupted sutures were completed extracorporeally and tightened with a knot pusher.

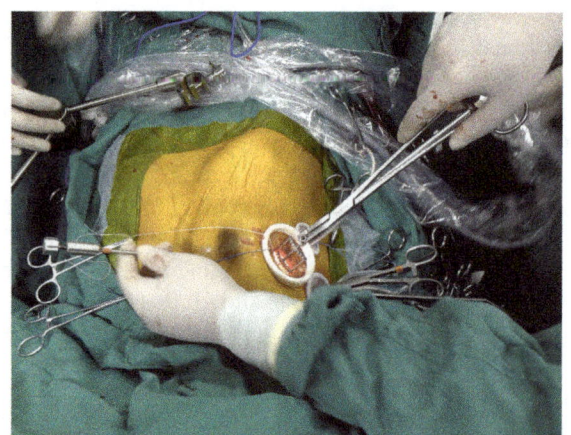

Fig. 2 Left atrium exposure by means of a blade retractor. The blade retractor was inserted through port 2 to raise the left atrium with a shaft. The blade retractor was fixed on a 2-mm shaft that penetrated parasternally in the fourth intercostal space and was held on the operating table

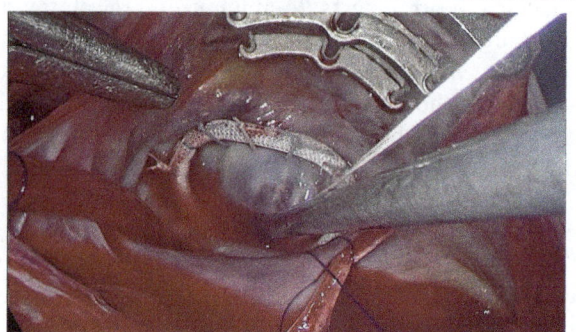

Fig. 3 Repair of mitral regurgitation under totally thoracoscopic visual guidance. The annuloplasty ring was implanted for mitral valve repair

Once the procedure was completed, the LA was closed, leaving the venting suction in place for deairing. If additional procedures on ASD and/or tricuspid regurgitation were performed, the RA was opened. The position and function of the MV prosthesis were confirmed by means of TEE analysis. For patients who suffered from difficulty in heart rebeating or severe arrhythmia after aortic crossclamp release, a pacing wire was introduced into the anterior surface of the right ventricle (RV).

Perioperative management

Following the operation, patients were monitored in a surgical intensive care unit overnight and were transferred to the wards as soon as they were haemodynamically stable. Additionally, chest X-ray and blood gas analysis were routinely performed to exclude complications in the lungs. Transthoracic echocardiography was performed before discharge, 3 months later and then annually after surgery to assess the postoperational condition.

Statistical analysis

The short-term outcome consisted of all major adverse events, including intraoperative conversion to sternotomy, re-exploration for bleeding, valve-related reoperation within the same hospital stay, and death. Statistical analysis was performed using SPSS 17.1 software (SPSS Inc., Chicago, IL). Categorical variables were presented as frequencies and percentages, and continuous variables were presented as the mean ± standard deviation.

Results

Baseline data and immediate technical feasibility

A total of 53 patients were included in this study. Two patients were excluded by severe indivisible plural adhesion and conversed to median sternotomy. The aetiologies of the mitral lesions and types of surgical procedures are shown in Table 1. The lesions of MV regurgitation happened on the anterior valve in 8 cases and on the posterior valve in 9 cases. Four cases were

Table 1 Baseline data

Characteristics	Totally video-assisted thoracoscopic MV procedure (n = 51)
Sex (female)	38
Age (years)	49 ± 14 [41, 60]
Height (cm)	159 ± 8 [154, 163]
Weight (kg)	59 ± 11 [50, 67]
BMI (kg/m²)	23.3 ± 3.3 [21.1, 25.9]
Left ventricular ejection fraction (%)	58.9 ± 7.2 [53, 65]
New York Heart Association functional class	2.7 ± 0.5
Coronary artery stenosis (< 50%)	7
Atrial fibrillation	25
Cerebral infarction history	2
Aetiology	51
Rheumatic valve disorder	27
Mitral regurgitation	17
Atrial septum defect (comorbidity)	4 (3)
Infective endocarditis	1
Myxoma	2

Values are given as median (interquartile range)

secondary to ASD, and two cases were concomitant with LA myxoma. There were 38 female patients, almost all of whom were small in stature. All patients underwent 16F cannulation on the SVC and 28F cannulation on the femoral vein. Cannula sizes ranged from 16 to 24F for the femoral artery. Only one patient received a 16F catheter on bilateral femoral arteries due to inadequate bypass flow from the right common femoral artery.

Operational data

Mitral valvuloplasty was the priority for all patients with MV regurgitation. Prosthetic rings were conventionally used for all patients if repair was possible. Two patients of these patients underwent mitral valve replacement (MVR) after attempted repair (repair success rate, 88%). Another 34 patients underwent scheduled MVR mainly for rheumatic lesions, only 4 patients received replacement of a biological prosthesis valve, and another 3 patients received concomitant ASD repair. Only 3 patients underwent the Maze procedure with a monopole radiofrequency device. A total of 28 patients (55%) suffered from tricuspid regurgitation and received tricuspid valve annuloplasty (TVP), which was corrected by insertion of an annuloplasty ring.

As shown in Table 2, total operation time, CPB time and ACC time were 251 ± 60 min, 144 ± 39 min and 80 ± 22 min, respectively. Two patients underwent

prosthesis valve replacement due to repair failure, and one of these patients underwent a second ACC. One patient experienced serious postoperative perivalvular leakage of a 2.5-cm peri-prosthetic jet under the TEE view, and this patient then completed a corrective procedure under a second ACC. A spontaneous heart beat resumed in 43 patients after the aortic clamp was released (84%). One patient experienced such troublesome haemostasis after sewing the temporary pacemaker wire that a second CPB was resumed, which led to the addition of a right minithoracotomy opposite of the bleeding site on the right ventricle. All of the operations were completed only after no abnormal blood flow kinetics were observed by TEE.

Postoperative events

There was only one operative death occurrence. The patient suffered from severe thrombosis on the MV mechanical prosthesis and TV annuloplasty ring and received a second MVR at 7 days after the operation. A low level of platelets while only receiving a half-dosage of low molecular weight heparin without warfarin anticoagulation could have been the cause of death. Transient third-degree atrioventricular conduction block was observed in three (5.8%) patients, who required epicardial temporary pacing. Four patients (8%) experienced postoperative atelectasis, and they recovered uneventfully after respiratory physiotherapy under the guidance of a specialized physical therapist. The New York cardiac function classification class was enhanced at discharge relative to its value before the operation at 2.7 ± 0.5 versus 1.9 ± 0.6, respectively (Table 3, P < 0.000).

Discussion

The totally video-assisted thoracoscopic procedure for MV disease is technically challenging, and its application is currently restricted to a handful of experienced operators because it entails the surgeon overcoming a lengthy learning curve [14]. In our department, the technique was performed on 51 cases by one experienced surgeon since the end of 2014. The result was technically feasible, required no transition to median sternotomy, and had a low rate of adverse events.

The totally video-assisted thoracoscopic procedure has been reported as a safe and effective method for repairing simple congenital heart defects with a rapid recovery of life quality and lower pain levels compared with both minithoracotomy and median sternotomy [15]. Meanwhile, lower systemic inflammatory reactions and myocardial damage were also observed after ASD repair with the method [16].

Compared with conventional median sternotomy, the sternum-exempt procedure could not only preserve the integrity of the osseous thoracic wall but also save time

Table 2 Operative details

Variable	Totally video-assisted thoracoscopic MV procedure ($n = 51$)
Conversion to minithoracotomy	1
Resumption procedure	2
MVP	17
Gore-Tex artificial chordae tendineae	9
MV Annuloplasty	17
MVR	34
Mechanical	30
Biological Concomitant procedure	4
TVP	28
ASD repair	7
Maze	3
Thrombus removal	3
Warden procedure	1
Operation time (minutes)	249 ± 60 [210, 275]
CPB (minutes)	144 ± 39 [122, 162]
ACC (minutes)	80 ± 22 [66, 86]
Cardiac defibrillation (cases)	8

on the formidable task of haemostasis as in median sternotomy. Compared with minithoracotomy, which requires a 6–8 cm skin incision in the right inframammary groove to create a small anterolateral "working port" [17], the totally video-assisted thoracoscopic MV procedure had an advantage in terms of minimal invasiveness. The totally thoracoscopic MV procedure,

Table 3 Postoperative results

Variable	Totally video-assisted thoracoscopic MV procedure ($n = 51$)
In-hospital mortality	1
Cerebrovascular complication	0
Atelectasis	4
Prolonged intubation (> 48 h)	2
Postoperation IABP implantation	0
Wound infection	0
Lung infection	3
Chest tube drainage (ml, 48 h)*	346 ± 316 [140, 445]
Mechanical ventilation time (hours)*	11 ± 11 [7, 12]
ICU stay (hours)*	23 ± 2 [15, 21]
New York Heart Association functional class at discharge	1.9 ± 0.6
Ejection fraction (%)*	58.5 ± 5.9 [55, 63]

*Values are given as number (interquartile range)

which offers fewer surgical incisions and improved cosmetics, was more attractive to patients than other approaches. The sparing of a rigid incision retractor rendered less injury to chest wall integrity. Nonetheless, high technical demands have impeded the popularization of minimally invasive endoscopic MV surgery.

It is too challenging to widely introduce this procedure because it is still difficult to perform for a large majority of surgeons. The survey of surgeons who were experienced in minimally invasive MV surgery showed that 90 % of the respondents believed that more than 20 cases were required to gain familiarity with the procedure [18]. Our department introduced a skilful cardiac surgeon who was well versed in performing the MV procedure with the guidance of a video-assisted thoracoscope instead of port-access minithoracotomy and robotic assistance. He had already carried out nearly 100 cases of MV repair/replacement from 2012 to 2014.

There were some disadvantages and pitfalls in terms of the characteristics of the totally video-assisted thoracoscopic MV procedure. Compared with the three-dimension vision under the totally direct open procedure, the manipulation zone lacked a stereoscopic experience. The field of vision during the operation was narrowed down by enlarged thoracoscope so that the surgeon had increased difficulty during manipulation. Each knotting entailed crossing of the sutures outside of chest cavity and then pulling down the knots with the assistance of a knot pusher.

There were some technical limitations in its clinical application. One of the key elements for procedural success was CPB establishment through femoral artery-vein bypass. Patients had a low body weight with smaller femoral blood vessels, which might hinder the insertion of venous or arterial cannulas for optimal CPB. As Table 1 indicates, the great majority of MV patients in our region were female and rheumatic, short in statue, with a BMI ranging from 18.1 to 30.8. Six patients received a 16F femoral artery cannula, and only one case underwent bilateral femoral artery cannulation due to hypoperfusion. The SVC was completely cannulated with a 16F cannula, which was inserted through the RJV during the initial phase of the programme. Due to the scar effect on the neck and the associated risk of penetrating into the pleural cavity, the plan was terminated after performing the first 11 cases in the middle of 2015. Instead, the operator completed the catheterization of the SVC directly through port 1 under the view of thoracoscopy. The femoral vein was successfully cannulated with a 28F cannula for IVC drainage. This satisfactory perfusion result could be due to the lower morbidity rate of peripheral artery disease in this population. Elective preoperative coronary angiography was often performed on the right radial artery, which avoided possible intima injury to the femoral artery.

The second element was heart arrest and cardiac protection. In our study, a lengthened cardioplegia perfusion cannula and transthoracic aortic clamp were introduced conventionally and smoothly. It was reported that intraluminal aortic clamping was applied by means of a sophisticated device consisting of a three-lumen catheter named an Endoclamp, which enabled simultaneous occlusion of the aorta, antegrade delivery of cardioplegia, and venting through the aortic root [19]. The minimally invasive approach should be excluded in patients with aortic regurgitation (AR) greater than grade I because of the risks of inadequate cardioplegia delivery and left ventricular distension [12]. No evidence in our study demonstrated that retrograde perfusion per se during minimally invasive MV surgery increased the incidence of cerebrovascular accidents [20].

The requirement of rethoracotomy for bleeding represented a major drawback of minimally invasive MV surgery because the entire operative field could not be directly visualized. In this study, there was one case undergoing transition to mini-thoracotomy for bleeding at the site of temporary pacemaker wire implantation, but no reexploration for bleeding happened after chest wall closure. This excellent outcome was attributable to overcoming the learning curve and innovative measure by the operator, who fixed the pacemaker wire with Teflon pressed with a titanium clip at both ends [21]. It was also routine for the operator to use a thoracoscope to inspect the inner thoracic wall thoroughly before closing the incision. It had been recorded that the rate of reexplorations for bleeding fell; it was reduced from 8.2 to 1.9% after 300 operations [11]. In contrast, we observed one case in which that patient died from prosthesis thrombosis because of insufficient anticoagulation. Due to fear of bleeding on the condition of thrombocytopenia and continuous excessive drainage, we did not regularly prescribe warfarin for prosthesis anticoagulation. The subsequent MV prosthesis replacement re-do procedure was ineffective, and the patient died from coagulation complications soon after the procedure. Granted that only two patients suffered reoperation after ACC release, the resultant operative quality of totally video-assisted thoracoscopic MV surgery could be on par with the conventional median sternotomy approach.

Regarding feasibility, chest wall deformity was restricted to perform the totally video-assisted thoracoscopic procedure to some extent. Due to case limitation and careful patient selection, we were not confronted with any cases of serious chest deformity or secondary port-access video-assisted thoracoscopic procedures.

Nevertheless, the mere presence of uncorrected congenital chest wall deformities should not deter surgeons from minimally invasive cardiac surgery [22]. Loose pleural adhesion did not restrict the feasibility unless indivisible adhesion existed. We also experienced several cases of painstaking synechiotomy and then completed the MV procedure under the guidance of thoracoscope. It had been shown that the outcomes in redo-port access surgery after previous port access surgery were favourable [23]. In our population, two cases required re-do surgery of a previous MV procedure were successfully completed in patients who underwent percutaneous balloon mitral valvuloplasty and MVR at median sternotomy. To some extent, the procedure from right thoracotomy access should be the optimal choice for re-do MV patients because post-sternum adhesion is avoided. The LA blade retractor used to pull up the LA anterior wall was held by a shaft that penetrated into chest cavity rather than through the main incision [24, 25]. This approach could minimize the size of the main incision, which merely allowed the prosthesis to enter into the port smoothly. Meanwhile, the additional penetrating point for the shaft did not increase the cosmetic burden.

Concomitant TVP was not associated with a risk-adjusted increase in mortality, regardless of TR severity. A more liberal approach to TVP at the time of MVR might be justified when long-term benefits are thought to outweigh incremental short-term morbidity risk [26]. In our study, we completed MV procedures associated with TVP in 28 cases. The operator also performed the Warden procedure in one case who suffered from ASD combined with supracardiac partial anomalous right upper pulmonary venous connection to SVC. A giant self-pericardium patch was added to the RA as an atrial septum to separate the total pulmonary venous connection into the LA [27].

Conclusions

We completed 51 cases of MV procedures totally by thoracoscopic visual guidance. The aetiology of these MV diseases was comprised of mitral regurgitation, rheumatic mitral disorders, congenital heart defect or left atrial myxoma. Through three incisions that were 2–4 cm length and one penetrating point in the right chest wall, mitral valve replacement or repair was successfully administered by an experienced surgeon. The additional procedures included LA thrombus removal, Cox-maze radiofrequency, ASD repair, and TV annuloplasty. Apart from its minimal invasiveness characteristics and wide range of clinical applications, the MV procedure under the assistance of thoracoscopic visual guidance and TEE surveillance was also a safe and effective operation approach. In total, the thoracoscopic procedure for conventional MV diseases is worth being advocated broadly, and more experienced surgeons should be trained on this procedure due to its high-demand in terms of manipulation skills and three-dimensional conception. In summary, the totally thoracoscopic procedure for MV disease by an experienced operator is feasible, safe, effective, and merits widespread adoption.

Abbreviations

ACC: aortic cross clamping; AR: aortic regurgitation; ASD: atrial septal defect; CPB: cardiopulmonary bypass; IVC: inferior vena cava; LA: left atrium; MV: mitral valve; MVR: mitral valve replacement; RA: right atrium; RJV: right jugular vein; RV: right ventricle; SVC: superior vena cava; TV: tricuspid valve; TVP: tricuspid valve annuloplasty

Acknowledgements

Not applicable.

Funding

No funding.

Authors' contributions

JQ analysed and interpreted the patient data and wrote the manuscript. ZXS performed all the procedures. YT and LLH were major contributors in data acquisition and edited the manuscript. HKL and HSS analysed and interpreted the results. All authors read and approved the final manuscript.

Competing interests

The authors declare that they have no competing interests.

Author details

[1]Department of Cardiac Surgery, Sichuan Provincial People's Hospital, Affiliated Hospital of University of Electronic Science and Technology, No.32, West Second Section First Ring Road, Chengdu, China. [2]Department of Cardiac Surgery, Affiliated Hospital of University of Jinan, Guangzhou, China. [3]Department of Cardiac Surgery, Fuwai Hospital, Chinese Academy of Medical Sciences and Peking Union Medical College, Beijing 100037, China.

References

1. Goldstone AB, Woo YJ. Is minimally invasive thoracoscopic surgery the new benchmark for treating mitral valve disease? Ann Cardiothorac Surg. 2016;5:567–72.
2. McClure RS, Athanasopoulos LV, McGurk S, Davidson MJ, Couper GS, Cohn LH. One thousand minimally invasive mitral valve operations: early outcomes, late outcomes, and echocardiographic follow-up. J Thorac Cardiovasc Surg. 2013;145:1199–206.
3. Miceli A, Murzi M, Canarutto D, Gilmanov D, Ferrarini M, Farneti PA, Solinas M, Glauber M. Minimally invasive mitral valve repair through right minithoracotomy in the setting of degenerative mitral regurgitation: early outcomes and long-term follow-up. Ann Cardiothorac Surg. 2015;4:422–7.
4. Mihos CG, Santana O, Lamas GA, Lamelas J. Outcomes of right minithoracotomy mitral valve surgery in patients with previous sternotomy. Ann Thorac Surg. 2011;91:1824–7.
5. Al Otaibi A, Gupta S, Belley-Cote EP, Alsagheir A, Spence J, Parry D, Whitlock RP. Mini-thoracotomy vs. conventional sternotomy mitral valve surgery: a systematic review and meta-analysis. J Cardiovasc Surg. 2017;58:489–96.
6. Lange R, Voss B, Kehl V, Mazzitelli D, Tassani-Prell P, Günther T. Right Minithoracotomy versus full sternotomy for mitral valve repair: a propensity matched comparison. Ann Thorac Surg. 2017;103:573–9.
7. Ma ZS, Dong MF, Yin QY, Feng ZY, Wang LX. Totally thoracoscopic repair of atrial septal defect without robotic assistance: a single-center experience. J Thorac Cardiovasc Surg. 2011;141:1380–3.
8. Ma ZS, Dong MF, Yin QY, Feng ZY, Wang LX. Totally thoracoscopic repair of ventricular septal defect: a short-term clinical observation on safety and feasibility. J Thorac Cardiovasc Surg. 2011;142:850–4.
9. Xiao C, Gao C, Yang M, Wang G, Wu Y, Wang J, Wang R, Yao M. Totally robotic atrial septal defect closure: 7-year single-institution experience and follow-up. Interact Cardiovasc Thorac Surg. 2014;19:933–7.
10. Casselman FP, Van Slycke S, Dom H, Lambrechts DL, Vermeulen Y, Vanermen H. Endoscopic mitral valve repair: feasible, reproducible, and durable. J Thorac Cardiovasc Surg. 2003;125:273–82.
11. Holzhey DM, Seeburger J, Misfeld M, Borger MA, Mohr FW. Learning minimally invasive mitral valve surgery: a cumulative sum sequential probability analysis of 3895 operations from a single high-volume center. Circulation. 2013;128:483–91.
12. Garbade J, Davierwala P, Seeburger J, Pfannmueller B, Misfeld M, Borger MA, Mohr FW. Myocardial protection during minimally invasive mitral valve surgery: strategies and cardioplegic solutions. Ann Cardiothorac Surg. 2013;2:803–8.
13. Okamoto K, Yozu R. Designing innovative retractors and devices to facilitate mitral valve repair surgery. Ann Cardiothorac Surg. 2015;4:364–9.
14. Casselman FP, Van Slycke S, Wellens F, De Geest R, Degrieck I, Van Praet F, Vermeulen Y, Vanermen H. Mitral valve surgery can now routinely be performed endoscopically. Circulation. 2003;108(Suppl 1):II48–54.
15. Ma ZS, Yang CY, Dong MF, Wu SM, Wang LX. Totally thoracoscopic closure of ventricular septal defect without a robotically assisted surgical system: a summary of 119 cases. J Thorac Cardiovasc Surg. 2014;147:863–7.
16. Liu X, Wu Y, Zhu J, Lv X, Tang Y, Sun J, Zhang S. Totally thoracoscopic repair of atrial septal defect reduces systemic inflammatory reaction and myocardial damage in initial patients. Eur J Med Res. 2014;19:13.
17. Raanani E, Spiegelstein D, Sternik L, Preisman S, Moshkovitz Y, Smolinsky AK, Shinfeld A. Quality of mitral valve repair: median sternotomy versus port-access approach. J Thorac Cardiovasc Surg. 2010;140:86–90.
18. Misfeld M, Borger M, Byrne JG, et al. Cross-sectional survey on minimally invasive mitral valve surgery. Ann Cardiothorac Surg. 2013;2:733–8.
19. Marullo AG, Irace FG, Vitulli P, et al. Recent developments in minimally invasive cardiac surgery: evolution or revolution? Biomed Res Int. 2015;483025:2015.
20. Modi P, Chitwood WR Jr. Retrograde femoral arterial perfusion and stroke risk during minimally invasive mitral valve surgery: is there cause for concern? Ann Cardiothorac Surg. 2013;2(6):E1. https://doi.org/10.3978/j.issn.2225-319X.2013.11.13.
21. Yu T, Zhang X, Huang K. Temporary epicardial pacing wire placement in totally endoscopic cardiac surgery. Asian Cardiovasc Thorac Ann. 2016;24:613–5.
22. van der Merwe J, Casselman F, Stockman B, Vermeulen Y, Degrieck I, Van Praet F. Endoscopic atrioventricular valve surgery in adults with difficult-to-access uncorrected congenital chest wall deformities. Interact Cardiovasc Thorac Surg. 2016;23:851–5.
23. van der Merwe J, Casselman F, Stockman B, Vermeulen Y, Degrieck I, Van Praet F. Late redo-port access surgery after port access surgery. Interact Cardiovasc Thorac Surg. 2016;22:13–8.
24. Ito T, Maekawa A, Hoshino S, Hayashi Y, Sawaki S, Yanagisawa J, Tokoro M. Three-port (one incision plus two-port) endoscopic mitral valve surgery without robotic assistance. Eur J Cardiothorac Surg. 2017.
25. Ishikawa N, Sun YS, Nifong LW, Watanabe G, Chitwood WR Jr. Port-access atrium retractors for totally endoscopic mitral valve surgery: theTornado Retractor, the Butterfly Retractor, and the Semiautomatic Butterfly Retractor. Surg Endosc. 2008;22:2088–90.
26. Badhwar V, Rankin JS, He M, et al. Performing concomitant tricuspid valve repair at the time of mitral valve operations is not associated with increased operative mortality. Ann Thorac Surg. 2017;103:587–93.
27. Zubritskiy A, Arkhipov A, Khapaev T, et al. The Warden procedure can be successfully performed using minimally invasive cardiac surgery without aortic clamping. Interact Cardiovasc Thorac Surg. 2016;22:225–7.

29

Treatment of malignant primary cardiac lymphoma with tumor resection using minimally invasive cardiac surgery

Yuki Endo[1*], Yoshitsugu Nakamura[1], Miho Kuroda[1], Yusuke Nakanishi[1], Yujiro Ito[1], Takaki Hori[1], Rumiko Okamoto[2] and Hiroshi Konishi[3]

Abstract

Background: Primary cardiac lymphoma (PCL) is extremely rare and progresses rapidly. The treatment of PCL has not yet been established. Unlike lymphoma that arises from other organs, PCL causes cardiovascular events. We report the complete remission (CR) of PCL after tumor resection using minimally invasive cardiac surgery (MICS) and chemotherapy.

Case presentation: The patient was a 79-year-old man who visited our hospital with chief complaints of weight loss and leg edema. A 40×30 mm mobile pedunculated tumor continuous with the right ventricular heart muscle was present in the right atrium upon echocardiography and extended cardiac surgery was difficult to perform. Tumor embolism-induced sudden death was prevented and a pathological diagnosis was obtained by making a 4-cm skin incision, and tumor resection with MICS was performed through a right fourth intercostal thoracotomy with a cardiopulmonary system. The histopathological diagnosis was diffuse large B cell malignant lymphoma. Eight cycles of postoperative rituximab plus cyclophosphamide, doxorubicin, vincristine, and prednisone (R-CHOP) therapy were performed. Three years after surgery, the tumor was not visible on imaging and CR was maintained.

Conclusions: This case highlights that tumor resection using MICS is effective for avoiding the risk of sudden death. This technique was useful for the diagnosis and treatment of a malignant cardiac tumor in an elderly patient that required a difficult extended cardiac surgery.

Keywords: Malignant primary cardiac lymphoma, Minimally invasive cardiac surgery, Tumor resection, Diffuse large B-cell malignant lymphoma, R-CHOP therapy

Background

Benign tumors such as myxomas account for a high percentage of primary cardiac tumors; however, primary malignant cardiac tumors (PMCTs) account for 5.1–28.7% of primary cardiac tumors. Primary cardiac lymphoma (PCL) is extremely rare, accounting for only 1.0–1.6% of PMCTs, but this tumor is difficult to diagnose and progresses rapidly [1, 2]. Moreover, the prognosis is poor because no consistent treatment has been established [1–3]. Unlike lymphoma that arises from other organs, PCL causes cardiovascular events. If a malignant cardiac tumor is suspected, biopsy is necessary to obtain a definitive diagnosis for chemotherapy and radiotherapy and can be achieved with either computed tomography (CT)-guided puncture or an intravenous approach. However, these methods are not able to prevent sudden death due to tumor embolism, can yield inaccurate samples due to tumor necrosis and fibrin clots, and cannot be used for mobile tumors because of the risk of embolus formation. Furthermore, cardiac surgery via a median sternotomy is very invasive, particularly in elderly patients. In addition, radiotherapy cannot be used with median sternotomy due to the risks of postoperative surgical site infections and mediastinitis. Therefore, mobile tumor resection by MICS without a median sternotomy was performed to reduce the risk of tumor embolism and to obtain an accurate pathological diagnosis. We report the CR of PCL after tumor resection using MICS and chemotherapy.

---

* Correspondence: endo.yuki@twmu.ac.jp
[1]Department of Cardiovascular Surgery, Chiba-Nishi General Hospital, 107-1, Kanegasaku, Matsudo-shi, Chiba 270-2251, Japan
Full list of author information is available at the end of the article

Case report

The patient was a 79-year-old man with chief complaints of exertional dyspnea, leg edema, and weight loss. On transthoracic echocardiography (TTE), a 25 × 40 mm mobile pedunculated mass continuous with the right ventricular heart muscle was detected in the right atrium and the patient was admitted to our department for close examination and treatment. At admission, his height was 162.0 cm, body weight was 61.1 kg, body temperature was 36.3 °C, pulse was 62 beats/min, blood pressure was 112/59 mmHg, and SpO_2 was 100% (room air). Pulmonary sounds were clear with no crackles, and heart sounds were regular with no murmur. Leg edema was present.

Plain chest radiography revealed a cardiothoracic ratio of 49% with no cardiac dilation. Electrocardiography revealed a sinus rhythm with a heart rate of 71 beats/min with nonspecific ST-T segment changes. Blood chemistry revealed the following: white blood cell (WBC) count of $51.9 × 10^4/\mu L$, hemoglobin (Hb) of 14.9 g/dL, platelet (Plt) count of $16.3 × 10^4/\mu L$, creatine kinase (CK) of 81 U/L, creatine kinase-MB (CKMB) of 8 ng/mL, lactate dehydrogenase (LDH) of 161 U/L, C-reactive protein (CRP) of 0.10 mg/dL, carcinoembryonic antigen (CEA) of 0.7 ng/mL, prostate-specific antigen (PSA) of 1.2 ng/mL, squamous cell carcinoma (SCC) antigen of 1.2 ng/mL, and soluble IL-2 receptor: 633 U/mL. Inflammatory parameters were within the normal range and the soluble IL-2 receptor level was slightly elevated, but the levels of other tumor markers were within their normal ranges. A coronary computed tomography (CT) scan showed no significant stenosis. It was deemed very difficult to completely excise, so we decided on partial tumor resection with MICS to reduce the risk of tumor embolism and to obtain an accurate pathology diagnosis. Therefore, we did not perform CAG. If we had performed a CAG, we may have seen arteries feeding the tumor.

TTE showed a 40 × 30-mm mobile pedunculated tumor in the right atrium that was continuous with the right ventricular heart muscle (Fig. 1a). Transesophageal echocardiography (TEE) showed a solid septated tumor with an irregular surface invading the free wall of the right atrium and surrounding the annulus of the anterior cusp and right and left coronary cusps of the aortic valve (Fig. 1b). Contrast-enhanced CT showed invasion based on soft tissue intensity near the tricuspid valve above the anterior right ventricle in the region between the aorta and pulmonary artery and around the pulmonary artery (Fig. 2a, b). Cardiac magnetic resonance imaging (MRI) showed a thickened anterior wall near the tricuspid valve and a mass protruding into the lumen and expanding into the region between the aorta and the pulmonary artery (Fig. 3a, b); in addition to the patient's advanced age, these features made it difficult to perform extended cardiac surgery. On fluorodeoxyglucose positron emission tomography (F-18 FDG-PET), there was

abnormal accumulation in the right atrium surrounding the aortic root (Fig. 4a).

Surgery was performed to prevent tumor embolism-induced sudden death and to obtain a pathological diagnosis. Anticoagulation was not performed preoperatively because it was unlikely that the tumor was a thrombus. A double-lumen tube was inserted during surgery and a Swan-Ganz catheter and 14-Fr cannula were inserted through the right internal jugular vein after draping. In a supine position with 30° elevation of the right side, a 4-cm skin incision was made in the fourth intercostal region at the medial aspect of the nipple. Meanwhile, the femoral artery (FA) and femoral vein (FV) were exposed. A pericardiotomy was performed 2 cm anterior to the phrenic nerve and the pericardium was elevated. After systemic heparinization, an 18-Fr blood supply tube was inserted through the right FA, and a 25-Fr cannula was inserted through the right FV to establish a cardiopulmonary bypass (CPB). The superior vena cava was blocked with a bulldog clamp and the heart rate was controlled at 40–50 bpm with a β-blocker. An oblique incision was made in the right atrium with the heart beating, and the lumen was observed. The tumor adhered to the anterior surface of the right atrium but not to the annular region and had marked mobility. The tumor was grasped with an Endocatch and the pedicle of 1-cm width was transected using electric cautery (Fig. 5a). The lack of any residual right atrial tumor or shunt was confirmed and the right atrium was closed in a double suture pattern; the patient was then weaned from CPB. The pericardium was closed as far as possible, the wound was closed by the standard method, and surgery was completed. The operative time was 1 h 56 min, and the duration of CPB was 38 min (Additional file 1).

Intraoperative macroscopic findings revealed a tumor with a smooth, greyish-white surface (Fig. 5b). A blackish-brown region suggestive of hemorrhage was present inside and on pathological examination (Fig. 6), a diffuse proliferation of round cells with a high nuclear-to-cytoplasmic (N/C) ratio were observed on hematoxylin and eosin staining. The tumor cells were mainly medium- and small-sized cells that contained nuclei with a shallow cut that were the same size or slightly smaller than the nuclei of vascular endothelial cells; large cells were also present. Broken nuclear products and histiocytes phagocytosing these products were also observed. Upon immunohistological staining, the tumor cells were CD79α-positive and CD3-negative. B-cell-derived cells were overwhelmingly predominant, which suggested that the lesion was a B-cell-derived tumor. Epithelial membrane antigen (EMA) immunostaining was negative. Based on these findings, the patient was diagnosed with diffuse large B-cell lymphoma (DLBCL).

Extubation was performed 6 h after surgery and the patient was transferred to a general ward 2 days after

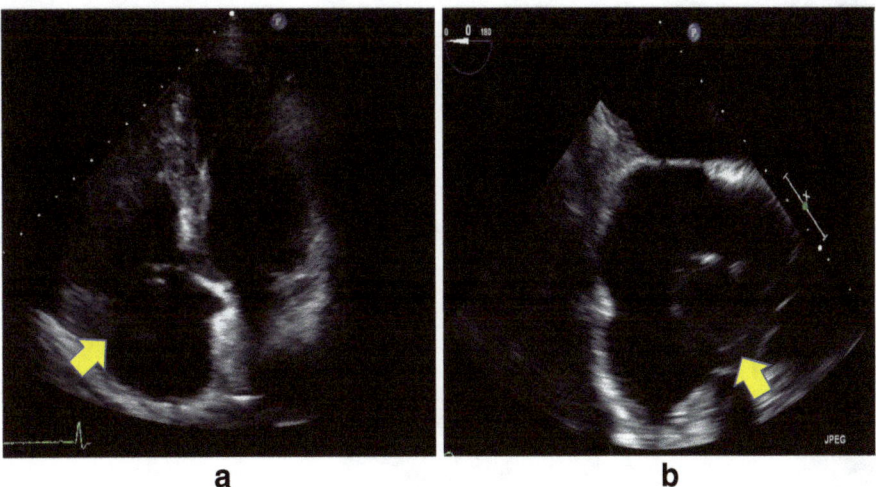

Fig. 1 Preoperative echocardiography. **a** Transthoracic echocardiography showed a mobile pedunculated tumor in the right atrium. **b** Transesophageal echocardiography showed a solid, septated tumor with an irregular surface invading the free wall of the right atrium and surrounding the annulus of the anterior cusp and right and left coronary cusps of the aortic valve

surgery. The disappearance of the tumor from the annular region was confirmed on TTE 5 days after surgery and the patient was discharged when he was able to independently walk 6 days after surgery. After observation at an outpatient clinic, rituximab plus cyclophosphamide, doxorubicin, vincristine, and prednisone (R-CHOP) therapy was initiated 37 days after surgery. After 8 cycles were administered in total, an FDG-PET scan performed 456 days after surgery showed no abnormal accumulation (Fig. 4b), indicating CR.

Discussion

PMCTs account for approximately 5.1–28.7% of primary cardiac tumors and diagnosis is difficult in many cases [1, 2]. PMCTs tend to occur in young patients with a mean age of 44 years and there was no difference in the ratio between the sexes [3]. The prognosis is poor, with a five-year survival rate of 19% [4]. Among PMCTs, although 75% is sarcoma, 1.0–1.6% is PCL. PCL is defined as extranodal lymphoma in which lesions only develop in the heart and pericardium or in which a giant tumor develops in the heart accompanied by an asymptomatic solitary extracardiac lesion or several localized lesions [5, 6]. Common sites are the right heart and epicardium, and the histological type is DLBCL in many cases [6]. Unlike lymphoma arising from other organs, PCL causes cardiovascular events such as heart failure, cardiac tamponade, arrhythmia, and embolism, leading to an acute presentation [1–7].

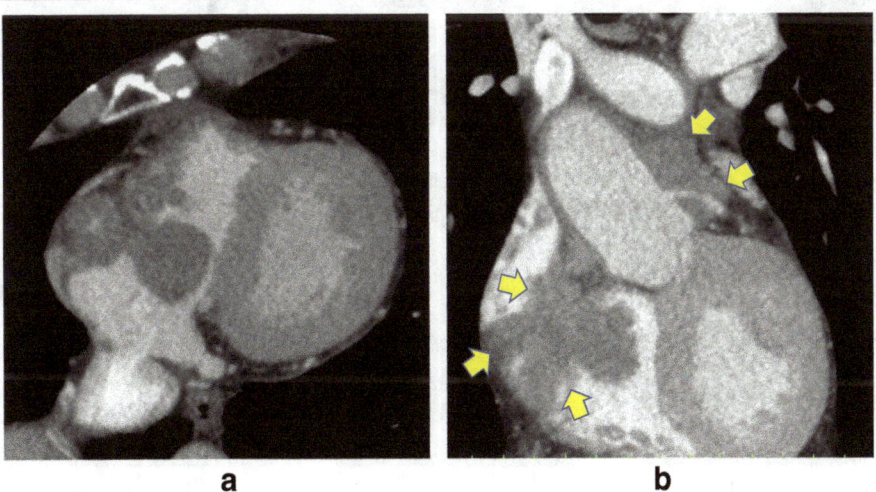

Fig. 2 Preoperative contrast-enhanced CT. The big tumor was existed in the right atrium with axial section (**a**). The right arrows show invasion based on soft tissue intensity near the tricuspid valve above the anterior right ventricle in the region between the aorta and pulmonary artery, and around the pulmonary artery with coronal section (**b**)

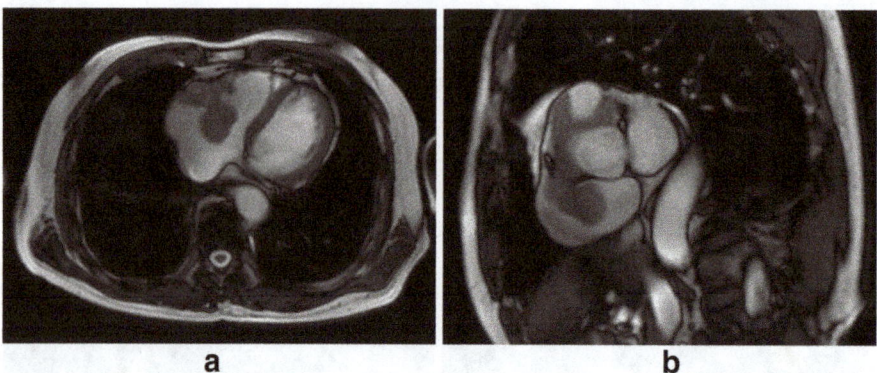

Fig. 3 Preoperative cardiac MRI. Cardiac MRI showed a thickened anterior wall near the tricuspid valve with axial section (**a**) and a mass protruding into the lumen and expanding into the region between the aorta and pulmonary artery with coronal section (**b**)

In our patient, a giant mobile pedunculated tumor in the right atrium with heart muscle invasion was evident on TTE and TEE performed to evaluate the causes of the patient's difficulty breathing and leg edema. An intracardiac tumor and invasion of the region between the aorta and pulmonary artery and near the pulmonary artery were observed without abnormalities in other organs on CT, which suggested a PMCT. In addition, PCL was suspected because of heart failure symptoms such as difficulty breathing and leg edema, and the development in the right heart.

There were three therapeutic options: 1. complete resection through median sternotomy, 2. CT-guided or intravenous biopsy followed by chemotherapy or radiotherapy, and 3. tumor resection of the mobile part with MICS followed by chemotherapy or radiotherapy. Regarding complete resection through median sternotomy, this was deemed too invasive for the patient because the cardiac invasion pattern of the tumor was complex, would require resection of the atrioventricular junction, and the patient was elderly. In addition, median sternotomy is associated with a high risk of surgical site infections and mediastinitis if radiotherapy on the mediastinum was necessary. Certainly, there was a case report in which the tumor was resected with an emergency median sternotomy; however, the results of enlargement surgery via a

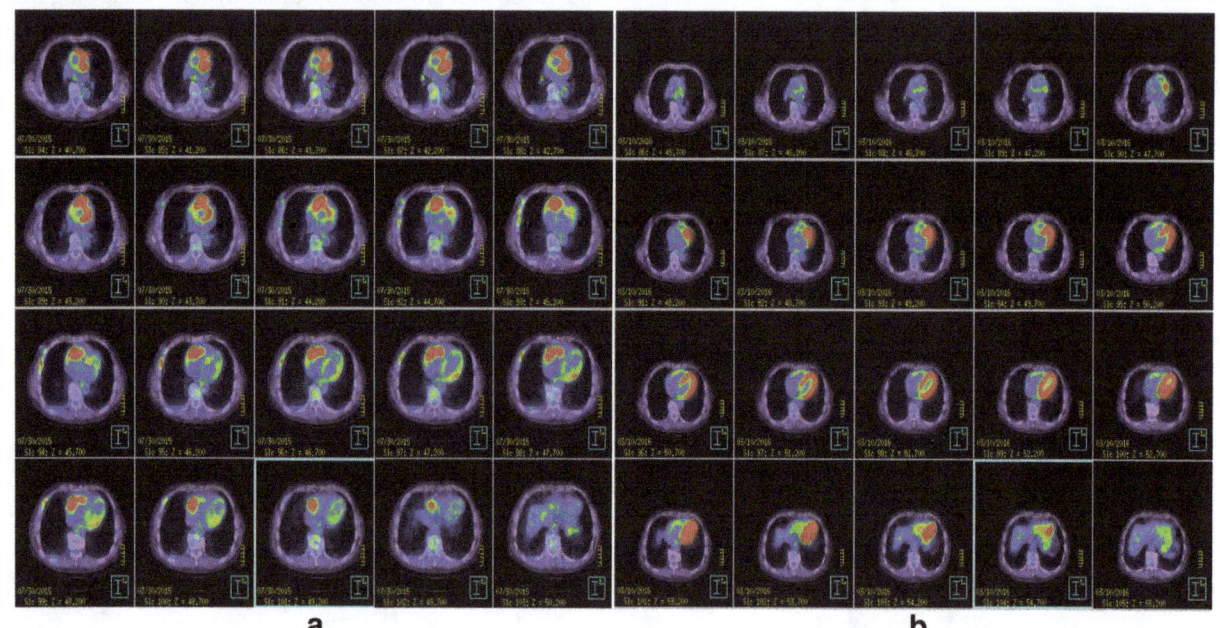

Fig. 4 F-18 FDG-PET. **a** Preoperative PET-CT showed abnormal accumulation in the right atrium surroundings the aortic root. **b** Postoperative PET-CT showed complete remission after completion of chemotherapy. Accumulation in the left ventricular myocardium was physiological, and the abnormal accumulation around the aortic root and pulmonary artery had disappeared

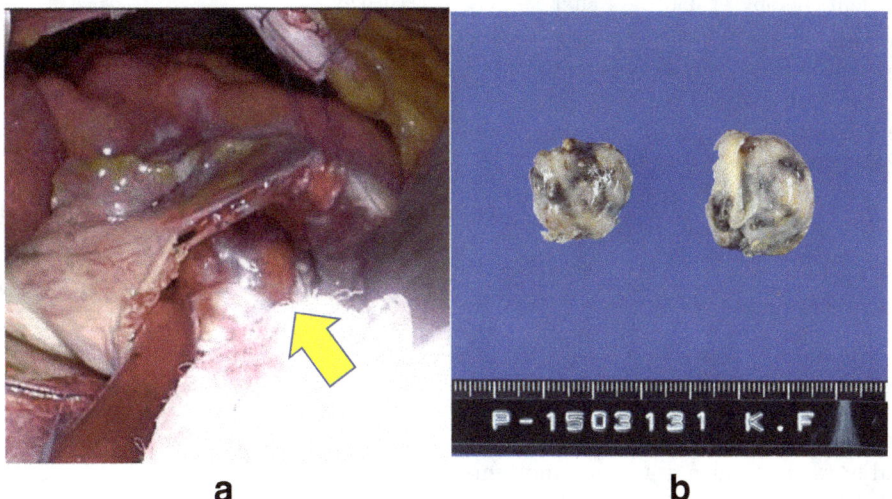

Fig. 5 Intraoperative photos and specimen. **a** An oblique incision was made in the right atrium with the heart beating, and the lumen was observed. The tumor adhered to the anterior surface of the right atrium but not to the annular region and had marked mobility. **b** Intraoperative macroscopic findings revealed a tumor with a smooth, greyish-white surface

median sternotomy incision are poor and there has never been a good report [8, 9]. Regarding CT-guided or intravenous biopsy, this could not prevent sudden death due to tumor embolism and atrioventricular valve obstruction. Generally, biopsy could have been achieved with a CT-guided or intravenous approach and some reports have shown these approaches' effectiveness [8–10]. However, these techniques were not possible in this case because the tumor was very mobile; in addition, these methods can yield inaccurate samples due to tumor necrosis and fibrin clots [10].

Based on these considerations, to avoid the risk of embolism and perform a biopsy in a minimally invasive manner, we decided to perform tumor resection using minimally invasive beating-heart surgery followed by

adjuvant therapy. Preoperative FDG-PET showed abnormal accumulation in the right atrium surrounding the aortic root and the pathological diagnosis was DLBCL. This disease responds to anthracycline-based chemotherapy regimens [11] and remission has been reported after chemotherapy alone or after chemotherapy used in combination with radiotherapy [12, 13] The DLBCL treatment algorithm for our patient recommended combined modality treatment with 3 cycles of R-CHOP therapy with involved-field radiotherapy (IFRT) or 6–8 cycles of R-CHOP therapy ± IFRT [14–16]. Early diagnosis and treatment intervention may determine the outcome [13], and 8 cycles of R-CHOP therapy were performed to avoid radiotherapy, beginning 37 days after MICS tumor resection. There was no abnormal accumulation on FDG-PET

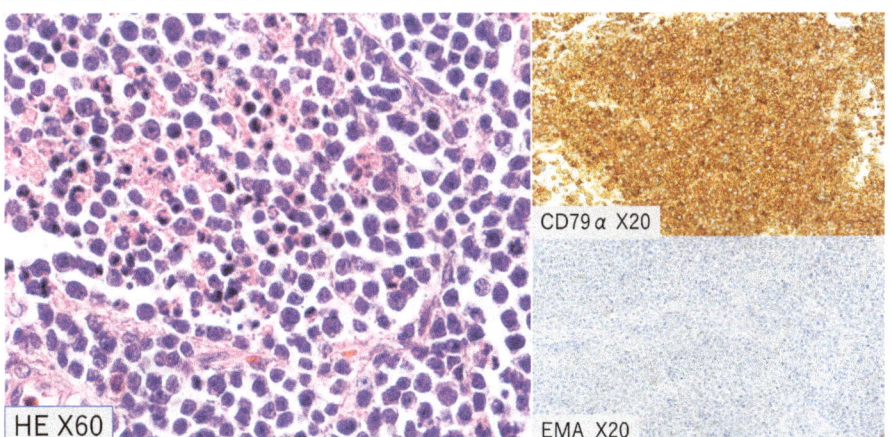

Fig. 6 Pathology. The tumor cells were CD79α-positive and CD3-negative. B-cell-derived cells were overwhelmingly predominant, suggesting that the lesion was a B-cell-derived tumor. Epithelial membrane antigen immunostaining was negative

after completing chemotherapy at 456 days after surgery and CR was achieved. IFRT was not performed because the radiation range was unclear and damage to the heart muscle by direct irradiation was possible. Careful observation has been recommended for patients with CR after R-CHOP therapy because there are no data showing improved survival with maintenance therapy [17]. Our patient has had no recurrence and careful follow-up is ongoing.

Conclusion

This case provides an example of a patient with an accurate pathological diagnosis who underwent successful chemotherapy and in whom sudden death by tumor embolism was avoided by tumor resection with MICS rather than by median sternotomy, which is associated with risks of delayed wound healing and mediastinitis if postoperative radiotherapy is required. As in this patient, tumor resection with MICS may be useful for patients in whom sudden death by tumor embolism is highly likely and in whom chemotherapy, radiotherapy, or both are necessary.

Funding
Funding from Chibanishi General Hospital is gratefully acknowledged.

Informed consent
We received explicit consent from the patient.

Author's contributions
YE is the corresponding author. YN conceived of the study and participated in its design and coordination. YE, MK, NY, YI, TH, RO and HK helped to draft the manuscript. All authors read and approved the final manuscript.

Competing interests
The authors declare that they have no competing interests.

Author details
[1]Department of Cardiovascular Surgery, Chiba-Nishi General Hospital, 107-1, Kanegasaku, Matsudo-shi, Chiba 270-2251, Japan. [2]Departments of Oncology, Chiba-Nishi General Hospital, 107-1, Kanegasaku, Matsudo-shi, Chiba 270-2251, Japan. [3]Departments of Hematology, Chiba-Nishi General Hospital, 107-1, Kanegasaku, Matsudo-shi, Chiba 270-2251, Japan.

References
1. Butany J, Nair V, Naseemuddin A, Nair GM, Catton C, Yau T. Cardiac tumors: diagnosis and management. Lancet Oncol. 2005;6:219–28.
2. Burazor I, Aviel-Ronen S, Imazio M, Markel G, Grossman Y, Yosepovich A, Adler Y. Primary malignancies of the heart and pericardium. Clin Cardiol. 2014;37:582–8.
3. Ramlawi B, Leja MJ, Abu Saleh WK, et al. Surgical treatment of primary cardiac sarcomas: review of a single-institution experience. Ann Thorac Surg. 2016;101:698–702.
4. Guilherme H, Al-Kindi SG, Hoimes C, Park SJ. Characteristics and survival of malignant cardiac tumors: a 40-year analysis of >500 patients. Circulation. 2015;132:2395–402.
5. HA MA, Fenoglio JJ. Tumors of the cardiovascular system. Atlas of tumor pathology, 2nd series. Fascicle 15. Washington: Armed Forces Institute of Pathology; 1978. p. 99–100.
6. Ceresoli GL, AJM F, Bucci E, Ripa C, Ponzoni M, Villa E. Primary cardialymphoma in immunocompetent patients: diagnostic and therapeutic management. Cancer. 1997;80:1497–506.
7. Patel J, Melly I, Sheppard MN. Primary cardiac lymphoma: B- and T-cell cases at a specialist UK centre. Ann Oncol. 2010;21:1041–5.
8. Anghel G, Zoil V, Remotti D, et al. Primary cardiac lymphoma: report of two cases occurring in immunocompetent subjects. Leuk Lymphoma. 2004; 45(4):781–8.
9. Sang-Bum Kang MD, Seung-Won Jin MD, Eun-Kyeong Lee MD, et al. A case of non-Hodgkin's lymphoma with massive involvement of the right atrium. Kor Circ J. 2000;(4):492–6.
10. Tanaka J, Takamoto S, Ryu T, Ichikawa K, Masuo M, Saito T. Primary cardiac lymphoma: a case report. J Cardiol. 2002;40:225–9.
11. Perich A, Cho SI, Billett H. Primary cardiac lymphoma: an analysis of presentation, treatment, and outcome patterns. Cancer. 2011;117:581–9.
12. Masaki Y, Hideaki N, Nobuo K, et al. Multidisciplinary approach for primary cardiac lymphoma associated with hemodynamic failure caused by tricuspid valve obstruction. J Cardiol Cases. 2016;13:189–92.
13. Miyashita T, Miyazawa I, Kawaguchi T, Kasai T, Yamaura T, Ito T, et al. A case of primary cardiac B cell lymphoma associated with ventricular tachycardia, success fully treated with systemic chemotherapy and radiotherapy. Jpn Circ J. 2000;64:135–8.
14. Persky DO, Unger JM, Spier CM, Stea B, LeBlanc M, McCarty MJ, et al. Phase II study of rituximab plus three cycles of CHOP and involved-field radiotherapy for patients with limited-stage aggressive B-cell lymphoma: southwest oncology group study 0014. J Clin Oncol. 2008;26:2258–63.
15. Miller TP, Dahlberg S, Cassady JR, Adelstein DJ, Spier CM, Grogan TM, et al. Chemotherapy alone compared with chemotherapy plus radiotherapy for localized intermediate and high-grade non-Hodgkin's lymphoma. N Engl J Med. 1998;339:21–6.
16. Pfreundschuh M, Trümper L, Osterborg A, Pettengell R, Trneny M, Imrie K, et al. CHOP-like chemotherapy plus rituximab versus CHOP-like chemotherapy alone in young patients with good-prognosis diffuse large-B-cell lymphoma: a randomised controlled trial by the MabThera international trial (MInT) group. Lancet Oncol. 2006;7:379–91.
17. Habermann TM, Weller EA, Morrison VA, Gascoyne RD, Cassileth PA, Cohn JB, et al. Rituximab-CHOP versus CHOP alone or with maintenance rituximab in older patients with diffuse large B-cell lymphoma. J Clin Oncol. 2006;24:3121–7.

30

Sutureless technique versus conventional surgery in the primary treatment of total anomalous pulmonary venous connection

Yuhao Wu[1,4,5,6†], Zhichao Wu[2†], Junmeng Zheng[2*], Yonggang Li[1,4,5,6], Yuehang Zhou[1,4,5,6], Hongyu Kuang[3,4,5,6], Xin Jin[1,4,5,6] and Chun Wu[1,4,5,6*]

Abstract

Backgroud: A meta-analysis was performed to compare the differences in outcomes between sutureless technique and conventional surgery for primary repair of Total Anomalous Pulmonary Venous Connection(TAPVC).

Methods: Electronic databases, including PubMed, EMbase, Medline, CNKI, Wanfang Data and Weipu Data were searched systematically for the literature aimed mainly at comparing the therapeutic effects for primary repair of TAPVC administered by sutureless technique and conventional surgery. Corresponding data sets were extracted and two reviewers independently assessed the methodological quality.

Results: Seven studies meeting the inclusion criteria were included, involving a total of 1293 subjects. It was observed that sutureless technique entailed a lower occurrence rate of post-operative Pulmonary Veins Obstruction (PVO) (OR, 0.52 95%CI, 0.32–0.86; $P = 0.01$) and re-operation due to PVO (OR, 0.28;95%CI, 0.09–0.87; $P = 0.03$). However, meta-analyses of hospitalization time (WMD, 5.92; 95%CI, − 7.97-19.80; $P = 0.40$) and post-operative mortality (OR, 0.65; 95%CI, 0.41–1.04; $P = 0.07$) showed no significant differences between sutureless technique and conventional surgery. Meta-analysis of Cardiopulmonary Bypass (CPB) time and aortic cross-clamp time also showed no significant differences between the two surgical approaches (WMD, 5.07; 95%CI, − 9.29-19.42; $P = 0.49$); (WMD, 5.73; 95%CI, − 7.76-19.23; $P = 0.40$), but the result remained inconclusive due to pooling result changes after sensitivity analysis.

Conclusions: Compared with conventional surgery, a lower occurrence rate of post-operative PVO and re-operation due to PVO were associated with sutureless technique. Meanwhile, hospitalization time and post-operative mortality were not statistically different between the two surgical approaches. Pooling result of CPB and aortic cross-clamp time between the two groups remained inconclusive.

Keywords: Congenital heart disease, Total anomalous pulmonary venous connection, Sutureless technique, Conventional surgery, Meta-analysis

* Correspondence: zhengjunmeng@126.com; 250734291@qq.com
†Yuhao Wu and Zhichao Wu contributed equally to this work.
2Department of Cardiovascular Surgery, Sun Yat-Sen Memorial Hospital, Sun Yat-Sen University, No.107 Yanjiang West Road, Yuexiu District, Guangzhou 510120, China
1Department of Cardiothoracic Surgery, Children's Hospital of Chongqing Medical University, No.136 Zhongshan Second Road, Yuzhong District, Chongqing 400014, China
Full list of author information is available at the end of the article

Background

Total Anomalous Pulmonary Venous Connection (TAPVC), a common congenital heart defect in which four pulmonary veins do not connect to the left atrium directly, occurres to 5.9–7.1 newborns per 100,000 neonates [1]. Traditionally, the main causes of death after conventional surgery for TAPVC are pulmonary hypertension and post-operative Pulmonary Venous Obstruction (PVO) [2]. In the 1990s, sutureless technique was employed to relieve the post-operative PVO [3, 4], in which the direct anastomosis between the left atrium and pulmonary veins was absent by creating a new left atrium by means of anastomosing the left atrium to the posterior pericardium. In recent years, this sutureless technique, utilized also for the primary repair of TAPVC, has been expanded for use in patients who had preoperative PVO or were at risk of developing PVO [5].

Although sutureless technique for primary repair of TAPVC was conducted by many advanced children's medical center, the safety and efficacy of sutureless technique remained controversial. This meta-analysis aimed to evaluate the outcomes of sutureless technique and conventional surgery for primary repair of TAPVC, as well as to provide explicit evidence to determine if sutureless technique in the treatment of TAPVC was superior to conventional surgery.

Methods

Literature search

We conducted the systematic search on the PubMed, EMbase, Medline, CNKI, Wanfang Data and Weipu Data for the relevant studies comparing the outcomes of applying sutureless technique and conventional surgery for priamry repair of TAPVC. The key words used for the search were *sutureless technique, sutureless surgery, conventional surgery, surgical repair, total anomalous pulmonary venous connection* and *total anomalous pulmonary venous drainage.* References from all the included studies and other relevant literature were also manually reviewed to identify additional eligible studies. This search was restricted to articles published in English and Chinese. The time period for the search was from January 1998 to March 2018. We contacted the authors through e-mail to acquire additional information as necessary.

Study selection

A study was included in this systematic review if it met both criteria as follow: 1) Cohort or case-controlled studies or Randomized Controlled Trials (RCTs); 2) The comparison of sutureless technique and conventional surgery for primary repair of TAPVC should be described in details. Specifically for sutureless technique, an incision was made on the posterior wall of the left atrium and the left atrial was anastomosed with the pericardium adjacent to the pulmonary vein, avoiding direct anastomosis with the pulmonary venous wall. For conventional surgery, the common pulmonary vein confluence was anastomosed to the left atrium directly for the supra-, infra- cardiac and mixed TAPVC. In the case of intracardiac TAPVC, an intra-atrial baffle technique between the atrial septal defect and the coronary sinus was created.

A study was excluded fromthis systematic review if any of the following was true: 1) Multiple studies were based on the same data; 2) Studies included sutureless technique for recurrent or post-operative PVO; 3) Studies only included patients with congenital or secondary pulmonary vein stenosis. 4) The clinical outcomes were not to our interest. Reviews, conference records, case reports and animal experiments were also excluded.

Two reviewers (W.Y.H and W.Z.C) screened all the studies independently and blindly. Any disagreements on the eligibility of studies were resolved by discussion with the third reviewer(K.H.Y).

Data extraction

Data extracted by two reviewers (W.Y.H and W.Z.C) independently and blindly were checked by the third reviewer(K.H.Y) for accuracy. A standardized extraction form in an Excel spreadsheet was used. The following information was extracted: 1) baseline characteristics of included studies: first author, publication year, study design, surgical approach, sample size, type of TAPVC, weight, age, occurrence of preoperative PVO, associated cardiac anomalies and follow-up time; 2) outcomes of both surgical approaches: cardiopulmonary bypass time, aortic cross-clamp time, post-operative mortality, total number of operation, occurrence rate of post-operative PVO and re-operation. Post-operative death was defined as death related to the surgery directly. Post-operative PVO was defined as obstruction in the anastomosis that occurred after initial surgery and diagnosed with cardiac echo. Re-operation was defined as surgery performed only for post-operative PVO that occurred after discharge. Total number of operation was defined as the sum of initial surgery plus re-operation.

Quality assessment

Quality assessment was performed by two reviewers (W.Y.H and W.Z.C) independently and bindly. Any disagreements on the assessed quality were resolved via consultation with the third reviewer(K.H.Y). The quality of the included studies was evaluated by using Newcastle-Ottawa Scale (NOS) scores. A study was judged on three dimensions with the Newcastle-Ottawa Scale (NOS) scale: the selection of the study groups; the comparability of the groups; and the ascertainment of the exposure [6].The maximum score of NOS was 9 and the minimum score was zero. Each study was graded as either low (scores 0–5) or high quality (scores 6–9).

Statistical analysis

All statistical analyses were conducted by using RevMan software (version 5.3; The Nordic Cochrane Centre, Copenhagen, Denmark), and $P < 0.05$ was considered statistically significant. Odds Ratio (OR) and Weighted Mean Difference (WMD) were adopted for dichotomous and continuous data. Heterogeneity was evaluated with the Cochrane Q test and the I^2 statistics, with $I^2 > 50\%$ indicating heterogeneity. If the I^2 statistic $> 50\%$, a random-effects model was adopted, and sensitivity analysis was used to detect the sources of heterogeneity; otherwise, a fixed-effects model of analysis was adopted. Sensitivity analyses were performed using the leave-one-out method in which the meta-analysis of outcomes was conducted with each study removed in turn until significant reduction in heterogeneity was observed. If the direction and magnitude of pooling estimates with respect to outcomes did not vary significantly with the removal of any given study, it indicated that the meta-analysis was confirmed and the data were not overly influenced by any study. Formulas provided by Hozo et al. [7] would be used to estimate the mean values and standard differences if only the median value and range were available. The publication bias was evaluated with Begg's test and Egger's test using Stata 12.0 (Stata Corp,Texas).

Results

A total of 50 studies were identified initially. After screening for duplicates and relevance in titles and abstracts, only 15 studies were eligible for the full-text evaluation. Eventually, this meta-analysis was based on 7 retrospective None-Randomized Controlled Trials(NRCTs). The literature search and study selection have been double checked by both reviewers (W.Y.H and W.Z.C), and the flowchart depicting the search strategy is shown in the Fig. 1.

Characteristics of included studies and quality assessments

All 7 studies [8–14] were retrospective NRCTs. A Total of 1293 patients were involved in this study, of whom 278 were in the sutureless technique group and 1015 in the conventional surgery group. Quality assessments of the included studies were carried out in accordance with the NOS. The NOS score of each of the 7 included studies [8–14] was higher than 6 (high quality). The characteristics of the included studies and quality assessments were described in detail in Table 1. All of the TAPVC patients were diagnosed with cardiac echo and combined with enhanced CT scan. The associated anomalies were shown in the Table 2.

The results of funnel plot could be considered accurate only when a minimum of 7 studies was included. Post-operative mortality were provided by all 7 NRCTs, therefore, we only conducted the funnel plot of post-operative mortality and no significant publication bias was found (Begg's test $P = 0.88$, Egger's test $P = 0.248$) (Fig. 2).

Cardiopulmonary bypass time (CPB)

Six of the 7 studies [8–10, 12–14] that analyzed the CPB time of both surgical approaches were included in this meta-analysis. Since a heterogeneity test

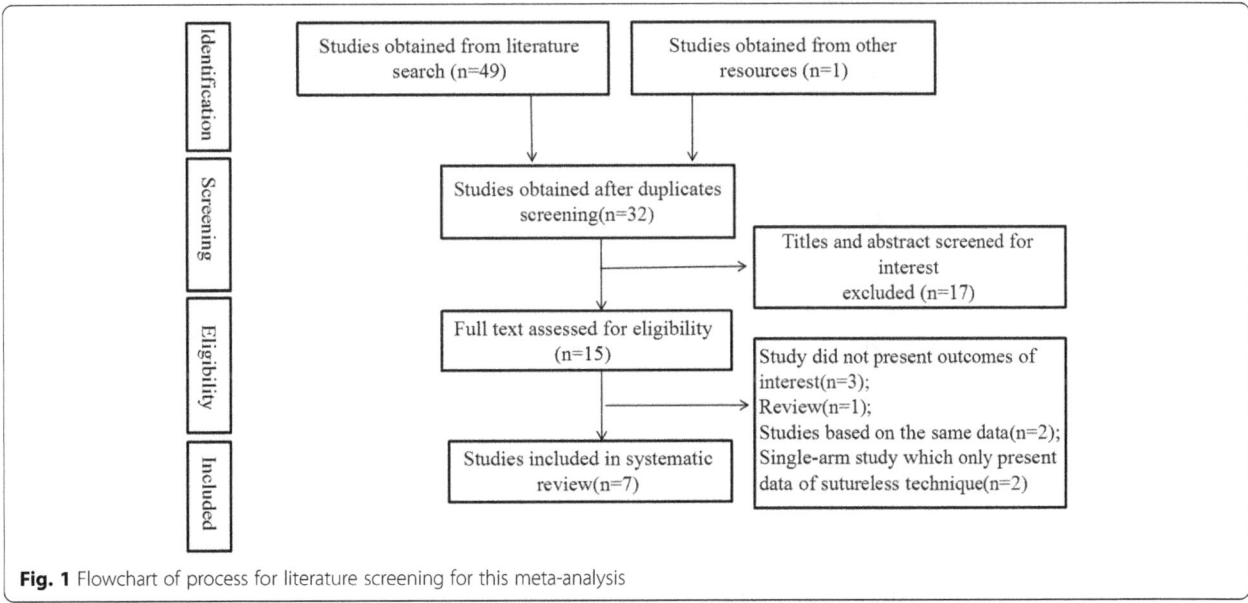

Fig. 1 Flowchart of process for literature screening for this meta-analysis

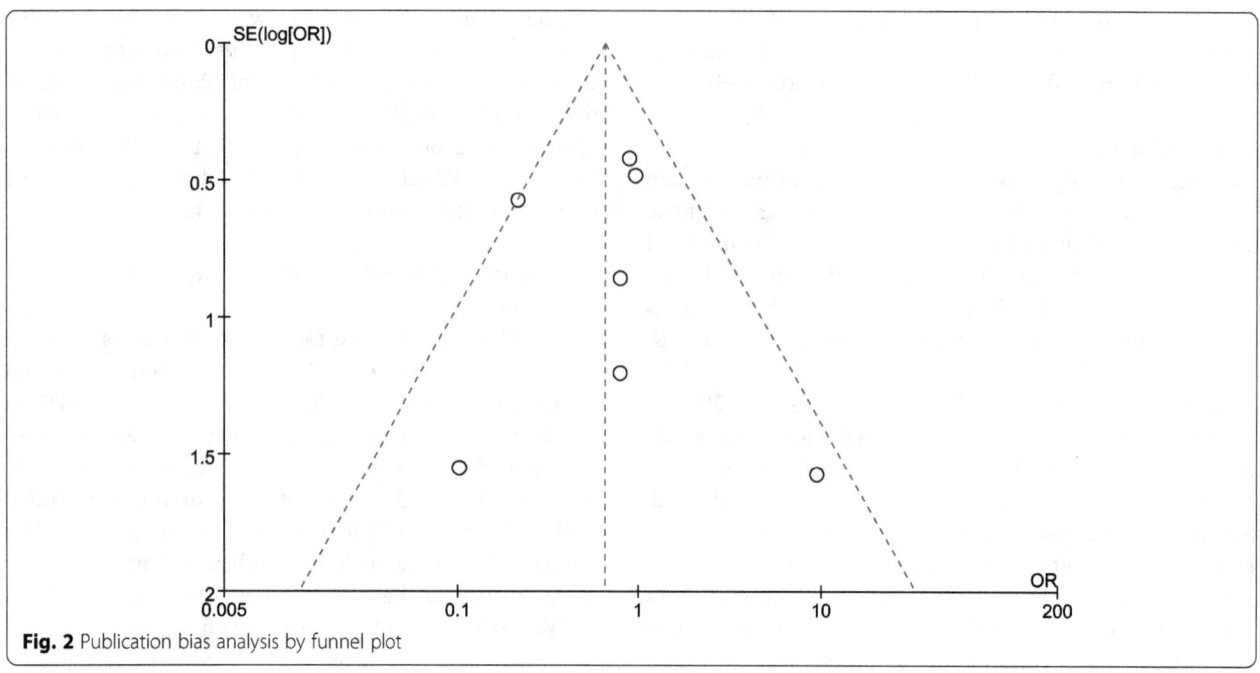

Fig. 2 Publication bias analysis by funnel plot

revealed Chi^2 = 253.05, $P < 0.001$, I^2 = 98%, therefore a randomized effects model was employed (Fig. 3). The result indicated that no statistically significant difference was observed between the two surgical approaches with respect to CPB time(WMD, 5.07; 95%CI, – 9.29-19.42; $P = 0.49$).

Aortic cross-clamp time

A total of 6 studies [8–10, 12–14] that analyzed the aortic cross-clamp time of both surgical approaches were included in this meta-analysis. A heterogeneity test revealed Chi^2 = 480.06, $P < 0.001$, I^2 = 99%, therefore a randomized effects model was employed (Fig. 4). The

Table 1 Characteristics and quality assessment of included studies

Author	Publication year	Study design	Surgical approach	Patients M/F (sex)	Type of TAPVC (supracardiac/ car-diac/ infracar-diac/ mixed)	Weight (Kg)	Age	Preoperative PVO (n)	Follow-up time	NOS
Gao [8]	2017	Retrospective	ST	56/25	63/0/14/4	4.3(3.3–5.3)^b	60(25.5–150)d	24	12 m^a	7
			CS	74/24	69/0/11/18	4.6(3.4–6)	60(29.3–180)d	28	12 m	(High)
Cui [9]	2016	Retrospective	ST	14	NA	3.5 ± 0.8	1.8 ± 0.4 m	NA	46 m^a	6
			CS	46		4.4 ± 1.2	2.4 ± 2.2 m		46 m	(High)
Shi [10]	2017	Retrospective	ST	78	59/2/13/4	NA	323.7 ± 23.8d	35	23.2(1–112)m	7
			CS	690	289/278/73/ 50		202.6 ± 41d	157	23.2(1–112)m	(High)
Yamashita [11]	2013	Retrospective	ST	5/2	4/0/2/1	3.4(3–8)	119(55–425)d	6	3.9 ± 2.8y	6
			CS	4/1	3/1/1/0	3.6(2.6–4.3)	93(42–147)d	2	7.2 ± 5.2y	(High)
Yanagawa [12]	2011	Retrospective	ST	12/9	12/4/5/0	3.3(1.9–5)	11(1–128)d	17	21.1(0.2–104.8)m	7
			CS	20/16	19/11/6/0	3.5(1.7– 11.7)	19(1–1157)d	18	45.8(0–143.1)m	(High)
Honjo [13]	2010	Retrospective	ST	2/6	0/0/0/8	3.8 ± 0.6	33 ± 26 d	7	50 ± 56 m	6
			CS	2/12	0/0/0/14	4.7 ± 3.2	70 ± 81 d	8	121 ± 110 m	(High)
Lo Rito [14]	2015	Retrospective	ST	37/32	32/6/16/15	3.6(3.1–4)	18(2–52)d	33	6.4y^c	7
			CS	81/45	59/33/20/14	3.6(3.1–4.6)	36(4–85)d	44	6.4y	(High)

a median value *b* median value and range *c* mean value

d days, *m* months, *y* years

ST Sutureles technique group, *CS* Conventional surgery group, *NOS* Newcastle-Ottawa scale, *NA* Not available

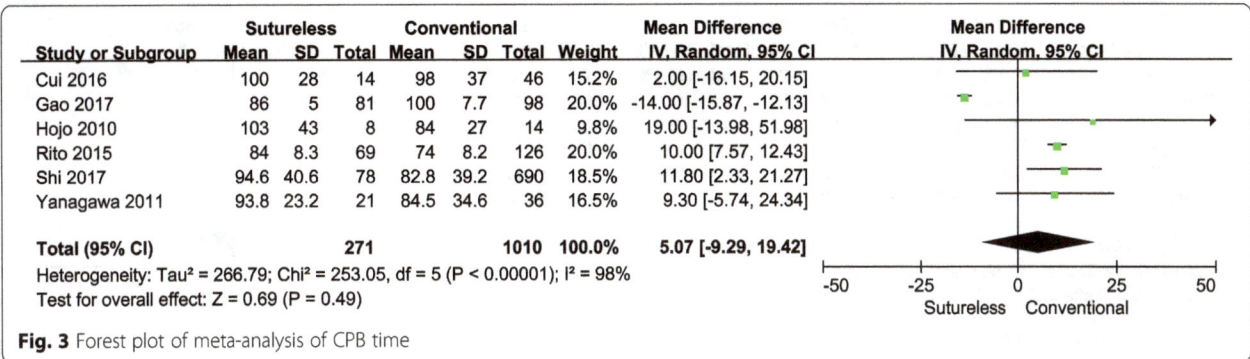

Fig. 3 Forest plot of meta-analysis of CPB time

result indicated that no statistically significant difference was observed with regard to aortic cross-clamp time (WMD, 5.73; 95%CI, − 7.76-19.23; $P = 0.40$).

Post-operative mortality

All 7 studies [8–14] that analyzed the post-operative mortality of both surgical approaches (Table 3) were included in this meta-analysis. A heterogeneity test revealed $Chi^2 = 9.31$, $P = 0.16$, $I^2 = 36\%$, so a fixed effects model was employed (Fig. 5). The test result indicated that no statistically significant difference existed between the two surgical approaches (OR, 0.65; 95%CI, 0.41–1.04; $P = 0.07$).

Hospitalization time

Three out of 7 studies [12–14] that analyzed the hospitalization time of both surgical approaches were included in this meta-analysis. A heterogeneity test revealed $Chi^2 = 110.25$, $P = 0.02$, $I^2 = 76\%$, so a randomized effects model was employed (Fig. 6). This result indicated that no statistically significant difference was observed between the two surgical approaches regarding

to the hospitalization time(WMD, 5.92; 95%CI, − 7.97-19.80; $P = 0.40$).

Post-operative obstruction (PVO), re-operation and total number of operation

A total of 6 studies [8, 10–14] analyzed the post-operative obstruction of both surgeries (Table 4). A heterogeneity test revealed $Chi^2 = 5.47$, $P = 0.36$, $I^2 = 9\%$, and a fixed effects model was employed (Fig. 7). The result indicated that sutureless technique, in comparison with with conventional surgery, was associated with a lower occurrence rate of PVO (OR, 0.52 95%CI, 0.32–0.86; $P = 0.01$).

A total of 5 studies [10–14] analyzed the re-operation due to post-operative PVO of both surgeries (Table 4). However, since the Shi et al. [10] study only recorded the overall re-operation of both approaches but without particular data in each group, therefore, only 4 studies were included in this meta-analysis. A heterogeneity test revealed $Chi^2 = 0.08$, $P = 0.99$, $I^2 = 0\%$, and a fixed effects model was employed (Fig. 8). This meta-analysis result indicated that sutureless technique, compared with conventional surgery, was associated with

Table 2 The associated anomalies of included TAPVC patients

Study	Associated anomalies(n)
Gao [8]	NA
Cui [9]	2 SV anatomy/PA stenosis; 2 unroofed coronary sinus syndrome; 1 DORV; 1 CoA; 1 VSD
Shi [10]	568 PDA; 19 VSD; 2 CoA; 1 TOF; 52 PA stenosis;
Yamashita [11]	8 PA stenosis;1 PV atresia/VSD; 1 Cor triatriatum; 1 Coronary artery fistula
Yanagawa [12]	NA[a]
Honjo [13]	2 DORV; 2 Cor triatriatum; 1 PV atresia/VSD; 1 RVOTO
Lo Rito [14]	5 VSD; 3 CoA; 3 DORV; 2 TA; 2 AVSD

[a] This study was based on isolated TAPVC and patients associated with cardiac lesions were excluded

SV Single ventricle anatomy, *PA* Pulmonary artery, *DORV* Double-outlet right ventricle, *CoA* Coarctation of the aorta, *TOF* Trilogy of fallot, *PV* Pulmonary vein, *RVOTO* Right ventricular outflow tract obstruction, *VSD* ventricular septal defect, *TA* Truncus arteriosus, *AVSD* Atrioventricular septal defect, *NA* Not available

Table 3 Post-operative death of included studies

Study	Post-operative death(n)
Gao [8]	NA[a]
Cui [9]	1 SVC thrombosis; 1 LCOS; 8 PVO
Shi [10]	10 LCOS; 10 PAH; 5 respiratory failure; 4 MODS; 1 intracranial hemorrhage; 1 sepsis; 10 PVO; 4 death with unknown causes; 2 none-cardiac death; 4 failed to recover from bypass
Yamashita [11]	3 PVO; 1 bleeding
Yanagawa [12]	1 none-cardiac death; 1 PVO
Honjo [13]	2 sudden cardiac arrest; 2 PVO; 1 LCOS
Lo Rito [14]	4 LCOS; 3 refractory arrhythmia; 3 PAH; 1 PE; 1 sepsis; 4 PVO; 5 comorbidities without evidence of PVO

[a] Only the numbers of death was available and the details of post-operative death were absent

SVC superior vena cava, *LCOS* Low cardiac output syndrome, *PVO* Pulmonary vein obstruction, *PAH* Pulmonary artery hypertension, *MODS* Multiple organs dysfunction syndrome, *PE* Pulmonary artery embolism, *NA* Not available

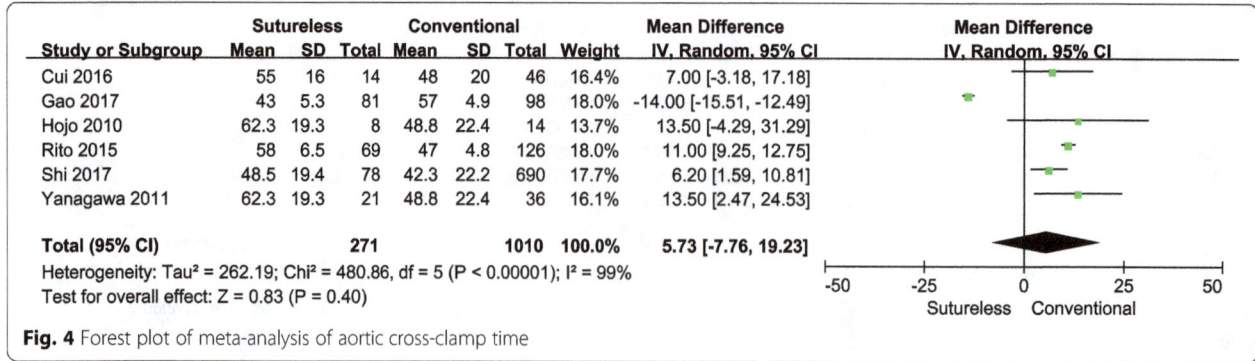

Fig. 4 Forest plot of meta-analysis of aortic cross-clamp time

a lower occurrence rate of re-operation (OR, 0.28;95%CI, 0.09–0.87; P = 0.03).

All the re-operated patients covered by the 5 studies [10–14] had only one re-operation. Referred to Table 4 for the total number of operation.

Sensitivity analysis

Sensitivity analyses using the leave-one-out method were adopted in the meta-analysis of CPB, aortic cross-clamp time and hospitalization time due to significant heterogeneity. In the meta-analysis of CPB and aortic cross-clamp time, the I^2 was reduced to 0 and 11% respectively when the Gao et al. [8] study was removed, whereas the pooling estimates became statistically significant respectively at (WMD, 10.01;95%CI, 7.71–12.30; P < 0.001) and (WMD, 10.00;95%CI,7.77–12.24; P < 0.001). In the meta-analysis of hospitalization time, the I^2 was reduced to 14% when the Yanagawa et al. [12] study was removed while the pooling esti-mate still remained statistically insignificant(WMD, 1.16; 95%CI, – 2.71-5.52; P = 0.50).

Discussion

Sutureless technique, initially employed for the recurrent PVO, was subsequently used for primarily 'prophylactic' repair in TAPVC patients who were at high risk of developing post-operative PVO [4, 13, 15] after tech-nique's efficacy was proven and widely applied. The risk of developing post-operative PVO was particularly high for the following scenarios: the existence of preoperative hypoplastic pulmonary veins, young age at initial surgery, TAPVC patients with right atrial isomerism, cardiac TAPVC with preexisting PVO and mixed type TAPVC [1, 2, 13]. Preexisting PVO could be difficult to diagnose with cardiac echo. However, in our study, 6 out of 7 included studies (Table 1) reported the the detection of pre-operative PVO. So it was noteworthy that surgeons should consider sutureless technique as a prior alternative for the primary repair of TAPVC in such condition. Yaganawa et al. [12] and Honjo [13] reported the circumstances under which sutureless technique was used for the primary repair of TAPVC: 1) all infracardiac TAPVC; 2) cardiac TAPVC with stenosis in the pulmon-ary veins or in the short confluence bridging between the pulmonary veins and the coronary sinus or the right atrium; 3) surgeons' preference for supracardiac TAPVC. Our study result was also consistent with that of previ-ous studies in that it indicated sutureless technique entailed a lower occurrence rate of post-operative PVO (OR, 0.52) and re-operation (OR, 0.28). We found post-operative PVO was one of the main causes of death (Table 3). Therefore, sutureless technique should be

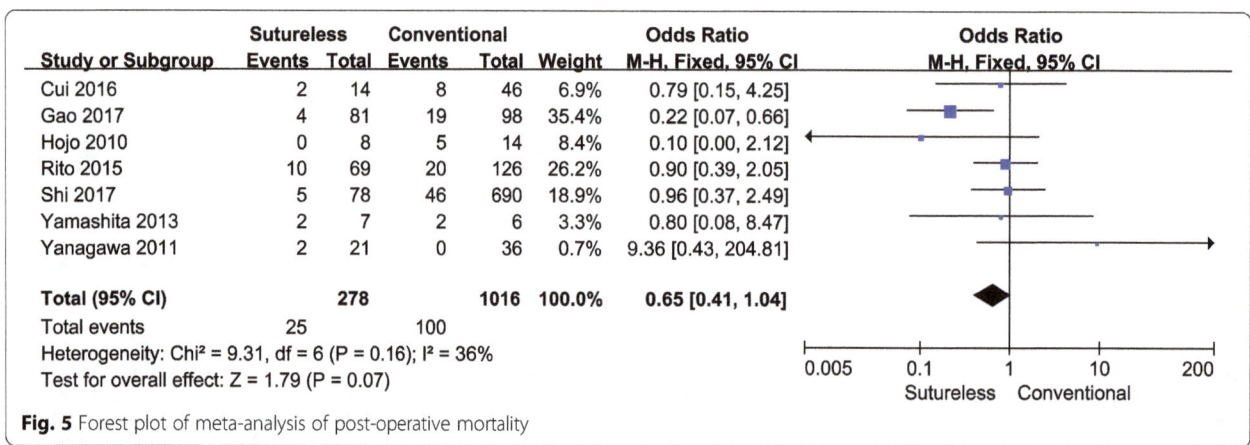

Fig. 5 Forest plot of meta-analysis of post-operative mortality

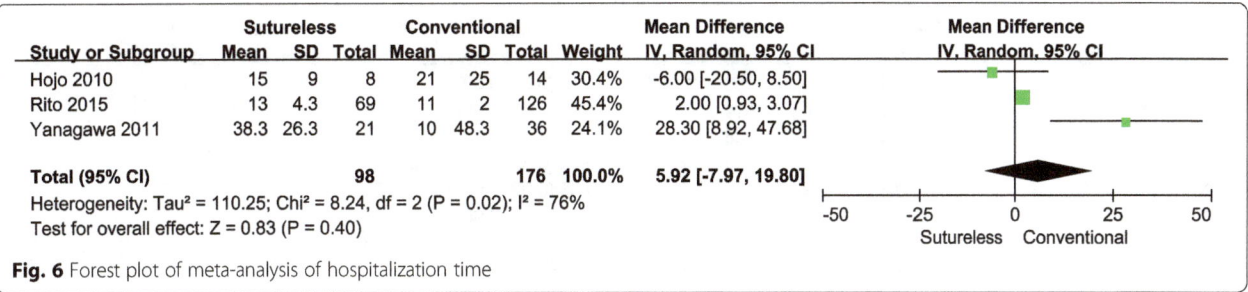

Study or Subgroup	Sutureless			Conventional			Weight	Mean Difference IV, Random, 95% CI
	Mean	SD	Total	Mean	SD	Total		
Hojo 2010	15	9	8	21	25	14	30.4%	-6.00 [-20.50, 8.50]
Rito 2015	13	4.3	69	11	2	126	45.4%	2.00 [0.93, 3.07]
Yanagawa 2011	38.3	26.3	21	10	48.3	36	24.1%	28.30 [8.92, 47.68]
Total (95% CI)			**98**			**176**	**100.0%**	**5.92 [-7.97, 19.80]**

Heterogeneity: Tau² = 110.25; Chi² = 8.24, df = 2 (P = 0.02); I² = 76%
Test for overall effect: Z = 0.83 (P = 0.40)

Fig. 6 Forest plot of meta-analysis of hospitalization time

recommended to patients with high risk of developing post-operative PVO. Even though sutureless technique was initially used for the recurrent PVO, surprisingly, the patch augmentation and fibrous resection were adopted as often as sutureless technique in the re-operation for PVO (Table 4) among our included studies. This practice could be due to the neoteric of the sutureless technique. A Cox proportional hazards analysis conducted by Yong et al. [16] suggested that operative weight < 2.5 kg and postoperative pulmonary hypertensive crisis were risk factors likely to trigger re-operation for post-operative PVO. However, the role of low body weight as a risk factor was far from conclusive as low body weight was found to be a high risk factor for every type of cardiac surgery. As such, the potentially complex interrelationship between low body weight and post-operative PVO warranted further investigation. But, tentatively, we postulated that relatively smaller pulmonary veins were generally associated with lower body weight. Therefore, to avoid distorsion of anastomosis in patients of low body weight with relatively smaller pulmonary veins, we suggested the use of sutureless technique in low weight infants with TAPVC.

The advantages for primary use of sutureless technique for TAPVC were obvious: 1) wide application to almost any type of pulmonary vein confluences, especially for patients with pulmonary vein stenosis [5, 13]; 2) better visualization of the edges of divided pulmonary veins to avoid Deep Hypothermic Circulatory Arrest (DHCA) [13, 15]; 3) avoided involving the vascular endothelium to reduce the scarring and distortion of pulmonary veins. The main disadvantage of the primary use of sutureless technique was potential bleeding from the gap between the pericardium and the confluence into the posterior mediastinum or pleural cavity. Yoshimura et al. [5] reported one case with intraoperative massive bleeding into the left pleural cavity. The four cases reported by Yun et al. [15] with similar complication could be managed by intrapleural hilar approximation. In our experience, as long as the integrity of the parietal pluera was kept intact, massive bleeding would not occur. The injury to the phrenic nerve in connection with sutureless technique was reported as well [13]. Other disadvantages such as thrombogenicity at the exposed pericardial surface, air embolism and soft tissue rupture were also reported [12]. Yaganawa et al. [12]

Table 4 Post-operative PVO and strategy of re-operation

Study	Surgical approach	Post-operative PVO(n)	Strategy of post-operative PVO underwent re-operation	Total number of operation(n)
Gao [8]	ST	2	NA[a]	NA
	CS	14		
Cui [9]	ST	NA	NA	NA
	CS			
Shi [10]	ST	10	12 sutureless technique; 7 patch augmentation; 5 fibrous resection[b]	792[b]
	CS	101		
Yamashita [11]	ST	1	1 sutureless technique	8
	CS	2	1 fibrous resection; 1 SI	8
Yanagawa [12]	ST	1	No patient required re-operation	21
	CS	2	NA[c]	38
Honjo [13]	ST	1	No patient required re-operation	8
	CS	6	3 fibrous resection	17
Lo Rito [14]	ST	5	1 fibrous resection; 1 sutureless technique	71
	CS	17	5 fibrous resection; 7 sutureless technique	138

[a] Only the numbers of PVO was available and lack of details of post-operative PVO
[b] Strategy of post-operative PVO underwent re-operation was presented totally
[c] Two patients in the conventional repair group underwent re-operation without description of details
ST Sutureles technique group, *CS* Conventional surgery group, *SI* Stent implantation, *NA* Not available

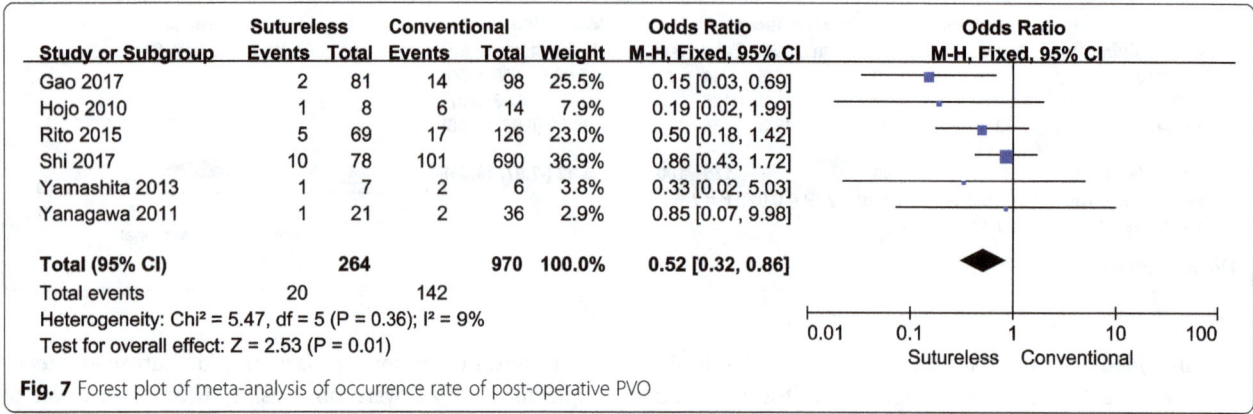

Fig. 7 Forest plot of meta-analysis of occurrence rate of post-operative PVO

reported primary sutureless repair to a neonate with mixed TAPVC involved the use of a distal incision into the individual pulmonary vein. Oscillation ventilation and ECMO were required postoperatively. And air bubbles found in the aorta during the ECMO initiation were probably related to the oscillation ventilation. However, we believe the air embolism was not caused by sutureless technique, but resulted from insufficient exhaust before weaning off CPB. In our center, we did not observe any patients with thrombogenicity or air embolism with the primary use of sutureless technique for TAPVC.

Sutureless technique enabled better visualization of pulmonary veins to avoid DHCA and also reduced the surgical exploration time of pulmonary veins. In addition, Yoshimura et al. [17] reported the suretureless technique was less technically demanding compared with conventional surgery. Therefore, the suretureless technique should theoretically reduce the CPB and aortic cross-clamp time. However, our study indicated that sutureless technique, contrary to conventional surgery, did not significantly reduce CPB and aortic cross-clamp time. In the meantime, in the sensitivity analysis of CPB and aortic cross-clamp time, we observed a significant heterogeneity reduction and the pooling estimates became statistically significant with the removal of the Gao et al. [8] study. It indicated that the meta-analysis of

CPB and aortic cross-clamp time were overly influenced by the Gao et al. [8] study and the pooling results could be inconclusive. Compared with other included studies, the Gao et al. [8] study entailed a significantly longer CPB and aortic cross-clamp time in the conventional surgery group than that in the sutureless technique group. Longer CPB and aortic cross-clamp time might be explained by the complexity of the surgical procedure or unstable patients requiring longer CPB support. As expected, we observed a higher percentage of mixed TAPVC patients in their conventional surgery group compared with other studies and could contribute to their longer CPB and aortic cross-clamp time.

Hospitalization time was related to post-operative recovery. Meta-analysis of hospitalization time indicated that compared with conventional surgery, sutureless technique did not reduce the hospitalization time significantly. In the sensitivity analysis of hospitalization time, we observed a statistically significant reduction in heterogeneity while the pooling estimate still remained statistically insignificant upon the removal of the Yanagawa et al. [12] study. However, hospitalization time was largely due to the era effect based on the evolution in ICU management and preoperative diagnosis. Therefore more standard evaluation of post-operative recovery should be conducted. Other endpoints connected to post-operative recovery such as ICU stay and ventilation

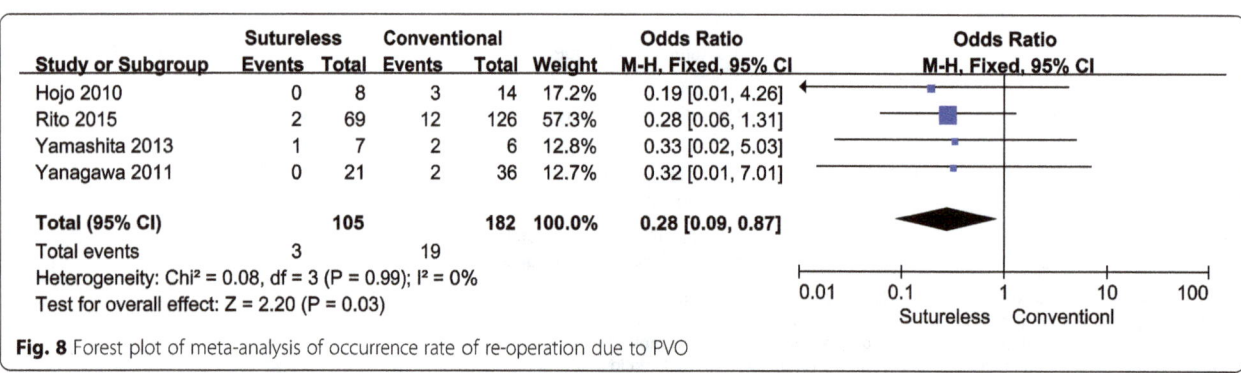

Fig. 8 Forest plot of meta-analysis of occurrence rate of re-operation due to PVO

time were not available for pooling estimates due to lack of relevant data.

Limitations

This was the first-ever study to-date to compare the outcomes between applying sutureless technique and conventional surgery for TAPVC patients. And several limitations to our study were identified as follows:

First, all 7 studies included were retrospective NRCTs. Consequently, the level of evidence was low;

Second, sutureless technique was generally adopted in higher risk patients of developing post-operative PVO. However, we only summarized the associated cardiac anomalies as baseline characteristics (Table 2) and failed to disclose the severity of preoperative PVO due to the divergent measurement method adopted in each study. Therefore, a high risk of selection bias of included patients might exist;

Third, the endpoints that we evaluated such as mortality and hospitalization time were largely influenced by the era effect. The transition from conventional to primary sutureless repair represented the evolution of surgical techniques over time, which occurred inevitably in parallel with other evolution including but not limited to ICU management and preoperative diagnosis;

Fourth, the only follow-up data we collected were post-operative PVO and mortality. The assessment of other long term outcomes of sutureless technique was absent in our study. The evaluation of cardiac-pulmonary function in the long term should have been included to augment the analysis of the benefits of each approach;

Finally, we only conducted meta-analysis of sutureless technique in the primary repair of TAPVC, and no conclusion could be drawn whether sutureless technique was effective and safe in the repair of secondary PVO. Further meta-analysis should be conducted to explore the effectiveness and safey of sutureless technique for secondary PVO. Another limitation was that 2 out of 7 included studies were written in Chinese only, reducing their accessibility to thethe rest of the world.

Conclusion

In conclusion, compared with conventional surgery, sutureless technique significantly reduced the occurrence rate of post-operative PVO and re-operation due to PVO. No significant statistical differences were observed between conventional surgery and sutureless technique with regard to mortality and hospitalization time. The initial meta-analysis of CPB and aortic cross-clamp time also found no statistical differences between the two surgical approaches. But the meta-analysis results could not be validated when highly heterogeneous studies were excluded

following sensitivity analysis yielded different results. In terms of the occurrence rate of post-operative PVO and re-operation, our study showed sutureless technique was superior to conventional surgery for primary repair of TAPVC, especially for TAPVC patients who were at a high risk of developing post-operative PVO. The level of evidence of our study was low and RCTs should be designed to evaluate and compare the safety and effectiveness of primary sutureless technique for TAPVC.

Abbreviations

CPB: Cardiopulmonary bypass time; ECMO: Extracorporeal membrane oxygenation; NOS: Newcastle-Ottawa Scale; NRCTs: None-randomized controlled trials; OR: Odds ratio; PVO: Pulmonary venous obstruction; TAPVC: Total anomalous pulmonary venous connection; WMD: Weighted mean difference

Authors' contributions

WYH and WZC participated in study design and manuscript writing. LYG, JX, WC, ZJM and KHY carried out data analysis. All authors read and approved the final manuscript.

Competing interests

The authors declare that they have no competing interests.

Author details

[1]Department of Cardiothoracic Surgery, Children's Hospital of Chongqing Medical University, No.136 Zhongshan Second Road, Yuzhong District, Chongqing 400014, China. [2]Department of Cardiovascular Surgery, Sun Yat-Sen Memorial Hospital, Sun Yat-Sen University, No.107 Yanjiang West Road, Yuexiu District, Guangzhou 510120, China. [3]Department of Cardiology, Children's Hospital of Chongqing Medical University, Chongqing 400014, China. [4]Ministry of Education Key Laboratory of Child Development and Disorders, Chongqing 400014, China. [5]China International Science and Technology Cooperation Base of Child Development and Critical Disorders, Chongqing 400014, China. [6]Chongqing Key Laboratory of Pediatrics, Chongqing 400014, China.

References

1. Seale AN, Uemura H, Webber SA, Partridge J, Roughton M, Ho SY, et al. Total anomalous pulmonary venous connection: morphology and outcome from an international population-based study. Circulation. 2010;122(25): 2718–26.
2. Mueller C, Dave H, Prêtre R. Primary correction of total anomalous pulmonary venous return with a modified sutureless technique. Eur J Cardiothorac Surg. 2013;43(3):635–40.
3. Lacour-Gayet F, Rey C, Planché C. Pulmonary vein stenosis. Description of a sutureless surgical procedure using the pericardium in situ. Arch Mal Coeur Vaiss. 1996;89(5):633.
4. Najm HK, Caldarone CA, Smallhorn J, Coles JG. A sutureless technique for the relief of pulmonary vein stenosis with the use of in situ pericardium. J Thorac Cardiovasc Surg. 1998;115(2):468–70.
5. Yoshimura N, Fukahara K, Yamashita A, Doki Y, Takeuchi K, Higuma T, et al. Surgery for total anomalous pulmonary venous connection: primary

sutureless repair vs. conventional repair. Gen Thorac Cardiovasc Surg. 2017;
65(5):1–7.

6.   Wells GA, Shea BJ, O'Connell D, Peterson J, Welch V, Losos M, et al. The
     Newcastle–Ottawa scale (NOS) for assessing the quality of non-randomized
     studies in meta-analysis. Appl Eng Agric. 2014;18(6):727–34.

7.   Hozo SP, Djulbegovic B, Hozo I. Estimating the mean and variance from the
     median, range, and the size of a sample. BMC Med Res Methodol. 2005;5:13.

8.   Gao XM, Nie ZQ, Ou YQ, He BC, Yuan HY, Qu YJ, et al. Comparison between
     two surgical techniques to repair total anomalous pulmonary venous
     connection using propensity score analysis. J Sun Yat-Sen Univ. 2017;38(1):
     143–50. (in Chinese)

9.   Cui HJ, Chen XX, Ma L, Xia YS, Yang SC, Zou MH, et al. Surgical treatment of
     total anomalous pulmonary venous connection under 6 months of age.
     Chin J Surg. 2016;54(4):276–80. (in Chinese)

10. Shi G, Zhu Z, Chen J, Ou YQ, Hong HF, Nie ZQ, et al. Total anomalous
     pulmonary venous connection: the current management strategies in a
     pediatric cohort of 768 patients. Circulation. 2016;135(1):48.

11. Yamashita K, Hoashi T, Kagisaki K, Kurosaki K, Shiraishi I, Yagihara T, et al.
     Midterm outcomes of sutureless technique for postoperative pulmonary
     venous stenosis. Gen Thorac Cardiovasc Surg. 2014;62(1):48–52.

12. Yanagawa B, Alghamdi AA, Dragulescu A, Viola N, Al-Radi OO, Mertens LL,
     et al. Primary sutureless repair for "simple" total anomalous pulmonary
     venous connection: midterm results in a single institution. J Thorac
     Cardiovasc Surg. 2011;141(6):1346–54.

13. Honjo O, Atlin CR, Hamilton BC, Al-Radi O, Viola N, Coles JG, et al. Primary
     sutureless repair for infants with mixed total anomalous pulmonary venous
     drainage. Ann Thorac Surg. 2010;90(3):862–8.

14. Rito ML, Gazzaz T, Wilder T, et al. Repair type influences mode of pulmonary
     vein stenosis in total anomalous pulmonary venous drainage. Ann Thorac
     Surg. 2015;100(2):654.

15. Yun TJ, Al-Radi OO, Adatia I, Caldarone CA, Coles JG, Williams WG, et al.
     Contemporary management of right atrial isomerism: effect of evolving
     therapeutic strategies. J Thorac Cardiovasc Surg. 2006;131(5):1108–13.

16. Yong MS, d'Udekem Y, Robertson T, Horton S, Dronavalli M, Brizard C, et al.
     Outcome of surgery for simple total anomalous pulmonary venous
     drainage in neonates. Ann Thorac Surg. 2011;91:1921–7.

17. Yoshimura N, Fukahara K, Yamashita A, Doki Y, Takeuchi K, Higuma T, et al.
     Current topics in surgery for isolated total anomalous pulmonary venous
     connection. Surg Today. 2014;44(12):2221.

31

The surgical management of non-malignant aerodigestive fistula

Yassar A. Qureshi[1*] iD, M. Muntzer Mughal[1], Sheraz R. Markar[2], Borzoueh Mohammadi[1], Jeremy George[3], Martin Hayward[4] and David Lawrence[4]

Abstract

Background: Acquired aerodigestive fistula (ADF) are rare, but associated with significant morbidity. Surgery affords the best prospect of cure. We present our experience of the surgical management of ADFs at a specialist unit, highlighting operative techniques, challenges and assess clinical outcomes following intervention. We also illustrate findings of a Hospital Episodes Statistics search for ADFs.

Methods: A prospectively-maintained database was searched to identify all patients diagnosed with an ADF who were managed at our institution. Of 48 patients with an ADF, eight underwent surgical intervention.

Results: Four patients underwent an exploration of the ADF with primary repair of the defect. Two of these patients had proximal ADFs, amenable to repair through a neck incision, and two required a thoracotomy. Two patients suffered fistulae secondary to endoscopic therapy and underwent oesophageal exclusion surgery, with subsequent staged reconstruction. Two patients with previous Tuberculosis had a lung segmentectomy and lobectomy respectively, and a further patient in remission after treatment for lymphoma underwent oesophageal resection with synchronous reconstruction. Three patients suffered a complication, with one post-operative mortality. The remaining seven patients all achieved normal oral alimentation, with no evidence of ADF recurrence at a median follow-up of 32 months.

Conclusions: Surgery to manage ADFs is effective in restoring normal alimentation and alleviates soiling of the airway, with a very low risk of recurrence. Several operative techniques can be utilised dependent on the features of the ADF. Early referral to specialist units is advocated, where the expertise to facilitate the complete management of patients is present, within a multi-disciplinary setting.

Keywords: Aerodigestive fistula, Tracheo-oesophageal fistula, Oesophageal cancer, Oesophageal surgery

Background

Surgical intervention affords the best prospect of long-term cure of aerodigestive fistulae (ADF). Although several operative techniques can be used to treat this debilitating condition, they can only be utilised in selected patients owing to both the underlying diagnosis and the risks associated with such surgery [1–4]. However, with ADFs becoming an increasing health problem, with improving diagnosis and evolving peri-operative care, it is likely that surgery will play a more important role in the management of ADFs.

The choice of operative technique to treat ADFs is dependent on several factors. However, the most important facet relates to the underlying oesophageal or airway disease, which determines the state of tissue and its amenability to repair and future surveillance, if required [1, 2, 5, 6]. Patients often present in a physiologically challenged state owing to the nature of the disease, and many will not be candidates for surgery. However, focused pre-operative intervention and nutritional support may enable some patients to proceed to surgery. For these reasons, a multi-disciplinary (MDT) approach is necessary, and underscores why these patients should be managed in dedicated centralised units. The range of operations include resection and reconstruction, exclusion and bypass of the affected segment of oesophagus, and exploration and repair of the ADF. The expertise of head

* Correspondence: yassar.qureshi.17@ucl.ac.uk
[1]Department of Oesophago-Gastric Surgery, University College London Hospital, 250 Euston Road, London NW1 2BU, UK
Full list of author information is available at the end of the article

and neck, thoracic and oesophago-gastric surgeons is required to manage these patients.

In this study, we present our experience of surgical intervention in patients diagnosed with an ADF. We explore the background leading to the development of an ADF, and relate how this can impact on the nature of surgery performed. Furthermore, we describe the operative technique, challenges and outcomes following intervention. We review the pertinent literature to enable an evidence-based approach to the surgical management of ADFs. We also illustrate findings of a Hospital Episodes Statistics (HES) search for ADFs, highlighting the challenges of diagnosis, management and reporting in contemporary practise.

Methods

We interrogated a prospectively-maintained database to identify patients diagnosed with an ADF and managed at our institution between January 2005 and January 2017. A total of 48 patients with an ADF were identified, of whom eight patients have undergone surgery to treat their fistula. All patients were discussed at a specialist MDT where a consensus on optimal management was reached. Of the 40 patients managed non-surgically, 31 were treated with endoscopic intervention (oesophageal or tracheal stent), mostly owing to the presence of advanced malignancy not amenable to curative treatment. Endoscopic treatment facilitated an alleviation of respiratory soiling, whilst allowing oncological treatment to be commenced. A further seven patients were managed in palliative setting after presenting *in extremis*, and two patients with very small asymptomatic ADFs were managed conservatively with regular surveillance. Follow-up refers to time from diagnosis of ADF (or underlying disease where specified) to last clinical engagement or death. Median follow-up was 32 months. Local ethical approval for retrieval and use of clinical data for this study was granted.

Operative technique

When considering surgery as treatment for ADF, several factors should be specifically assessed for. It is imperative that a careful search for malignancy is performed prior to surgery, particularly as many patients will have a preceding history of proximal oesophageal squamous cell carcinoma (SCC) treated with chemo-radiotherapy. If active malignancy is present in the context of an ADF, this represents locally advanced disease with poor outcome, rarely amenable to curative surgical intervention. In these patients, endocopic treatment should be considered to alleviate symptoms, coupled with chemo-radiotherapy if appropriate. The physiological state of the patient must also be thoroughly assessed, to ensure that the risks of major morbidity and mortality after surgery are minimised, and

that the patient would be able to recover from such intervention. Patients should be carefully optimised, and where indicated, the pre-operative placement of a feeding jejunostomy and a venting gastrostomy to improve the nutritional and metabolic state, and to minimise continued soiling of the airway, should be performed.

Once a patient is deemed to have an ADF curable by surgery, secondary factors relating to the ADF and surrounding tissue become important considerations. A larger defect, a history of previous local radiotherapy and endoscopic intervention are all factors which make surgery more challenging. Also, the location of the ADF is important, as more proximally sited fistulae are amenable to repair through a neck incision, yet for distal ADF a thoracotomy is mandated, carrying a greater risk of major morbidity and mortality. If there has been significant local contamination, then it may be prudent not perform a synchronous reconstruction, as the likelihood of an anastomotic dehiscence increases. In these patients, a delayed reconstruction confers improved chances of better recovery. However, given the heterogenous aetiology of ADF, each case should be considered with a view to an individualised treatment plan.

At induction, for tracheo-oesophageal fistulae (TOF), it is important that the endotracheal tube balloon is sited distal to the fistula. This will avoid inadvertent damage to the cuff whilst dissecting and exposing the fistula, and negate the possibility of ventilatory embarrassment intra-operatively. Furthermore, this manoeuvre minimises further contamination of the respiratory tract by manipulation of the affected structures during surgery.

ADF exploration and repair

This may involve either an incision in the neck for proximal fistulae, or a thoracotomy for more distal ADFs. In the neck, dissection must proceed to mobilise the thyroid with careful identification and preservation of the recurrent laryngeal nerves and parathyroid glands. The oesophagus should be circumferentially mobilised, as this manoeuvre will allow the pharyngo-laryngeal complex to be gently pulled superiorly and away from the thoracic inlet, to provide good access to the fistula. Once the fistula has been identified, it can be dissected free and a primary repair of the oesophagus and trachea with absorbable sutures can be performed. It is critical that the fistula is accessible from both sides of the neck to ensure complete control of the airway during the repair, whilst also facilitating a pedicled strap muscle interposition flap. This reinforces the repair by providing a physical barrier between the two suture lines.

In the thorax, a similar approach is used with an intercostal flap which is carefully prepared at the time of thoracotomy. Once the fistula has been identified, again, it is dissected free and a primary repair performed, with the intercostal flap placed between the suture lines.

Exclusion

Exclusion surgery involves isolating the oesophagus from alimentary tract continuity, both proximal and distal to the fistula. This involves an incision in the neck to access the proximal oesophagus, where, once circumferentially mobilised, it is transected above the fistula and brought to the skin as an oesophagostomy. If the fistula is very proximal, then the superior oesophagus may be left in situ, and a large T-tube placed in the lumen with the distal limb of the tube brought to the skin.

Next, a laparotomy is performed where the oesohagogastric junction (OGJ) is mobilised and the stomach transected below this, from the lesser curve through to the fundus. This manoeuvre excludes the oesophagus from the GI tract entirely, whilst preserving the majority of the stomach for future reconstruction. The small stomach remnant attached to the OGJ is brought to the abdominal wall, where a generous gastrostomy is fashioned. This allows retrograde access to the excluded oesophagus, for both endoscopic surveillance and therapy, and facilitates venting of oesophageal mucous.

Our unit policy is to defer reconstruction as a second, staged procedure. This allows the patient a period of recovery, whilst respiratory and nutritional optimisation continues. Furthermore, by fashioning an anastomosis at the index operation in a potentially contaminated surgical field, there is a higher chance of a leak. If this were to occur, there is substantial risk of fistula recurrence. Where possible, the stomach is used a conduit, and is brought to the neck through the retrosternal space, thus avoiding the need for a repeat thoracotomy. If there is insufficient proximal oesophagus, the stomach may be anastomosed directly to the inferior pharyngeal constrictors.

Resection

This is normally reserved for large or recurrent fistulae. For proximally sited ADF - those affecting the trachea, this will involve resection of the oesophagus, via a transthoracic approach. The fistula is identified, and the oesophagus dissected away around it. However, the oesophageal tissue intimately involved with the fistula is left in situ, thus avoiding direct dissection of the trachea and minimising the risk of an air leak. The tracheal defect with the overlying oesophageal tissue is then primarily closed, with the latter acting as a buttress reinforcing the tracheal repair. Typically, a gastric conduit is utilised for reconstruction, necessitating a laparotomy.

For more distal ADF, those affecting the bronchus intermedius and more distal, a thoracotomy is performed to identify the fistula. A segmentectomy or lobectomy of the lung can be performed, dependent on the size of the defect and the quality of the surrounding parenchyma. Thus, the affected distal airway and the fistula are excised *en*

bloc. The oesophageal defect can be repaired primarily, utilising an intercostal flap to reinforce the repair, or an oesophageal resection is performed if the defect is very large and unlikely to heal. In these instances, given the anastomosis will be at a distinct site from the ADF, a synchronous reconstruction can be performed safely.

In our experience, tracheal resection is a very challenging operation, with the risk of significant short and long-term complications [2, 3]. Owing to the limited vascularity of the trachea, healing, particularly in this cohort of patients, may be protracted, necessitating prolonged mechanical ventilation. Thus, we have preferred to avoid such an operative intervention. However, for very large TOFs, or those where a circumferential injury to the trachea is present (such as cuff related fistulae), or where other intervention has failed, tracheal resection and reconstruction may be indicated. Mathisen et al provide an operative description and experience of this technique [3].

Results

Preceding history and previous intervention

The median age at diagnosis of ADF was 56 years (range 29–73 years). Three patients had a previous diagnosis of oesophageal malignancy; all were treated with chemo- and/or radiotherapy, and one with surgical resection in addition. Two patients had a prior diagnosis of Tuberculosis (TB) and had received anti-microbial therapy in the past, and one patient previously had surgical intervention following a post-emetic oesophageal leak. In two patients, no obvious cause of ADF was identified, likely representing congenital fistulae that had persisted into adulthood. Of these cases, two patients (1 and 6) developed oesophageal strictures after their initial treatment. Patient 1 had undergone several balloon dilations and stent placements, with the stent subsequently eroding into the airway (Fig. 1). Similarly, patient 6 also received a stent which directly caused the fistula. Table 1 summarises key patient factors.

ADF characteristics

The two patients with an unknown cause of fistula had a very long history of symptoms, and had been managed in the community with a diagnosis of asthma (Table 2). The median time to ADF development for the three patients with a malignancy was 15 months (range 3–21), with the shortest time affecting a patient who had an oesophageal lymphoma (Patient 7). She had a complete response to chemotherapy, with a residual fistula persisting (Fig. 2). Both patients with TB had a long interval after curative medical therapy, although they had suggestive symptoms for some time prior to referral. Most patients presented with recurrent chest infections and symptoms suggestive of aspiration. Of these, one patient

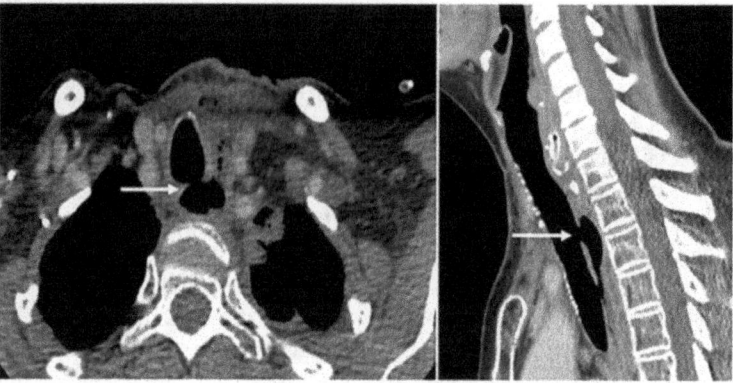

Fig. 1 CT scan of Patient 1 demonstrating the aerodigestive fistula (arrows)

(4) presented with acute respiratory failure owing to overwhelming infection caused by aspiration. Of interest, he had a fistula affecting the very proximal trachea (Fig. 3).

The size of the fistula ranged from 3 to 16 mm, with the larger defects affecting those who had a prior diagnosis of carcinoma or who underwent surgical treatment. The location of the fistula in relation to the airway too was variable, reflecting the site of underlying disease. Those thought to be congenital were very proximal. Those secondary to TB were both distal, involving the smaller bronchi and lung parenchyma at the original Ghon focus. Patient 6 presented with Boerhaave's Syndrome, and was initially managed with surgery to repair the oesophageal defect. However, he subsequently re-leaked, which again was managed surgically with a repair over a T-tube, but then developed a stricture at the site of injury, which was treated with an oesophageal stent. This eroded into the airway at its proximal extent, causing a fistula at 24 cm, with subsequent referral to our unit (Fig. 4).

After the diagnosis of ADF, three patients underwent further endotherapy in an attempt to manage the fistula prior to referral to our unit. Patient 1 had 3 oesophageal stents placed, but given the proximal location of the ADF, these all slipped distally. Patient 3, who had developed an ADF between the airway and a gastric conduit, most likely after a sub-clinical leak, had endoclips placed via flexible gastroscopy which failed to close the ADF. Patient 6 too had a stent[s] placed to treat the fistula without the desired effect.

Surgical intervention for ADF treatment

Three patients (3, 4, 8) underwent a primary repair of their ADF. Patient 3 required a thoracotomy given that the ADF was communicating with a gastric conduit and Patients 4 and 8 had proximally-sited fistulae approached through the neck. For the former case, an intercostal flap was interposed between the suture lines and for the latter two, the strap muscles were similarly utilised. These fistulae were small and the quality of tissue was sufficiently good to enable primary repair. Patient 4 presented as an acute emergency following aspiration -intubated- and a laparotomy was performed prior to repair, in order to place a feeding jejunostomy and venting gastrostomy (Table 3).

Table 1 Preceding history and intervention, prior to the diagnosis of ADF

Patient	Age at ADF Diagnosis (years)	Sex	Preceding Diagnosis	Preceding Intervention	Chemo-Radiotherapy	Preceding Treatment Related Complication	Previous Endotherapy
1	60	F	SSC[a] Proximal Oesophagus	Definitive chemo-radiotherapy	Chemo-radiotherapy	Radiotherapy related stricture	-×2 stents -×3 dilations
2	57	M	TB[b]	Medical therapy	–	–	–
3	59	M	Adenocarcinoma Distal Oesophagus	Ivor-Lewis Oesophagectomy	Neo-adjuvant chemotherapy	Anastomotic leak	–
4	73	M	Unknown	–	–	–	–
5	32	F	TB[b]	Medical Therapy	–	–	–
6	33	M	Boerhaave's Syndrome	Repair of leak	–	Re-leak; stricture	-× 1 stent
7	55	F	Oesophageal B Cell lymphoma	Chemotherapy	Chemotherapy	–	–
8	29	F	Unknown	–	–	–	–

[a]SCC- Squamous Cell Carcinoma; [b] TB- Tuberculosis

Table 2 Anatomical and Clinical Features of the ADFs

Patient	Time to ADF Development (months)	Fistula Site	Fistula Size (mm)	Main Symptoms	Endotherapy to Treat ADF
1	15	Proximal trachea 20 cm	12	Aspiration	×3 stents
2	> 30 years	Oesophagus-right bronchus intermedius 30 cm	12	Recurrent chest infections	–
3	21	Gastric conduit-lung 25 cm	16	Recurrent chest infections	Endoclip
4	> 30 years	Proximal trachea 17 cm	5	Aspiration; Respiratory embarrassment	–
5	144	Distal oesophagus-lung 38 cm	15	Haemoptysis	–
6	3	Oesophagus-carina 24 cm	15	Recurrent chest infections	×3 stents
7	3	Oesophagus- left main bronchus 26 cm	5	Recurrent chest infections	–
8	> 20 years	Proximal trachea 17 cm	3	Recurrent chest infections	–

Two patients (1 and 6) underwent an oesophageal exclusion operation. These were both performed as staged procedures with delayed reconstruction. The reason for performing this operation was that in both patients there was sufficient concern regarding the state of tissue. Patient 1 had previous radiotherapy for an oesophageal SCC, on a background of achalasia requiring a myotomy via thoracotomy several years previously. The degree of tissue inflammation, scarring and adhesions precluded a transthoracic resection. Thus, through a neck incision, the oesophagus was transected above the fistula and an oesophagostomy fashioned with a synchronous repair of the fistula. Distally, the oesophagus and OGJ was transected and a venting gastrostomy fashioned. After a period of optimisation and treatment of longstanding respiratory disease, the patient underwent reconstruction utilising a gastric conduit through the retrosternal space. Patient 6 too had severe inflammation and adhesions in

the chest following his surgical management of Boerhaave's syndrome. Exclusion and subsequent reconstruction with a colonic conduit (he had previously undergone a distal gastrectomy for benign ulcer disease) was performed. In both cases, the native tissues were poor enough to carry a high risk of leak with primary anastomosis at index surgery.

Patient 2 had a distal ADF, approached through a thoracotomy. The right bronchus intermedius was involved, and the ADF and affected parenchyma was excised as a segmentectomy, with oesophageal repair. Patient 5 underwent an exploration of the fistula through a thoractomy with a lobectomy. The fistula, along with associated necrotic parenchyma was excised *en bloc*, with a subsequent suture repair of the oesophagus. Patient 7, after chemotherapy for lymphoma, underwent an oesophageal resection. Again, severe residual inflammation was noted at the time of the surgery precluding repair of a small (5 mm) fistula. In addition, our oncology colleagues felt there was

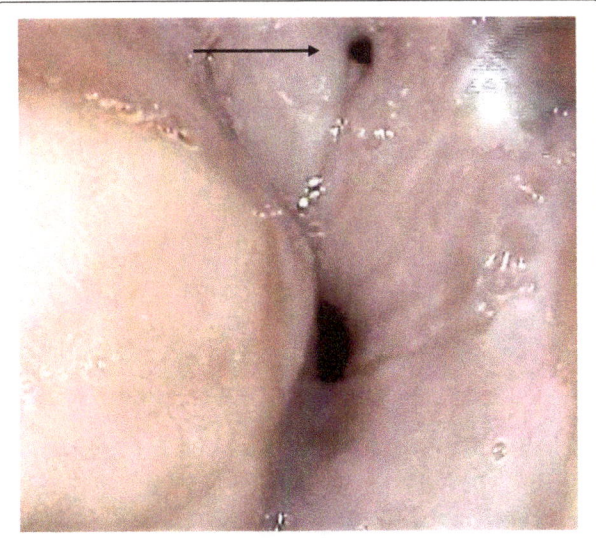

Fig. 2 Residual ADF (arrow) following treatment for oesophageal lymphoma

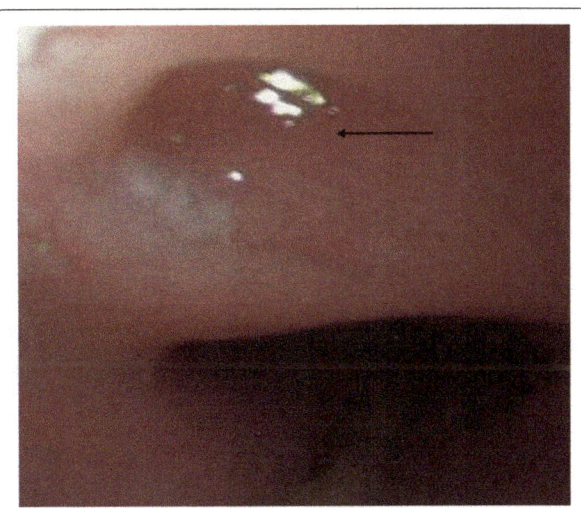

Fig. 3 ADF (arrow) in a proximal location, as seen by oesophagoscopy

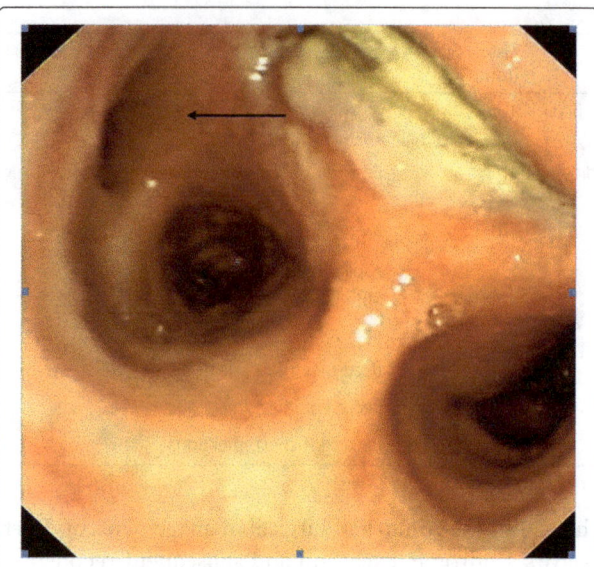

Fig. 4 A bronchoscopic image of the ADF (arrow) close to the carina

7 weeks confirmed complete healing of the leak, after which gradual oral feeding was commenced.

Patient 4, who presented with respiratory failure, was affected by severe post-operative recurrent chest infections, and an inability to wean off mechanical ventilation. This had been anticipated, and hence a tracheostomy had been placed at the time of surgery. Despite 4 months of intensive management, he passed away with respiratory failure and multiple organ dysfunction. He represents the only mortality in this series.

Normal oral alimentation following surgery was achieved in all patients, bar patient 4. The time to attain this milestone ranged from 2 to 3 weeks in all cases, with the exception of patient 7 who had suffered a leak. She required supplemental enteral feeding at home for a short period. We reserve the use of contrast studies and formal swallow assessment for the very proximal fistulae, where the risk of leak and aspiration is highest. At the time of last follow-up, no patient demonstrated clinical evidence of recurrent ADF.

Hospital episodes statistics (HES)

We performed a search of the English national HES database to assess the reported incidence of ADFs in the UK between 2000 and 2012 (Table 4). Only 71 cases were found. However, we noted that the terms used in the HES system to record an episode or event related to an ADF were difficult to identify and, we suspect, many patients with an ADF were not coded correctly and thus not recorded. Of the 71 cases, 17 (23.9%) underwent documented treatment: 9 (12.7%) were treated surgically and 8 (11.3%) underwent oesophageal stent placement. Most patients (56.4%) presented with respiratory symptoms. The 30-day and 90-day mortality rates were 32.4 and 42.3% respectively, although for cases

a reasonable risk of future recurrence of lymphoma, thus a resection was advocated. A primary repair of the left main bronchus was performed, utilising a flap muscle graft. A single-phase operation was performed as the anastomosis was at a distinct site to the fistula.

Morbidity and mortality

Three patients suffered from complications following surgery. Patient 2 developed a severe respiratory infection on Day 4 following surgery, requiring bronchoscopic washout. Patient 7 suffered a small anastomotic leak, necessitating prolonged nil oral alimentation. Her nutrition was maintained with jejunal feeding, and a contrast swallow at

Table 3 Surgical Intervention for the Correction of ADF, and Post-Operative Complications

Patient	Operation	Incision	Phases	Reconstruction	Complications
1	Oesophageal Exclusion and fistula repair with strap muscle	Left collar Right PL[a] thoracotomy Laparotomy	2 phase	Retrosternal Gastric conduit	–
2	Fistula Repair with intercostal muscle	Right PL[a] thoracotomy	1 phase	n/a	Respiratory infection
3	Fistula Repair with intercostal muscle	Right PL[a] thoracotomy	1 phase	n/a	–
4	Fistula Repair with strap muscle	Bilateral collar Laparotomy	1 phase	n/a	Respiratory failure RIP
5	Right lower lobe resection and fistula repair	Right PL[a] mini-thoracotomy	1 phase	n/a	–
6	Oesophageal Exclusion and fistula repair	Left collar Right PL[a] thoracotomy Laparotomy	2 phase	Retrosternal Colonic conduit	–
7	Oesophagectomy and fistula repair with intercostal muscle	Left collar Right PL[a] thoracotomy Laparotomy	1 phase	Retrosternal Gastric conduit	Anastomotic leak
8	Fistula Repair with strap muscle	Bilateral collar	1 phase	n/a	–

[a]PL- Postero-lateral

Table 4 HES data search for ADFs between 2000 and 2012 ([a] denotes hospitals that perform ≥20 oesophageal cancer resections per year)

HES data (2000–2012)	n	%	p
Age ≥ 70 years	35	49.3	
Sex			
Female	35	49.3	
Male	36	50.7	
Treatment	17	24	
Surgery	9	12.7	
Stenting of oesophagus	8	11.3	
Unknown	54	76	
Presenting Clinical Feature			
Pneumonia	18	25.4	
Pleural effusion	22	31	
Pulmonary embolus	1	1.4	
Ischaemic cardiac event	1	1.4	
Unknown	29	40.8	
All Hospitals			
30-day mortality	23	32.4	
90-day mortality	30	42.3	
Specialist Centres[a]	16	22.5	
30-day mortality	4	25	0.473
90-day mortality	5	31.3	0.311

managed in high-volumes centres this fell to 25 and 31.3% respectively.

Discussion

This series demonstrates the techniques, challenges and strategies utilised in the surgical management of ADFs. The key aspect in the approach to such intervention is the multi-disciplinary nature of care, utilising the experience of several distinct surgical specialities. Pre-operative respiratory optimisation should be aggressive, and ideally patients should be weaned off artificial ventilation prior to surgery [2, 3]. As the HES data demonstrates, apart from being rare, there is a deficiency in accurate diagnosis, coding and documentation of this condition.

The range of operations that can be utilised reflect the nature of underlying disease [1–4]. The determinants of which operation will be performed are mainly the site and size of the ADF, and the state of the affected tissue-itself a reflection of the preceding disease and treatment. For the most proximal ADFs, an approach through a neck incision is the most desirable. A pivotal stratagem here involves mobilising the oesophagus circumferentially. This manoeuvre allows the more distal structures to be brought superiorly into the wound, making further

surgery easier and away from the rigid confines of the thoracic inlet. If necessary, the medial clavicle and sternoclavicular joint can be excised, a procedure which does not cause future disability [7]. Distal ADFs necessitate a thoracotomy. These ADFs can cause significant damage to the lung parenchyma, affecting the compliance by causing fibrosis [8]. Thus, where necessary, we advocate a lobar or segmental resection, with closure of the associated distal bronchi. Where an oesophagectomy is indicated, we favour leaving a cuff of oesophageal tissue around the trachea. This enables a dissection plane away from the airway, and the remnant tissue can be incorporated into the repair. This manoeuvre also lessens the future risk of tracheal stenosis [3].

Although not universally favoured, we have found the oesophageal exclusion operation a beneficial option in specific patients. Gross contamination of the airway, or in patients who have had a previous leak or radiotherapy, results in significant inflammation and adhesions in the thorax. Attempting a resection in this circumstance is hazardous, and if there is no definite indication to resect, the oesophagus can be safely left in situ. It is important that a generous venting gastrostomy is sited, from where the oesophagus can be accessed. We have successfully performed a retrograde endoscopy through this, and administered therapeutic agents required for treatment of disuse oesophagitis. Most importantly, it enables venting of oesophageal mucous. Some authors favour a single operation rather than a staged approach for resection or repair and reconstruction [3, 7]. In our experience, fashioning an anastomosis in a contaminated field increases the chance of a leak. In such an event, the fistula has a high chance of recurrence. Most importantly, however, a significant leak may necessitate a far more morbid operative intervention. Indeed, any resultant fistula is likely to be more difficult to treat, if this remains at all possible.

Several other series also demonstrate the complexity of surgical intervention [1–4, 9]. A feature of these reports is that experience is limited to a few specialist units where an expertise in ADF management is present. This results in better outcomes, and facilitates an environment where management is continually improved. In our series, there was one post-operative death. The remaining patients all achieved normal alimentation soon after surgery, with no evidence of ADF recurrence at a median of 32 months. These results are comparable to other dedicated units. Mathisen et al demonstrated a mortality rate of 10.5% in a series of 38 patients, many of whom underwent tracheal reconstruction, with excellent long-term outcomes [3]. In a subsequent report, highlighting 35 years' experience in the management of ADFs, the operative mortality rate fell to 2.8%, reflecting the effect of concentrating cases in specialist units [1].

Shen et al similarly report a low mortality rate of 5.7%, with a post-operative complication rate of 54.3%, and an oesophageal leak rate of 11.4% [9]. Baisi et al reported on 31 patients, of whom 26 underwent simple closure of the oesophageal and tracheal defects. Operative mortality was 3.2%, with a recurrence rate of 6.4% [10].

Non-operative techniques can be used to manage ADFs. Oesophageal stenting is the most common intervention, and although it plays a key role in some patients, they can themselves *cause* fistulae and may affect future surgical intervention [11, 12]. Newer endoscopic techniques utilising endoscopic suturing, clip placement or tissue glue, may have an increasing role in the management of ADFs in the future. Thus, early referral to a dedicated unit is advocated, as the *whole* management of the patient can be pursued where the complete skill-set, including access to novel treatments, is present. By focusing care in specific units, the expertise in all facets of management and outcomes can continually improve.

Conclusion

In summary, for a select group of patients an operative approach can be a truly life-saving intervention. Although surgery is not without risk, it offers the best chance of cure of ADF with a very low risk of recurrence and a return to normal oral alimentation.

Abbreviations

ADF: Aerodigestive Fistula; HES: Hospital Episodes Statistics; MDT: Multidisciplinary Team; OGJ: Oesophago-Gastric Junction; TB: Tuberculosis; TOF: Tracheo-Oesophageal Fistula

Acknowledgements

N/A

Funding

No funding to declare

Authors' contributions

Each author has participated sufficiently in the work to take public responsibility for this manuscript as per the guidelines of the International Committee of Medical Journal Editors (ICMJE) criteria. YQ and MM designed the study, acquired and analysed the data and drafted the manuscript; SM collected HES data and assisted in writing the manuscript; BM, JG, MH and DL assisted in interpretation of the data and critically revising the intellectual content. All authors approved the final version of the manuscript and are accountable for all aspects of accuracy and integrity related to this work.

Competing interests

The authors declare that they have no competing interests.

Author details

Department of Oesophago-Gastric Surgery, University College London Hospital, 250 Euston Road, London NW1 2BU, UK. [2]Department of Surgery and Cancer, Imperial College London, London, UK. [3]Department of Thoracic Medicine, University College London Hospital, London, UK. [4]Department of Thoracic Surgery, University College London Hospital, London, UK.

References

1. Muniappan A, Wain JC, Cameron D, et al. Surgical treatment of nonmalignant tracheoesophageal fistula: a thirty-five year experience. Ann Thorac Surg. 2013;95:1141–6.
2. Macchiarini P, Verhoye J-P, Chapelier A, et al. Evaluation and outcome of different surgical techniques for postintubation tracheoesophageal fistulas. J Thorac Cardio Vasc Surg. 2000;119(2):268–76.
3. Mathisen DJ, Grillo HC, Wain JC, et al. Management of Acquired Nonmalignant Tracheoesophageal Fistula. Ann Thorac Surg. 1991;52:759–65.
4. Meunier B, Stasik C, Raoul JL, et al. Gastric bypass for malignant esophagotracheal fistula: a series of 21 cases. Eur J Card Thorac Surg. 1998; 13:184–98.
5. Grillo HC. Acquired tracheoesophageal fistula and bronchoesophageal. In: Frillo HC, ed. Surgery of the Trachea and Bronchi. New York: BC Dekker Inc., 2003, 341–356.
6. Bartels HE, Stein HJ, Siewert JR. Tracheobronchial lesions following oesophagectomy: prevalence, predisposing factors and outcome. Br J Surg. 1998;85:403–6.
7. Barkley C, Orringer MB, Iannettoni MD, Yee J. Challenges in reversing esophageal discontinuity operations. Ann Thorac Surg. 2003;76:989–95.
8. Diddee R, Shaw IH. Acquired trachea-oesophageal fistula in adults. BJA: CEACCP. 2006;6(3):105–8.
9. Shen KR, Allen MS, Cassivi SD, et al. Surgical management of acquired nonmalignant tracheoesophageal and Bronchoesophgageal fistulae. Ann Thorac Surg. 2010;90:914–9.
10. Baisi A, Bonavina L, Narne S, et al. Benign trachea-esophageal fistula: results of surgical therapy. Dis Esoph. 1999;12:209–11.
11. Desiree van den Bongard HJ, Boot H, Baas P, Taal BG. The role of parallel stent insertion in patients with esophagorespiratory fistulas. Gastointest Endosc. 2002;55:110–5.
12. Ellul JP, Morgan R, Gold D, et al. Parallel self-expanding covered metal stents in the trachea and oesophagus for the palliation of complex high tracheo-oesophageal fistula. Br J Surg. 1996;83:1767–8.

Permissions

The contributors of this book come from diverse backgrounds, making this book a truly international effort. This book will bring forth new frontiers with its revolutionizing research information and detailed analysis of the nascent developments around the world.

We would like to thank all the contributing authors for lending their expertise to make the book truly unique. They have played a crucial role in the development of this book. Without their invaluable contributions this book wouldn't have been possible. They have made vital efforts to compile up to date information on the varied aspects of this subject to make this book a valuable addition to the collection of many professionals and students.

This book was conceptualized with the vision of imparting up-to-date information and advanced data in this field. To ensure the same, a matchless editorial board was set up. Every individual on the board went through rigorous rounds of assessment to prove their worth. After which they invested a large part of their time researching and compiling the most relevant data for our readers.

The editorial board has been involved in producing this book since its inception. They have spent rigorous hours researching and exploring the diverse topics which have resulted in the successful publishing of this book. They have passed on their knowledge of decades through this book. To expedite this challenging task, the publisher supported the team at every step. A small team of assistant editors was also appointed to further simplify the editing procedure and attain best results for the readers.

Apart from the editorial board, the designing team has also invested a significant amount of their time in understanding the subject and creating the most relevant covers. They scrutinized every image to scout for the most suitable representation of the subject and create an appropriate cover for the book.

The publishing team has been an ardent support to the editorial, designing and production team. Their endless efforts to recruit the best for this project, has resulted in the accomplishment of this book. They are a veteran in the field of academics and their pool of knowledge is as vast as their experience in printing. Their expertise and guidance has proved useful at every step. Their uncompromising quality standards have made this book an exceptional effort. Their encouragement from time to time has been an inspiration for everyone.

The publisher and the editorial board hope that this book will prove to be a valuable piece of knowledge for researchers, students, practitioners and scholars across the globe.

List of Contributors

Hailong Cao, Qing Zhou, Fudong Fan, Yunxing Xue, Jun Pan and Dongjin Wang
Department of Thoracic and Cardiovascular Surgery, the Affiliated Drum Tower Hospital of Nanjing, University Medical School, 321 Zhongshan RD, Nanjing 210008, China

Takuma Yamasaki, Shuhei Fujita, Yuji Kaku, Junko Katagiri and Takeshi Hiramatsu
Department of Cardiovascular Surgery, Japanese Red Cross Kyoto Daini Hospital, Kamanza-Dori, Marutamachi-Agaru, Kamigyo-Ku, Kyoto 602-8026, Japan

Xu Ma, Guofeng Liu, Qingchun Li, Daping Yang, Yingbo Zhang and Ning Li
Department of Plastic Surgery, The Second Affiliated Hospital of Harbin Medical University, 246 Xuefu Road, Nangang District, Harbin, Heilongjiang 150086, China

Zhijuan He
Department of Obstetrics and Gynecology, The First Affiliated Hospital of Harbin Medical University, 23 Youzheng Street, Nangang District, Harbin, Heilongjiang 150086, China

Ling Li
Department of Cardiology, The Second Affiliated Hospital of Harbin Medical University, 246 Xuefu Road, Nangang District, Harbin, Heilongjiang 150086, China

Marco Zanobini, Sabrina Manganiello, Giorgia Bonalumi, Raoul Biondi and Francesco Alamanni
Department of Cardiac Surgery, IRCCS - Centro Cardiologico Monzino, Università degli Studi di Milano, Via C. Parea 4, 20138 Milano, Italy

Matteo Saccocci
Department of Cardiac Surgery, IRCCS - Centro Cardiologico Monzino, Università degli Studi di Milano, Via C. Parea 4, 20138 Milano, Italy
Department of CardioVascular Surgery, Heart Center - University Hospital of Zurich, Zurich, Switzerland

Marco Russo
Department of CardioVascular Surgery, Heart Center - University Hospital of Zurich, Zurich, Switzerland

Massimo Mapelli
Department of Cardiology -IRCCS – Centro Cardiologico Monzino, Università degli Studi di Milano, Milano, Italy

Fernando Teiichi Costa Oikawa, Whady Hueb, Cesar Higa Nomura, Alexandre Ciappina Hueb, Alexandre Volney Villa, Leandro Menezes Alves da Costa, Rodrigo Morel Vieira de Melo, Paulo Cury Rezende, Carlos Alexandre Wainrober Segre, Cibele Larrosa Garzillo, Eduardo Gomes Lima, Jose Antonio Franchini Ramires and Roberto Kalil Filho
Instituto do Coracao (InCor), Hospital das Clinicas HCFMUSP, Faculdade de Medicina, Universidade de São Paulo, São Paulo, SP, Brazil

Tia R. Pilikian
Department of Surgery, Division of Cardiothoracic Surgery, University of Arizona, Tucson, AZ, USA

Katie M. Marsh
Department of Surgery, Division of Cardiothoracic Surgery, University of Arizona, Tucson, AZ, USA College of Medicine – Tucson, University of Arizona, Tucson, AZ, USA

Toshinobu Kazui
Department of Surgery, Division of Cardiothoracic Surgery, University of Arizona, Tucson, AZ, USA College of Medicine – Tucson, University of Arizona, Tucson, AZ, USA
Division of Cardiohracic Surgery, Banner University Medical Center Tucson, 1501 N Campbell Ave., Rm 4302A, Tucson, AZ 85724-5071, USA

Zain I. Khalpey
Department of Surgery, Division of Cardiothoracic Surgery, University of Arizona, Tucson, AZ, USA
College of Medicine – Tucson, University of Arizona, Tucson, AZ, USA
Department of Physiological Sciences, University of Arizona, Tucson, AZ, USA
Department of Biomedical Engineering, University of Arizona, Tucson, AZ, USA
Artificial Heart Program, Banner University Medical Center, Tucson, AZ, USA
Division of Cardiohracic Surgery, Banner University Medical Center Tucson, 1501 N Campbell Ave., Rm 4302A, Tucson, AZ 85724-5071, USA

Phat L. Tran
College of Medicine – Tucson, University of Arizona, Tucson, AZ, USA
Artificial Heart Program, Banner University Medical Center, Tucson, AZ, USA

Raymond Runyan and John Konhilas
Department of Physiological Sciences, University of Arizona, Tucson, AZ, USA

Richard Smith
Artificial Heart Program, Banner University Medical Center, Tucson, AZ, USA

Anna Gomes and Bhanu Sinha
Department of Medical Microbiology, University of Groningen, University Medical Center Groningen, Groningen, Netherlands

Jayant S. Jainandunsing
Department of Anesthesiology, University of Groningen, University Medical Center Groningen, Groningen, Netherlands

Sander van Assen
Department of Internal Medicine, Infectious Diseases, Treant Care Group, Hoogeveen, Netherlands

Peter Paul van Geel
Department of Cardiology, University of Groningen, University Medical Center Groningen, Groningen, Netherlands

Sandro Gelsomino and Daniel M. Johnson
Department of Thoracic Surgery, Maastricht University Medical Center, Maastricht, Netherlands

Ehsan Natour
Department of Thoracic Surgery, Maastricht University Medical Center, Maastricht, Netherlands
Department of Cardio-Thoracic Surgery, University of Groningen, University Medical Center Groningen, Groningen, Netherlands

Ai Kojima, Toru Okamura, Shunji Uchita, Kenji Namiguchi, Takumi Yasugi and Hironori Izutani
Department of Cardiovascular Surgery, Ehime University, Shitsukawa, Toon, Ehime 7910295, Japan

Fumiaki Shikata and Yujiro Kawanishi
Department of Cardiovascular Surgery, Ehime University, Shitsukawa, Toon, Ehime 7910295, Japan
Department of Cardiothoracic Surgery, St Vincent's Hospital, Sydney, NSW, Australia

Takashi Higaki
Department of Pediatric Cardiology, Children's Medical Center, Ehime University, Ehime, Japan

Seiko Ohno and Minoru Horie
Department of Cardiovascular and Respiratory Medicine, Shiga University of Medical Science, Shiga, Japan

Pierre Gianello and Daela Xhema
Pôle de Chirurgie Expérimentale et Transplantation (CHEX), Institut de Recherche Expérimentale et Clinique (IREC), Secteur des Sciences de la Sante, Université Catholique de Louvain, Avenue Hippocrate 55/B1.55.04, B-1200 Brussels, Belgium

Mathieu van Steenberghe
Pôle de Chirurgie Expérimentale et Transplantation (CHEX), Institut de Recherche Expérimentale et Clinique (IREC), Secteur des Sciences de la Sante, Université Catholique de Louvain, Avenue Hippocrate 55/B1.55.04, B-1200 Brussels, Belgium
Service de chirurgie cardiaque et vasculaire, Clinique Cecil, avenue Louis Ruchonnet 53, 1003 Lausanne, Switzerland

Hitoshi Ogino and Toshiki Fujiyoshi
Cardiovascular Surgery, Tokyo Medical University, 6-7-1 Nishishinjuku Shinjuku-ku Tokyo, 160, Tokyo -0023, Japan

Thomas Schubert
Service d'orthopédie et de traumatologie de l'appareil locomoteur, Cliniques universitaires Saint-Luc, Avenue Hippocrate 10, B-1200 Brussels, Belgium
Unité de thérapie tissulaire et cellulaire de l'appareil locomoteur, Cliniques universitaires Saint Luc, Avenue Hippocrate 10, B-1200 Brussels, Belgium

Sébastien Gerelli
Service de chirurgie cardiaque, Centre hospitalier Annecy-Genevois, site Annecy, 1 Avenue de l'Hopital, F-74370 Pringy, France

Caroline Bouzin
Institut de Recherche Expérimentale et Clinique (IREC), IREC Imaging Platform (2IP), Université catholique de Louvain, Avenue Hippocrate 55/ B1.55.20, B-1200 Brussels, Belgium

Yves Guiot
Service d'anatomie pathologique, Cliniques universitaires Saint Luc, Avenue Hippocrate 10, B-1200 Brussels, Belgium

Xavier Bollen
Institute of Mechanics, Materials and Civil Engineering, Mechatronic, Electrical Energy, and Dynamic Systems (MEED), Secteur des Sciences et Technologies, Université Catholique de Louvain, Place du Levant 2/L5.04.02, B-1348 Louvain-la-Neuve, Belgium

Karim Abdelhamid
Service d'oncologie, Centre hospitalier universitaire vaudois, Rue du Bugnon 46, CH-1011 Lausanne, Vaud, Switzerland

Kenji Minatoya
Departments of Cardiovascular Surgery, National Cerebral and Cardiovascular Center, Osaka, Japan

Yoshihiko Ikeda and Hatsue Ishibashi-Ueda
Departments of Pathology, National Cerebral and Cardiovascular Center, Osaka, Japan

Takayuki Morisaki and Hiroko Morisaki
Departments of Bioscience and Genetics, National Cerebral and Cardiovascular Center, Osaka, Japan

Sohsyu Kotani, Yoshito Inoue, Mio Kasai and Satoru Suzuki
Department of Cardiovascular Surgery, Hiratsuka City Hospital, Kanagawa, Japan

Takashi Hachiya
Department of Cardiovascular Surgery, Kawasaki City Hospital, Kanagawa, Japan

Jerry Easo, Michael Horst and Alexander Weymann
Department of Cardiac Surgery, European Medical School Oldenburg-Groningen, University Hospital Oldenburg, Carl von Ossietzky University Oldenburg, Rahel Straus Str. 10, 26133 Oldenburg, Germany

Bernhard Schmuck and Rohit Philip Thomas
Department of Diagnostic and Interventional Radiology, European Medical School Oldenburg-Groningen, University Hospital Oldenburg, Carl von Ossietzky University Oldenburg, Oldenburg, Germany

Steffen Saupe
University Department of Obstetrics and Gynaecology, European Medical School Oldenburg-Groningen, University Hospital Oldenburg, Carl von Ossietzky University Oldenburg, Oldenburg, Germany

Malte Book
Department of Anaesthesiology, Critical Care, Emergency Medicine and Pain Therapy, European Medical School Oldenburg-Groningen, University Hospital Oldenburg, Carl von Ossietzky University Oldenburg, Oldenburg, Germany

Po-Sung Li
Department of Emergency Medicine, Taichung Veterans General Hospital, Taichung, Taiwan

Chung-Lin Tsai
Division of Cardiac Surgery, Cardiovascular Center, Taichung Veterans General Hospital, Taichung, Taiwan

Sung-Yuan Hu
Department of Emergency Medicine, Taichung Veterans General Hospital, Taichung, Taiwan
School of Medicine, Chung Shan Medical University, Taichung, Taiwan
Institute of Medicine, Chung Shan Medical University, Taichung, Taiwan
Department of Nursing, College of Health, National Taichung University of Science and Technology, Taichung, Taiwan
Department of Nursing, Central Taiwan Univeristy of Science and Technology, Taichung, Taiwan
1650 Taiwan Boulevard Sect. 4, Taichung 40705, Taiwan

Yao-Tien Chang
Department of Emergency Medicine, Taichung Veterans General Hospital, Taichung, Taiwan
School of Medicine, Chung Shan Medical University, Taichung, Taiwan
Department of Nursing, College of Health, National Taichung University of Science and Technology, Taichung, Taiwan

Tzu-Chieh Lin
Department of Emergency Medicine, Taichung Veterans General Hospital, Taichung, Taiwan
School of Medicine, Chung Shan Medical University, Taichung, Taiwan
Department of Nursing, College of Health, National Taichung University of Science and Technology, Taichung, Taiwan
College of Public Health, China Medical University, Taichung, Taiwan

Ryan Avery and Kevin Day
Department of Medical Imaging, Banner - University Medical Center, 1501 N. Campbell Ave, Tucson, AZ 85724, USA

Clinton Jokerst
Department of Radiology, Mayo Clinic Hospital – Phoenix, Phoenix, AZ, USA

Toshinobu Kazui and Zain Khalpey
Department of Surgery, Division of Cardiothoracic Surgery, Banner – University Medical Center, Tucson, AZ, USA

Elizabeth Krupinski
Department of Radiology and Imaging Science, Emory University Hospital, Atlanta, US, Georgia

Yasushi Tsutsumi, Osamu Monta, Hisazumi Uenaka, Kenji Tanaka, Takaaki Samura and Hirokazu Ohashi
Department of Cardiovascular Surgery, Fukui Cardiovascular Center, 2-228Shinbo, Fukui 910-0833, Japan

Ryohei Matsuura
Department of Cardiovascular Surgery, Fukui Cardiovascular Center, 2-228Shinbo, Fukui 910-0833, Japan
Department of Cardiovascular Surgery, Osaka University Graduate School of Medicine, 2-2 E1, Yamadaoka, Suita-shi, Osaka 565-0871, Japan

Seung Hyun Lee, Byung Chul Chang, Young-Nam Youn, Hyun Chel Joo, Kyung-Jong Yoo and Sak Lee
Division of Thoracic and Cardiovascular Surgery, Severance Cardiovascular Hospital, Yonsei Cardiovascular Research Institute, Yonsei University, College of Medicine, 250 Seongsanno, Seodaemun-gu, Seoul 03722, Republic of Korea

Jesper Park-Hansen, Anders M. Greve, Johan S. R. Clausen, Anne S. Nørskov and Helena Dominguez
Department of Cardiology, Bispebjerg and Frederiksberg University Hospital, Nordre Fasanvej 57, DK-2000 Frederiksberg, Denmark
Department of Biomedicine, University of Copenhagen, Copenhagen, Denmark

Susanne J. V. Holme and Christian L. Carranza
Department of Thoracic Surgery, Rigshospitalet, Copenhagen, Denmark

Akhmadjon Irmukhamedov
Department of Thoracic Surgery, Odense University Hospital, Odense, Denmark

Gina Al-Farra
Department of Radiology, Herlev Gentofte University Hospital, Herlev, Denmark

Robert G. C. Riis
Department of Radiology, Bispebjerg and Frederiksberg Hospital, Frederiksberg, Denmark

Brian Nilsson
Department of Cardiology, Hvidovre University Hospital, Copenhagen, Denmark

Christina R. Kruuse
Department Neurology, Neurovascular Research Unit, Herlev Gentofte Hospital, Herlev, Denmark

Egill Rostrup
Mental Health Center Glostrup, Copenhagen, Denmark

Hiroshi Kubota, Hidehito Endo, Hikaru Ishii, Hiroshi Tsuchiya, Yusuke Inaba, Yu Takahashi and Katsunari Terakawa
Department of Cardiovascular Surgery, Kyorin University, 6-20-2, Shinkawa, Mitaka, Tokyo 181-8611, Japan

Yuki Takahashi, Masahiro Miyajima, Taijiro Mishina, Ryunosuke Maki, Makoto Tada, Kodai Tsuruta and Atsushi Watanabe
Department of Thoracic Surgery, Sapporo Medical University, School of Medicine and Hospital, South 1, West 16, Chuo-ku, Sapporo, Hokkaido 060-8556, Japan

Gopichand Mannam
Department of cardiac surgery, Star Hospital Banjara Hills, 8-2-596/5, Road No.10, Banjara Hills, Hyderabad, Telangana 500034, India

Yugal Mishra
Department of cardiac surgery, Escorts Heart Institute and Research Centre, New Delhi, India

Rajan Modi
Department of cardiac surgery, SAL Hospital, Ahmedabad, India

Alla Gopala Krishna Gokhale
Department of cardiac surgery, Yashoda Hospital, Secunderabad, India

Rajan Sethuratnam
Department of cardiac surgery, The Madras Medical Mission, Chennai, India

Kaushal Pandey
Department of cardiac surgery, P. D. Hinduja National Hospital & Medical Research Center, Mumbai, India

Rajneesh Malhotra
Department of cardiac surgery, Max Super Speciality Hospital, New Delhi, India

Sumit Anand and Anushreeta Borah
Abbott Pvt. Ltd, New Delhi, India

Sushan Mukhopadhyay
Department of cardiac surgery, Apollo Gleneagles Hospitals, Kolkata, India

Dhiren Shah
Department of cardiac surgery, Care Institute of Medical Sciences, Ahmedabad, India

Tek Singh Mahant
Department of cardiac surgery, Fortis Hospital, Mohali, India

Armah M Akuffu, Haige Zhao, Junnan Zheng and Yiming Ni
Department of Cardiothoracic Surgery, the First Affiliated Hospital of Zhejiang University, No.79 Qingchun Road, Hangzhou 310003, China

Arnar B. Ingason
Department of Medicine, University of Iceland, Vatnsmyrarvegur 16, 101 Reykjavik, Reykjavik, Iceland

Bjarni Torfason
Department of Medicine, University of Iceland, Vatnsmyrarvegur 16, 101 Reykjavik, Reykjavik, Iceland

Gunnlaugur Sigfusson
Children's Hospital, Landspitali University Hospital, Reykjavik, Iceland

Hiroyuki Nakajima, Akitoshi Takazawa, Akihiro Yoshitake, Masato Tochii, Chiho Tokunaga, Jun Hayashi, Hiroaki Izumida, Daisuke Kaneyuki, Toshihisa Asakura and Atsushi Iguchi
Department of Cardiovascular Surgery, Saitama Medical University, International Medical Center, 1397-1 Yamane Hidaka, Saitama 350-1298, Japan

Leo M Nherera and Paul Trueman
Smith & Nephew Advanced Wound Management, Global Market Access, 101 Hessle Road, Hull HU3 2BN, UK

Michael Schmoeckel
Vascular and Diabetic Centre Department of Heart Surgery, Asklepios Klinik St. Georg Cardiac, Lohmühlenstr 5, 20099 Hamburg, Germany

Francis Λ Fatoye
Department of Health Professions, Manchester Metropolitan University, Manchester, UK

Likui Fang, Luming Wang, Yiqing Wang, Wang Lv and Jian Hu
Department of Thoracic Surgery, the First Affiliated Hospital, Zhejiang University School of Medicine, Hangzhou 310003, China

Zhibing Qiu, L. Auchoybur Merveesh, Yueyue Xu, Yinshuo Jiang, Liming Wang, Ming Xu and Fei Xiang
Department of Thoracic and Cardiovascular Surgery. Nanjing First Hospital, Nanjing Medical University, Changle Rd 68, Nanjing 210006, Jiangsu, China

Xin Chen
Department of Thoracic and Cardiovascular Surgery. Nanjing First Hospital, Nanjing Medical University, Changle Rd 68, Nanjing 210006, Jiangsu, China
Department of Cardiothoracic and vascular Surgery, Nanjing First Hospital, Nanjing Medical University, 68 Changle Rd, Nanjing 210006, China

Jing Guo, Chenwei Li and Xinjian Li
Department of Thoracic Surgery, Ningbo First Hospital, Ningbo 315010, China

Qiuyuan Li
Department of Thoracic Surgery, Ningbo First Hospital, Ningbo 315010, China
Department of Thoracic Surgery, Shanghai Pulmonary Hospital Tongji University, Shanghai, China

Qin Jiang, Tao Yu, Keli Huang and Lihua Liu
Department of Cardiac Surgery, Sichuan Provincial People's Hospital, Affiliated Hospital of University of Electronic Science and Technology, No.32, West Second Section First Ring Road, Chengdu, China

Xiaoshen Zhang
Department of Cardiac Surgery, Affiliated Hospital of University of Jinan, Guangzhou, China

Shengshou Hu
Department of Cardiac Surgery, Fuwai Hospital, Chinese Academy of Medical Sciences and Peking Union Medical College, Beijing 100037, China

Yuki Endo, Yoshitsugu Nakamura, Miho Kuroda, Yusuke Nakanishi, Yujiro Ito and Takaki Hori
Department of Cardiovascular Surgery, Chiba-Nishi General Hospital, 107-1, Kanegasaku, Matsudo-shi, Chiba 270-2251, Japan

Rumiko Okamoto
Departments of Oncology, Chiba-Nishi General Hospital, 107-1, Kanegasaku, Matsudo-shi, Chiba 270-2251, Japan

Hiroshi Konishi
Departments of Hematology, Chiba-Nishi General Hospital, 107-1, Kanegasaku, Matsudo-shi, Chiba 270-2251, Japan

Yuhao Wu, Yonggang Li, Yuehang Zhou, Xin Jin and Chun Wu
Department of Cardiothoracic Surgery, Children's Hospital of Chongqing Medical University, No.136 Zhongshan Second Road, Yuzhong District, Chongqing 400014, China
Ministry of Education Key Laboratory of Child Development and Disorders, Chongqing 400014, China
China International Science and Technology Cooperation Base of Child Development and Critical Disorders, Chongqing 400014 Chongqing Key Laboratory of Pediatrics, Chongqing 400014, China

Zhichao Wu and Junmeng Zheng
Department of Cardiovascular Surgery, Sun Yat-Sen Memorial Hospital, Sun Yat-Sen University, No.107 Yanjiang West Road, Yuexiu District, Guangzhou 510120, China

Hongyu Kuang
Department of Cardiology, Children's Hospital of Chongqing Medical University, Chongqing 400014, China
Ministry of Education Key Laboratory of Child Development and Disorders, Chongqing 400014, China
China International Science and Technology Cooperation Base of Child Development and Critical Disorders, Chongqing 400014, China
Chongqing Key Laboratory of Pediatrics, Chongqing 400014, China

Yassar A. Qureshi, M. Muntzer Mughal and Borzoueh Mohammadi
Department of Oesophago-Gastric Surgery, University College London Hospital, 250 Euston Road, London NW1 2BU, UK

Sheraz R. Markar
Department of Surgery and Cancer, Imperial College London, London, UK

Jeremy George
Department of Thoracic Medicine, University College London Hospital, London, UK

Martin Hayward and David Lawrence
Department of Thoracic Surgery, University College London Hospital, London, UK

Index

CPSIA information can be obtained
at www.ICGtesting.com
Printed in the USA
LVHW061629080222
710591LV00005B/372